Hot Topics in Acute Care Surgery and Trauma

Ari Leppaniemi, Helsinki, Finland

Ron Maier, Seattle, USA

Ernest E. Moore, Fort Collins, USA

Lena Napolitano, Ann Arbor, USA

Andrew Peitzman, Pittsburgh, USA

Patrick Reilly, Philadelphia, USA

Sandro Rizoli, Toronto, Canada

Boris E. Sakakushev, Plovdiv, Bulgaria

Massimo Sartelli, Macerata, Italy

Thomas Scalea, Baltimore, USA

David Spain, Stanford, USA

Philip Stahel, Denver, USA

Michael Sugrue, Letterkenny, Ireland

George Velmahos, Boston, USA

Dieter Weber, Perth, Australia

This series covers the most debated issues in acute care and trauma surgery, from perioperative management to organizational and health policy issues. Since 2011, the founder members of the World Society of Emergency Surgery's (WSES) Acute Care and Trauma Surgeons group, who endorse the series, realized the need to provide more educational tools for young surgeons in training and for general physicians and other specialists new to this discipline: WSES is currently developing a systematic scientific and educational program founded on evidence-based medicine and objective experience. Covering the complex management of acute trauma and non-trauma surgical patients, this series makes a significant contribution to this program and is a valuable resource for both trainees and practitioners in acute care surgery.

More information about this series at http://link.springer.com/series/15718

Federico Coccolini · Mauro Podda
Robert B. Lim · Massimo Chiarugi
Editors

Mini-invasive Approach in Acute Care Surgery

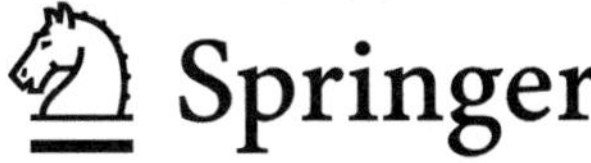

Editors
Federico Coccolini (iD)
General, Emergency and Trauma Surgery
Department
Pisa University Hospital
Pisa, Pisa, Italy

Robert B. Lim
Oklahoma Univ. School of Med. at Tulsa
Tulsa, OK, USA

Mauro Podda
Emergency Surgery Department, Cagliari
University Hospital
A.O.U. di Cagliari
Monserrato, Cagliari, Italy

Massimo Chiarugi
General, Emergency and Trauma Surgery
Department
Pisa University Hospital
Pisa, Pisa, Italy

ISSN 2520-8284   ISSN 2520-8292   (electronic)
Hot Topics in Acute Care Surgery and Trauma
ISBN 978-3-031-39003-6   ISBN 978-3-031-39001-2   (eBook)
https://doi.org/10.1007/978-3-031-39001-2

This Springer imprint is published by the registered company Springer Nature Switzerland AG
The registered company address is: Gewerbestrasse 11, 6330 Cham, Switzerland

Series Foreword

Research is fundamentally altering the daily practice of acute care surgery (trauma, surgical critical care, and emergency generally surgery) for the betterment of patients around the world. Management for many diseases and conditions is radically different than it was just a few years ago. For this reason, concise up-to-date information is required to inform busy clinicians. Therefore, since 2011 the World Society of Emergency Surgery (WSES), in partnership with the American Association for the Surgery of Trauma (AAST), endorses the development and publication of the "Hot Topics in Acute Care Surgery and Trauma," realizing the need to provide more educational tools for young in-training surgeons and for general physicians and other surgical specialists. These new forthcoming titles have been selected and prepared with this philosophy in mind. The books will cover the basics of pathophysiology and clinical management, framed with the reference that recent advances in the science of resuscitation, surgery, and critical care medicine have the potential to profoundly alter the epidemiology and subsequent outcomes of severe surgical illnesses and trauma.

General, Emergency and Trauma Surgery
University Hospital of Pisa, Pisa, Italy

Federico Coccolini

Riverside University Health System Medical Center
Riverside, CA, USA

Raul Coimbra

Department of Surgery and Critical Care Medicine,
Foothills Medical Centre
Calgary, AB, Canada

Andrew W. Kirkpatrick

Department of Surgery, Madonna del Soccorso Hospital
San Benedetto del Tronto, Italy

Salomone Di Saverio

Contents

The History of Minimally Invasive Techniques in Acute Care Surgery. . . .   1
Robert B. Lim, Freeman Condon, and Robert Conrad

History of Thoracoscopy in Emergency Surgery and Trauma.   17
Morgan M. Sellers, Fredric M. Pieracci, and Clay Cothren Burlew

**Role and Limitations of Mininvasive Approach in Abdominal
Emergencies and Trauma**.   23
Marcelo A. F. Ribeiro Jr, Gabriela Karabachian Tebar,
José Lucas Rodrigues Salgueiro, and Gabriel Franco de Camargo Galindo

Role of MIS Approaches in Thoracic Emergencies and Trauma   33
Daniel VanDerPloeg, Clay Cothren Burlew, and Fredric M. Pieracci

Acute Appendicitis   45
Andrea Pakula and Ruby Skinner

Acute Cholecystitis and Emergency Common Bile Duct Exploration.   51
Simone Frassini, Paola Fugazzola, Matteo Tomasoni, and Luca Ansaloni

Acute Colonic Diverticulitis.   69
Dario Tartaglia, Federico Coccolini, Alessio Mazzoni, Valerio Genovese,
Camilla Cremonini, Enrico Cicuttin, and Massimo Chiarugi

**Complicated Inflammatory Bowel Disease and Colonic Non-diverticular
Emergencies**.   87
Francesco Maria Carrano, Antonino Spinelli, and Hayato Kurihara

Gastroduodenal Perforation   103
Amit Sharma and Mansoor Ali Khan

Adhesive Small Bowel Obstruction (ASBO).   111
Gabriele Luciano Petracca, Vittoria Pattonieri, Concetta Prioriello,
Gennaro Perrone, Antonio Tarasconi, and Fausto Catena

Large Bowel Obstructions   127
Elisa Reitano, Aleix Martínez-Pérez, and Nicola de'Angelis

Minimally Invasive Approach to Treatment of Acute Pancreatitis 139
Christopher Goljan, Jesse Bandle, and Matthew J. Martin

Complicated Hiatal Hernia 157
Siobhan Rooney, Victoria Hudson, and Stavros Gourgiotis

Inguinal and Incisional Hernia Emergency Management 171
Dario Parini, Roberta La Mendola, and Monica Zese

Internal and Congenital Hernias 185
Giovanni D. Tebala, Emanuela Ceriati, Roshneen Ali, Sonia Battaglia,
Francesco De Peppo, Frances Dixon, Mahul Patel, Amanda Shabana,
and Valerio Voglino

Post-traumatic Diaphragmatic Hernia 215
Camilla Cremonini, Enrico Cicuttin, Dario Tartaglia, Silvia Strambi,
Serena Musetti, Massimo Chiarugi, and Federico Coccolini

Minimally Invasive Approach to Intestinal Bleeding 227
Aditi M. Kapil and Kimberly A. Davis

Bowel Ischemia 239
Francesco Pata, Antonio Pata, Gianluca Pellino, Gaetano Gallo,
and Giancarlo D'Ambrosio

General Surgery Emergencies in Pregnancy 253
Goran Augustin

Nonspecific Abdominal Pain 271
Gaetano Gallo, Monica Ortenzi, Mario Guerrieri, Francesco Virdis,
Marta Goglia, and Salomone Di Saverio

Management of Bariatric Surgery Early and Delayed Complications 281
Uri Kaplan

Gynecological Emergencies 301
J. L. Kilkenny and M. S. J. Wilson

Role of Emergency Laparoscopy in Pediatric Patients 319
Robert B. Laverty and Margaret E. Gallagher

**Minimally Invasive Surgery for Emergency General Surgery
in Elderly** 331
Kenji Okumura, Matthew McGuirk, and Rifat Latifi

**Role of Emergency Laparoscopy in Surgical and Endoscopic
Complications** 343
Aleix Martínez-Pérez, Carmen Payá-Llorente, Álvaro Pérez-Rubio,
and Nicola de'Angelis

Role of Bedside Laparoscopy. 355
Rhiannon Bradshaw, Heather M. Grossman Verner, Rachel Krzeczowski,
and Michael S. Truitt

**Anesthesia Considerations for MIS in Emergency
and Trauma Surgery**. 361
Hillary Prince and Michael W. Cripps

**Utility of Video-Assisted Thoracoscopic Surgery (VATS) in Acute Care
Surgery**. 375
Ariel W. Knight and Andre R. Campbell

The History of Minimally Invasive Techniques in Acute Care Surgery

Robert B. Lim, Freeman Condon, and Robert Conrad

1   Background

It is widely accepted that a patient has "healed from surgery" once their incisions or wounds have sufficiently closed. It natrurally follows that minimizing the size of surgical incisions and the trauma from an operation would ultimately help a patient heal more rapidly, hence, the birth of minimally invasive surgery (MIS), a field which includes laparoscopic and endoscopic surgery.

Laparoscopy named from the Ancient Greek words *lapara* (flank) and *skopeo* (to see) allows for minimally invasive operations to be performed with the use of a camera. Traditionally, exploratory laparotomy was considered the goal standard for both diagnosis and therapeutic intervention. However, laparoscopic surgery used in the correct setting allows for both diagnosis and therapeutic intervention with the advantages of smaller incisions, reduced pain, minimal hemorrhage, and shorter recovery. Today, the use of minimally invasive surgery (MIS) is widely accepted in a multitude of specialties including bariatric, thoracic, abdominal, gastrointestinal, obstetric, urologic, orthopedic, and gynecologic surgery.

R. B. Lim (✉)
Wake Forest University, Charlotte, NC, USA
e-mail: Robert-Lim@ouhsc.edu

F. Condon · R. Conrad
United States Army, Honolulu, HI, USA

F. Coccolini et al. (eds.), *Mini-invasive Approach in Acute Care Surgery*,
Hot Topics in Acute Care Surgery and Trauma,
https://doi.org/10.1007/978-3-031-39001-2_1

2   History

Over 120 years ago, in 1901, German physician George Kelling pioneered the use of laparoscopy based on animal experiments using a cystoscope in dogs to evaluate the effect of the pneumoperitoneum [1]. Kelling is credited with inventing the technique of the *celioscopy* and later applied his techniques on human patients.

In 1910, Hans Christian Jacobaeus became the first physician to use laparoscopic surgery in the clinical setting, publishing his results in *Münchner Medizinischen Wochenschrift* under the title "The Possibilities For Performing Cystoscopy In Examinations Of Serous Cavities." Jacobaeus is credited with coining the term laparothorakoskopie or laparoscopy [2]. His work helped demonstrate the enormous diagnostic and therapeutic potential of laparoscopic surgery [1, 2]. He also outlined some of its limitations and technical challenges and advocated for specialized surgical training—a tenet of modern surgical training.

Over the next century, technological advancements such as the advent of chip-based cameras and fiber optic cables have allowed numerous surgeons to refine and popularize laparoscopic surgery. Between 1950 and 1970, modern-day laparoscopic surgery began to take shape. The earliest adopters of laparoscopic surgery were gynecologists. The use of modern diagnostic laparoscopy was first published by French gynecologist Raoul Palmer in 1947. In the 1970s, Palmer along with German gynecologist Kurt Semm would go on to publish on the use of CO_2 for hysteroscopy and the use of thermocoagulation and intracorporeal knotting for hemostasis [3].

In 1981, Semm performed the first laparoscopic appendectomy. As with many pioneers of new technology, he was initially criticized. The German Gynecological Society even went as far as to suggest the suspension of Semm from medical practice. While subsequently published in the journal *Endoscopy*, Semm's manuscript on laparoscopic appendectomy was initially rejected by the *American Journal of Obstetrics and Gynecology* [3, 4]. Over the next decade, laparoscopic surgery gained traction and became widely popularized. Semm, a leader in the field of laparoscopic surgery, published over 1000 papers and in 1985 even developed the early *laparo-trainer*. The first laparoscopic cholecystectomy was performed in 1985 by German surgeon Erich Mühe. It was after Mühe's success that laparoscopic surgery garnered widespread acceptance across a multitude of surgical specialties [5, 6].

3   Advantages

It did not take long for surgeons to recognize the numerous advantages of minimally invasive laparoscopic surgery to the patient. Numerous studies suggest that laparoscopic approaches can minimize bleeding risk and transfusion requirement. A minimally invasive pancreaticoduodenectomy or Whipple procedure remains one of the most challenging general surgery abdominal procedures; but a metanalysis of this approach for the pancreaticoduodenectomy demonstrated the safety of this approach and a reduced transfusion requirement [7].

Another well-established benefit of minimally invasive laparoscopic surgery is the reduction in pain. Less pain translates into shorter recovery periods and a faster return to previous activities, although this is not well defined. In the age of the narcotic epidemic, reduction in pain via the use of minimally invasive approaches has allowed for minimal to narcotic-free postoperative pathways [8]. It even facilitates the performance of a transversus abdominis plane block by the operative surgeon which greatly decreases postoperative opiate requirements [9].

The use of laparoscopy in bariatric surgery has revolutionized the use of minimally invasive techniques in obese patients and garnered more acceptance of bariatric surgery as a result. In the 1990s, obesity was considered a relative contra-indication for the use of laparoscopy. Now laparoscopic surgery can often be technically easier than conventional surgery in the obese population, regardless of the procedure being performed.

Intra-abdominal adhesions are a risk associated with both open and laparoscopic surgery. Postoperative adhesions remain a significant problem causing complications such a chronic pain, bowel obstructions, and female infertility. There is some evidence to suggest less adhesive scar formation occurs after laparoscopic surgery when compared to open surgery. Techniques such as films or gels to separate tissues during the postoperative healing period have been suggested as ways to prevent adhesions in open procedures, but none have proven to completely prevent adhesions. Laparoscopic procedures, though, have fewer readmissions related to adhesions compared to open operations [10]. MIS techniques also reduce the physiologic stress response with lower IL-6 levels, which is an acute phase reactant partially responsible for the inflammatory response after surgery [11]. This would support the notion that laparoscopy is a better option for the more frail patients who would not tolerate operative stress well.

Finally, there are several studies that demonstrate laparoscopy results in fewer surgical site infections [12, 13]. Ultimately, this means that the patient undergoing a laparoscopic procedure has less physiologic stress, less adhesive disease, less bleeding, fewer infections, and less pain while at times providing better visualization even in the most challenging procedures like a Roux-en-Y gastric bypass or emergency general surgery procedures where the anatomy is distorted and the tissue is friable.

4   Disadvantages

MIS can also often be technically challenging, with limited range of motion and a perceived limited field of view. Conventional laparoscopic surgery is also limited by lack of depth perception, tactile feedback, and instrument dexterity. Because surgeons must perform the procedure with instruments rather than their hands, the ability to manipulate tissues, judge the amount of force being applied, and evaluate vital structures such as tumors or vascular tissues is significantly diminished. Similarly, laparoscopic instruments function by the fulcrum effect and therefore move in the opposite direction of the surgeon's hands. MIS requires learning difficult nonintuitive motor skills. A graduating general surgery resident is required to perform 75 cases in advanced laparoscopy, and it is not clear if this affords them the ability to handle the complex patients or diseases with laparoscopy. As increasingly challenging procedures are performed with laparoscopy, additional fellowship training is often required as is the case with bariatric/metabolic surgery.

Some of these limitations can be overcome with newer camera technology and robot-assisted surgery. The use of the robot platform allows greater dexterity, and it may also allow the ability to perform complex maneuvers by surgeons who are not as proficient with traditional laparoscopic techniques. It could, therefore, allow the acute care surgeon to operate as if the procedure was open while still having the advantages of MIS. Robot-assisted surgery, though, comes with its own disadvantages in the context of acute care surgery. These include the need for equipment familiarity on the part of the operating team. The nonelective nature of ACS cases means that these cases are often handled by a nonspecialized OR team which may have limited training in robot-assisted surgery. Additionally, operative times in robotic vs. laparoscopic surgery are highly dependent on surgeon experience suggesting there is a learning curve [14]. Finally, hospitals are likely to be reluctant to utilize a robot platform after hours because of cost concerns.

There is a significant risk of injury from trocar insertion into the abdominal or thoracic cavities [15]. Regardless of technique of insertion, there is a component of blind insertion. Injuries vary from abdominal wall hematomas and hernias to bowel and major vascular injuries. The risk of complication from initial trocar placement increased with low body mass index and prior abdominal surgeries. The incidence of these injuries is quite low but should be recognized as early as possible. Vascular injuries can result in massive hemorrhage and be life-threatening as they can be harder to recognize and not easily controlled via a minimally invasive technique. Likewise, hollow viscus injuries may go undetected and result in delayed peritonitis.

Injuries can also occur from stray surgical energy. The use of surgical electricity transfers energy to tissue, which can result in cutting through or coagulating the tissue. Unfortunately, the energy does not always go where it is directed and injuries can even occur out of the laparoscope's field of vision. This accounts for roughly 40,000 burns annually and 70% of the burns that occur with laparoscopy are not detected at the time of the initial operation [16]. Consequently, surgeons who operate with MIS techniques must know how to properly use these different electrosurgical devices. The Fundamental Use of Surgical Energy (FUSE) program was designed to do exactly this, but it is not a requirement for credentialing or board certification [17]. As a result, most surgeons on not familiar with this knowledge may be risking injury to their patients when operating laparoscopically [18].

Laparoscopic surgery also requires a pneumoperitoneum, which causes cardiopulmonary physiologic changes such as decreased preload, systemic CO_2 absorption and subsequent metabolic acidosis, and a possible gas embolism [19]. Some patients with underlying cardiopulmonary comorbidities may not tolerate the pneumoperitoneum required for laparoscopic procedures. The exact trade-off of less physiologic stress from MIS approaches against the cardiopulmonary compromise from the pneumoperitoneum is not known.

Another area of controversy in minimally invasive surgery is its role in oncologic procedures. Laparoscopic surgery has been suggested to potentially risk port site and intra-abdominal metastases after ovarian, gastric, gallbladder, and appendiceal cancer. The feared risk being tumor rupture leads to peritoneal carcinomatosis. Specialized training, trocar site protection devices, and morselization devices have all been used to decrease the incidence of iatrogenic dissemination of cancer during minimally invasive surgery. Ultimately, however, the use of laparoscopy has not been proven to increase cancer spread via the trocar sites.

There is also a theoretical risk to the surgical team during laparoscopic surgery as the gas used to create working space and the smoke generated from the procedure itself may aerosolize in the operating room. The plume from minimally invasive surgery has been suggested to spread cancer particles, bacteria, and even viral particles, such as SARS-CoV-2, the pathogen responsible for the COVID-19 disease. There is no data published to substantiate this concern, so it remains only theoretical.

5   History of Adoption

Following the doubt of Semm's work, the routine use of laparoscopy for appendicitis was slow to be applied. In 1996, Bonanni et al. published their experience of 300 open appendectomies versus 66 laparoscopic ones in the Journal of the American Medical Association [20]. The authors found that patients who had complicated appendicitis did much worse with the laparoscopic approach including a 45% readmission rate in patients who were found to have gangrene, perforation with an abscess, or peritonitis. Additionally, there were longer operative times and operating room costs. The author recommended that the laparoscopic approach not be used for complicated appendicitis.

A decade later, the concern for laparoscopy was still being debated for complicated appendicitis. The same journal published a report by Yau et al. that showed that even in complicated appendicitis, the laparoscopic approach had shorter operative times, fewer wound infections, and shorter hospital stays [21]. In their study, the patients did not have a higher incidence of postoperative intra-abdominal abscesses than those that had an open approach. Conversely and around the same time, another study claimed that the intra-abdominal abscess rate after laparoscopic appendectomy was 14% compared to 0% in patients who had an open approach [22]. Both of these studies showed, however, that the concern for extra cost of the MIS approach was offset by fewer overall complications and a shorter length of hospital stay.

Over the next decade, several studies compared the two approaches for complicated appendicitis [23–26]. These studies include systematic reviews, a meta-analysis, and a randomized control trial which show that the rate of intra-abdominal abscess is not higher with the laparoscopic approach. Today, the presence of complicated appendicitis should not be a reason to convert to an open procedure. The inflammation or abscess can be treated with washout and drainage done laparoscopically along with the appendectomy. Further, the advantages to the laparoscopic approach such as fewer surgical site infections, less morbidity, and a shorter length of hospital stay are still present.

In contrast to appendectomy, the use of the laparoscopic approach for gallbladder disease gained acceptance a little faster. This is perhaps due to the fact that an open cholecystectomy (OC) incision was much more painful and morbid compared to those of the laparoscopic cholecystectomy (LC). In this sense, surgeons were looking for reasons to do an LC as opposed for looking for reasons not to do an LA. As a result, the frequency of all cholecystectomies done increased as more surgeons became comfortable with performing them laparoscopically [27]. Studies also showed that the increased use of the LC corresponded with an increased incidence of major bile duct injuries, though these injuries seemed to lessen after more experience with the technique [28].

It also became clear that the LC approach fared worse if the indication for removal was acute cholecystitis. In the 1990s, if a patient presented with acute cholecystitis with a more than 72-h history of pain, surgeons would put these patients on a short antibiotic course and then would wait 4–6 weeks before performing an LC to allow the inflammation to subside. This would enable the surgeons to perform a LC without converting. In the early 2000s, several studies showed that this waiting period resulted in another bout of acute cholecystitis about 35% of the time and that an LC done initially did not have a higher rate of injury or need for a conversion to an open procedure [29, 30]. Today, most surgeons advocate for an early LC done during the index admission. There is also data that suggests operating within 24 hours of the admission improves outcomes [31].

To help prevent bile duct injuries and to assist with identification of the biliary anatomy, surgeons began routinely using intraoperative cholangiography (IOC). This also had the benefit of identifying common bile duct stones. Despite these theoretical benefits, the routine use of an IOC has not decreased the bile duct injury rate, and a positive IOC for choledocholithiasis results in a not insignificant rate of negative common bile duct exploration [32, 33]. Laparoscopic ultrasound has also been utilized as a substitute for IOC, and while effective, it has a steep learning curve [33]. Immunofluorescence using indocyanine green (ICG) and near-infrared cameras has also been touted for identifying biliary anatomy. Unlike laparoscopic ultrasound, it is easy to implement and appears to aid in the detection of biliary anatomy including variants [34]. ICG cholangiography has not proven to prevent bile duct injury, however, and it does not necessarily detect common bile duct stones. It also requires laparoscopes that have near-infrared imaging capability.

Today, the Tokyo Guidelines can predict difficult cholecystectomies and account for the patient's physiologic response to identify those better treated by percutaneous drainage [35] (see Table 1).

Additionally, the Society of Gastrointestinal and Endoscopic Surgeons (SAGES) has published guidelines for prevention of bile duct injuries. The guidelines advocate for establishing the critical view of safety (see Fig. 1).

If this view cannot be achieved, even if using a top-down technique, then a subtotal cholecystectomy with drain placement should be performed. Additionally,

Table 1 The Tokyo guidelines for acute cholecystitis [35]

Grade	Definition	Recommendation
Grade I—mild	Cholecystitis in a healthy patient with mild inflammatory changes and without organ dysfunction	Cholecystectomy
Grade II—moderate	WBC > 18,000/mm³ Palpable tender mass in the RUQ Duration of complaints >72 h Marked local inflammation (gangrenous cholecystitis, pericholecystitis, abscess, bile peritonitis, emphysematous cholecystitis	If patient can withstand surgery and resources are appropriate, then can proceed with cholecystectomy. If not, then biliary drainage is preferred
Grade III—severe meaning organ dysfunction of one of the following	Cardiovascular—hypotension requiring pressor support Neurologic—decreased level of consciousness Respiratory—PaO_2/FiO_2 ratio < 300 Renal—oliguria or Cr > 2.0 mg/dL Hepatic—INR > 1.5 Hematological—platelet count <100,000/mm³	Biliary drainage is preferred but if physiology can be corrected and the cholecystectomy can be performed by an experienced surgeon and ICU care is available, then a cholecystectomy can be considered

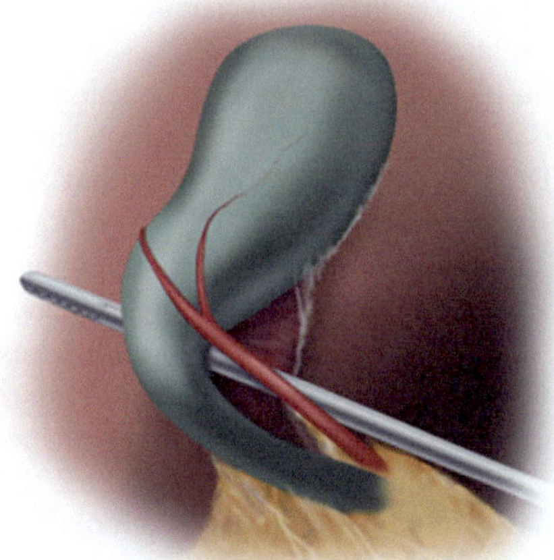
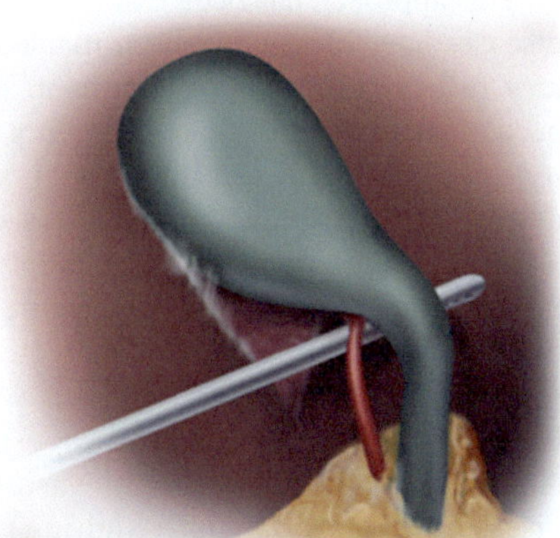

Critical view of safety anterior view   Critical view of safety posterior view

Fig. 1 Critical views of safety. This view should be achieved before ligating and dividing any duct (*Reproduced with permission from SAGES*)

every effort should be made to remove all the stones from the gallbladder [36]. Recent national trends highlight a rising number of laparoscopic subtotal cholecystectomies, suggesting the acceptance of this strategy versus traditional conversion to open surgery [37].

Since the beginning of the twenty-first century, there is no doubt that MIS techniques are being utilized more frequently for several other diseases. A review of the NSQIP data from 2007 to 2016 shows the use of MIS to treat perforated peptic ulcers increased from 0 to 37% and small bowel obstructions from 6 to 11% [13]. There is more and more data available that suggests the laparoscopic approach for small bowel obstructions from adhesive disease fares much better than do open ones. The LASSO trial is a prospective, randomized, multicenter trial that shows fewer complications and a shorter length of stay with the laparoscopic approach for patients with a small bowel obstruction [38].

An additional role for the minimally invasive approach in acute care surgery is that of damage control. Damage control surgery (DCS) was first described in the context of wartime management of severe polytrauma and physiologic derangement. Its principals are to stop hemorrhage, limit contamination, and exit the operating room as quickly as possible to allow ongoing resuscitation in a critical care environment. These tenets are now being more broadly applied to civilian trauma and emergency general surgery. The DCS approach allows the surgeon to prevent contamination and progression of disease while at the same time minimizing the initial surgical physiologic insult. It can also allow the acute care surgeon to temporize surgical disease and buy time for the involvement of the specialist more germane to that disease, like a colorectal, hepatobiliary, or bariatric surgeon.

This approach has been examined in Hinchey Grade 3 and 4 diverticulitis. These diseases have classically been managed with a laparotomy, resection, and temporary ostomy placement (Hartmann's procedure). Laparoscopy has traditionally been avoided due to a feared inability to clear all contamination and degraded ability to assess tissue viability. Laparoscopic DCS to perform only a washout and drainage of perforated diverticulitis disease has been described. This technique, along with antibiotics, has been employed to avoid an initial extensive surgery and the creation of an ostomy with requirement of a subsequent takedown. After recovery, the patient can be taken for an elective resection of the diseased colon. Studies show that this method does not necessarily mean the formation of fewer ostomies because of the need for an ileostomy to protect the colonic anastomosis. Additionally, the laparoscopic washout does not seem to adequately control the disease with more patients requiring reoperations, more secondary procedures like radiology-guided drainage, and without an improved quality of life. There is also a concern for missed carcinoma [39–41]. On the other hand, a laparoscopic Hartmann's with subsequent laparoscopic reversal after recovery has also been described [42]. So in this instance, laparoscopic washout is an option that may benefit the extremely frail patient, but if possible, a laparoscopic Hartmann's may be a better option.

Another surgical emergency, which lends itself to a DCS approach, is that of a strangulated paraesophageal hernia with or without a gastric volvulus. Initial reduction of the herniated contents and gastric detorsion are a surgical emergency to prevent ischemia and perforation with subsequent overwhelming sepsis. In the elective setting, this is best facilitated by a laparoscopic approach due to the limited working space at the diaphragmatic hiatus and the morbidity of an upper midline or thoracic incision. In elective cases, formal repair of the hernia is mandated to prevent recurrence. In the emergent setting and for surgeons with limited expertise with crural repairs, reduction and detorsion can be followed by anterior gastropexy with a plan to return for formal hernia repair either by the index surgeon or an MIS expert [43]. Ischemic gastric tissue can be removed with a stapler and wedge resection. In frail patients who have limited physiologic reserve, a formal repair can be a long and risky operation, so even for surgeons with extensive foregut experience, a reduction and pexy may be the more prudent goal at the initial presentation.

In the bariatric surgery patient with a leak, laparoscopic DCS can again be performed by the acute care surgeon. First and foremost, hemodynamically unstable patients need surgical intervention to visualize the leak, the involved bowel, and to rule out internal herniation. Even in the cases of negative preoperative imaging, a high index of suspicion must be maintained in those patients who do not improve with resuscitation [44]. The exploration can be done laparoscopically. Repairs can be done with an omental patch; but at times, the leak site is so diseased with inflammation that any attempt at repair is unlikely to hold. Additionally, even with the use of intraoperative endoscopy, the leak site may be hard to locate. In those cases, laparoscopic washout, drain placement, and distal enteric access can suffice as a damage control strategy [45, 46]. Further control of the leak can be done endoscopically or with an elective revision by an experienced bariatric surgeon.

6 Today

Success with EGS is as much dependent on the surgeon as it is on the patient's physiology and the disease itself. For EGS patients, about 3,000,000 cases are done annually, and these patients are *eight times* more likely to die than elective patients and 50% of EGS patients will have at least one complication [47]. Eighty percent of the procedures, mortality, cost, and complications from EGS come from seven relatively common surgeries to include appendectomies, cholecystectomy, colectomies, lysis of adhesions, repair of a perforated peptic ulcer, small bowel resection, and an emergent laparotomy, most likely done for an acute abdomen of unclear etiology, like mesenteric ischemia [47]. Appendectomies and cholecystectomies account for a significant percentage of the cost mostly due to their frequency, while the very high mortality from a laparotomy comes from the fact that these patients are likely very sick and more likely to be hemodynamically unstable. The four remaining diseases benefit from the laparoscopic approach with lower mortality, fewer wound infections, and a shorter length of stay. In fact, in the same study regarding the national burden of emergency general surgery, the laparoscopic partial colectomies were seven times less likely to die and 50% less likely to have a complication [47]. Clearly, there are benefits to the laparoscopic approach and when possible, this approach should be attempted. Robot-assisted laparoscopic surgery has the potential to allow more acute care surgeons to perform complex laparoscopic procedures without formal laparoscopic training. As such, it should be utilized in acute settings because it may allow less experienced laparoscopic surgeons to provide the benefits of laparoscopy without needing formal laparoscopic training.

7   MIS in Trauma

Currently, the MIS approach for the trauma patient is only indicated for hemodynamically stable patients regardless of the mechanism. As in the world of EGS, there is considerable debate regarding the role for laparoscopy in trauma. Its benefit, though, is documented in four key areas:

1. To rule out occult diaphragmatic injury in patients otherwise without indication for laparotomy
2. To rule out peritoneal violation in low-energy penetrating abdominal trauma
3. To intervene on an injury identified on imaging despite a normal clinical presentation
4. To investigate a concerning abdominal exam that has normal radiologic studies

Asymptomatic diaphragm injuries can be difficult to diagnosis in the stable trauma patient following thoracoabdominal injury. Blunt injury tends to cause larger defects which are less likely to be radiographically or clinically occult [48]. Penetrating injury, however, has been shown to cause smaller defects which nonetheless require repair to prevent long-term sequelae. Diagnostic laparoscopy has proven a useful adjunct to both screen for these injuries and, when present, repair them [49, 50].

In the setting of penetrating abdominal wounds with unclear violation of the peritoneum, laparoscopy can serve as a useful adjunct. Negative or nontherapeutic laparotomy has a significant burden of morbidity without therapeutic gain in trauma patients. Rates of negative laparotomy have declined with improved imaging and resuscitative techniques yet remain a small but significant contributor to morbidity in trauma [51]. The use of laparoscopy to detect peritoneal violation in these cases is effective and decreases rates of negative laparotomy [52]. Additionally, if peritoneal violation is found, the surgeon can elect to convert to laparotomy or perform the repairs laparoscopically [53]. Critics of therapeutic laparoscopy after detection of peritoneal violation have argued that the MIS approach leads to missed additional injuries, but systematic schema for evaluating the peritoneal contents have been shown to be highly effective for detecting additional injuries in the hands of experienced laparoscopists [54].

8   Endoscopy

Any discussion of the evolution of MIS in acute care must include a discussion of the evolution of endoscopic therapies. Endoscopy has supplanted open surgery for many indications in a similar manner to laparoscopy. Endoscopic therapies can further limit the physiologic insult placed on patients by anesthesia and in many cases provide incisionless therapies that might previously have required laparotomy.

Much like laparoscopy, the technology behind flexible endoscopy stops and starts with sometimes lukewarm interest in its adoption. Open specula for peering into natural offices date to Galen's time, and Hippocrates described their use in the assessment of fistulae. In the early 1800s, German-Italian physician Philipp Bozzini added mirror-reflected candlelight and, much like Kurt Semm's early work, was met with derision from the academic establishment [55]. Over the next century, light condensers, telescopic lenses, and insufflators were added. A breakthrough was achieved in 1898 when the first gastroscopy was performed using an articulating, lighted scope designed by the same aforementioned George Kelling of early celiotomy fame [55]. The use of flexible glass fibers for both light transmission and image return developed in the 1950s and heralded an explosion in the utility and adoption of truly flexible endoscopy. Remote cameras and televisions replaced eye pieces in the 1980s, and computer chip-based cameras have since drastically improved image quality. The development of novel therapeutic attachments and devices remains ongoing today.

In the case of gastrointestinal bleeding, endoscopy established itself as a useful diagnostic tool as early as the 1940s [56]. Nonetheless, even a decade later, proponents of endoscopy were still lobbying the medical community to advocate for more routine use [57]. In 1979, the use of "endoscopic electrohemostasis" was described, ushering in the era of therapeutic endoscopy for GI hemorrhage [58]. Today, electrosurgical energy, epinephrine injection, endoscopic clipping, and even endoscopic suturing to treat many lesions would have been managed with open surgery and morbid resections 40 years ago.

In addition to endoscopic adjuncts for bleeding, the ability to endoscopically place stents offers another tool in the armamentarium of the acute care surgeon. The first use of a colonic stent to decompress a malignant large bowel obstruction was performed in 1994 [59]. Previously, an acute, complete, large bowel obstruction necessitated prompt resection, often without the time for staging and in an unprepped colon. Stenting allows prompt relief of obstruction allowing for more workup, an appropriate mechanical bowel prep, the use of chemo and radiation therapy when appropriate, and time for a frank discussion with the patient and family. Even more recently, foregut use of endoscopic stenting in the case of leak following bariatric surgery highlights the utility of this adjunct as a tool for the acute care surgeon [60].

The endoscope, much like the laparoscope and for many of the same reasons, has demonstrated its utility as a diagnostic, therapeutic, and adjunctive tool. As this technology continues to improve, the acute care surgeon must also be a competent therapeutic endoscopist to effectively treat patients with the lowest possible morbidity.

9   Summary

Many of the concepts here are discussed in more detail in other chapters of this textbook, but it is safe to say the laparoscopic and endoscopic techniques have improved outcomes and patient safety in the many acute care surgical diseases. In many of these instances, patients have shorter hospital stays, lower overall costs, less morbidity, and even less mortality. The poor physiologic health of the EGS patients that present acutely cannot be understated, and it often dictates how and when surgical intervention takes place. The frail patient should have the least amount of surgical stress possible. Sometimes that means utilizing interventional radiology or endoscopic techniques, and other times, it means doing damage control procedures laparoscopically. As laparoscopy extends to other diseases like trauma, so too should the use of the robot platform in the acute setting. It allows the surgeon more options in cases where the anatomy is compromised and the tissue is poor. Endoscopy also has many benefits in the acute setting, and therapeutic endoscopy should be part of the acute care surgeon's skill set. Finally, damage control principles can be employed to control laparoscopically the bleeding, ischemia, or infection to allow time for adequate resuscitation and physiologic optimization of the patient with less physiologic stress and fewer complications than that of an open procedure. It behooves surgical educators to make sure these skills are part of the training of residents, and it is incumbent on practicing surgeons to add these MIS techniques to their work.

References

1. Hatzinger M, et al. Hans Christian Jacobaeus: inventor of human laparoscopy and thoracoscopy. J Endourol. 2006;20(11):848–50. https://doi.org/10.1089/end.2006.20.848.
2. Kelley WE Jr. The evolution of laparoscopy and the revolution in surgery in the decade of the 1990s. JSLS. 2008;12(4):351–7.
3. Bhattacharya K. Kurt Semm: a laparoscopic crusader. J Minim Access Surg. 2007;3(1):35–6. https://doi.org/10.4103/0972-9941.30686.
4. Semm K. Endoscopic appendectomy. Endoscopy. 1983;15(2):59–64. https://doi.org/10.1055/s-2007-1021466.
5. Litynski GS. Erich Mühe and the rejection of laparoscopic cholecystectomy (1985): a surgeon ahead of his time. JSLS. 1998;2(4):341–6.
6. The minimally invasive operations that transformed surgery. www.facs.org/-/media/files/archives/shg-poster/2017/10_minimally_invasive.ashx?la=en.
7. Wang S, Shi N, You L, Dai M, Zhao Y. Minimally invasive surgical approach versus open procedure for pancreaticoduodenectomy: a systematic review and meta-analysis. Medicine (Baltimore). 2017;96(50):e8619. https://doi.org/10.1097/MD.0000000000008619.
8. Bertleff MJ, Halm JA, Bemelman WA, van der Ham AC, van der Harst E, Oei HI, et al. Randomized clinical trial of laparoscopic versus open repair of the perforated peptic ulcer: the LAMA trial. World J Surg. 2009;33(7):1368–73.

9. Fields AC, Gonzalez DO, Chin EH, Nguyen SQ, Zhang LP, Divino CM. Laparoscopic-assisted transversus abdominis plane block for postoperative pain control in laparoscopic ventral hernia repair: a randomized controlled trial. J Am Coll Surg. 2015;221(2):462–9.
10. Krielen P, Stommel MW, Pargmae P, Bouvy ND, Bakkum EA, Ellis H, et al. Adhesion-related readmissions after open and laparoscopic surgery: a retrospective cohort study (SCAR update). Lancet. 2020;395(10217):33–41.
11. Sammour T, Kahokehr A, Chan S, Booth RJ, Hill AG. The humoral response after laparoscopic versus open colorectal surgery: a meta-analysis. J Surg Res. 2010;164(1):28–37. https://doi.org/10.1016/j.jss.2010.05.046.
12. Kulkarni N, Arulampalam T. Laparoscopic surgery reduces the incidence of surgical site infections compared to the open approach for colorectal procedures: a meta-analysis. Tech Coloproctol. 2020;24(10):1017–24. https://doi.org/10.1007/s10151-020-02293-8.
13. Arnold M, Elhage S, Schiffern L, Lauren Paton B, Ross SW, Matthews BD, Reinke CE. Use of minimally invasive surgery in emergency general surgery procedures. Surg Endosc. 2020;34(5):2258–65. https://doi.org/10.1007/s00464-019-07016-1.
14. Pernar L, Robertson FC, Tavakkoli A, Sheu EG, Brooks DC, Smink DS. An appraisal of the learning curve in robotic general surgery. Surg Endosc. 2017;31(11):4583–96. https://doi.org/10.1007/s00464-017-5520-2.
15. Ahmad G, Baker J, Finnerty J, Phillips K, Watson A. Laparoscopic entry techniques. Cochrane Database Syst Rev. 2019;1(1):CD006583. https://doi.org/10.1002/14651858.CD006583.pub5.
16. Lee J. Update on electrosurgery. Outpatient Surg. 2002;2(2):44–53.
17. Fuchshuber P, Schwaitzberg S, Jones D, Jones SB, Feldman L, Munro M, Robinson T, Purcell-Jackson G, Mikami D, Madani A, Brunt M, Dunkin B, Gugliemi C, Groah L, Lim R, Mischna J, Voyles CR. The SAGES fundamental use of surgical energy program (FUSE): history, development, and purpose. Surg Endosc. 2018;32(6):2583–602. https://doi.org/10.1007/s00464-017-5933-y.
18. Ha A, Richards C, Criman E, Piaggione J, Yheulon C, Lim R. The safe use of surgical energy devices by surgeons may be overestimated. Surg Endosc. 2018;32(9):3861–7. https://doi.org/10.1007/s00464-018-6116-1.
19. Atkinson TM, Giraud GD, Togioka BM, Jones DB, Cigarroa JE. Cardiovascular and ventilatory consequences of laparoscopic surgery. Circulation. 2017;135(7):700–10. https://doi.org/10.1161/CIRCULATIONAHA.116.023262.
20. Bonanni F, Reed J 3rd, Hartzell G, Trostle D, Boorse R, Gittleman M, Cole A. Laparoscopic versus conventional appendectomy. J Am Coll Surg. 1994;179(3):273–8.
21. Yau KK, Siu WT, Tang CN, Yang GP, Li MK. Laparoscopic versus open appendectomy for complicated appendicitis. J Am Coll Surg. 2007;205(1):60–5. https://doi.org/10.1016/j.jamcollsurg.2007.03.017.
22. Pokala N, Sadhasivam S, Kiran RP, Parithivel V. Complicated appendicitis—is the laparoscopic approach appropriate? A comparative study with the open approach: outcome in a community hospital setting. Am Surg. 2007;73(8):737–42.
23. Asarias JR, Schlussel AT, Cafasso DE, Carlson TL, Kasprenski MC, Washington EN, Lustik MB, Yamamura MS, Matayoshi EZ, Zagorski SM. Incidence of postoperative intraabdominal abscesses in open versus laparoscopic appendectomies. Surg Endosc. 2011;25(8):2678–83. https://doi.org/10.1007/s00464-011-1628-y.
24. Quah GS, Eslick GD, Cox MR. Laparoscopic appendectomy is superior to open surgery for complicated appendicitis. Surg Endosc. 2019;33(7):2072–82. https://doi.org/10.1007/s00464-019-06746-6.
25. Talha A, El-Haddad H, Ghazal AE, Shehata G. Laparoscopic versus open appendectomy for perforated appendicitis in adults: randomized clinical trial. Surg Endosc. 2020;34(2):907–14. https://doi.org/10.1007/s00464-019-06847-2.
26. Yu MC, Feng YJ, Wang W, Fan W, Cheng HT, Xu J. Is laparoscopic appendectomy feasible for complicated appendicitis? A systematic review and meta-analysis. Int J Surg. 2017;40:187–97. https://doi.org/10.1016/j.ijsu.2017.03.022.

27. Orlando R 3rd, Russell JC, Lynch J, Mattie A. Laparoscopic cholecystectomy. A statewide experience. The Connecticut Laparoscopic Cholecystectomy Registry. Arch Surg. 1993;128(5):494–9. https://doi.org/10.1001/archsurg.1993.01420170024002.
28. Russell JC, Walsh SJ, Mattie AS, Lynch JT. Bile duct injuries, 1989-1993. A statewide experience. Connecticut Laparoscopic Cholecystectomy Registry. Arch Surg. 1996;131(4):382–8. https://doi.org/10.1001/archsurg.1996.01430160040007.
29. Gurusamy KS, Davidson C, Gluud C, Davidson BR. Early versus delayed laparoscopic cholecystectomy for people with acute cholecystitis. Cochrane Database Syst Rev. 2013;(6):CD005440. https://doi.org/10.1002/14651858.CD005440.pub3.
30. Gurusamy KS, Koti R, Fusai G, Davidson BR. Early versus delayed laparoscopic cholecystectomy for uncomplicated biliary colic. Cochrane Database Syst Rev. 2013;(6):CD007196. https://doi.org/10.1002/14651858.CD007196.pub3.
31. Ford JA, Soop M, Du J, Loveday BP, Rodgers M. Systematic review of intraoperative cholangiography in cholecystectomy. Br J Surg. 2012;99(2):160–7. https://doi.org/10.1002/bjs.7809.
32. Donnellan E, Coulter J, Mathew C, Choynowski M, Flanagan L, Bucholc M, Johnston A, Sugrue M. A meta-analysis of the use of intraoperative cholangiography; time to revisit our approach to cholecystectomy? Surg Open Sci. 2020;3:8–15. https://doi.org/10.1016/j.sopen.2020.07.004.
33. Dili A, Bertrand C. Laparoscopic ultrasonography as an alternative to intraoperative cholangiography during laparoscopic cholecystectomy. World J Gastroenterol. 2017;23(29):5438–50. https://doi.org/10.3748/wjg.v23.i29.5438.
34. Dip F, LoMenzo E, Sarotto L, Phillips E, Todeschini H, Nahmod M, Alle L, Schneider S, Kaja L, Boni L, Ferraina P, Carus T, Kokudo N, Ishizawa T, Walsh M, Simpfendorfer C, Mayank R, White K, Rosenthal RJ. Randomized trial of near-infrared incisionless fluorescent cholangiography. Ann Surg. 2019;270(6):992–9. https://doi.org/10.1097/SLA.0000000000003178.
35. Okamoto K, Suzuki K, Takada T, Strasberg SM, Asbun HJ, Endo I, Iwashita Y, Hibi T, Pitt HA, Umezawa A, Asai K, Han HS, Hwang TL, Mori Y, Yoon YS, Huang WS, Belli G, Dervenis C, Yokoe M, Kiriyama S, et al. Tokyo guidelines 2018: flowchart for the management of acute cholecystitis. J Hepatobiliary Pancreat Sci. 2018;25(1):55–72. https://doi.org/10.1002/jhbp.516.
36. Michael Brunt L, Deziel DJ, Telem DA, Strasberg SM, Aggarwal R, Asbun H, Bonjer J, McDonald M, Alseidi A, Ujiki M, Riall TS, Hammill C, Moulton CA, Pucher PH, Parks RW, Ansari MT, Connor S, Dirks RC, Anderson B, Altieri MS, et al. Safe cholecystectomy multi-society practice guideline and state-of-the-art consensus conference on prevention of bile duct injury during cholecystectomy. Surg Endosc. 2020;34(7):2827–55. https://doi.org/10.1007/s00464-020-07568-7.
37. Sabour AF, Matsushima K, Love BE, Alicuben ET, Schellenberg MA, Inaba K, Demetriades D. Nationwide trends in the use of subtotal cholecystectomy for acute cholecystitis. Surgery. 2020;167(3):569–74.
38. Sallinen V, Di Saverio S, Haukijärvi E, Juusela R, Wikström H, Koivukangas V, Catena F, Enholm B, Birindelli A, Leppäniemi A, Mentula P. Laparoscopic versus open adhesiolysis for adhesive small bowel obstruction (LASSO): an international, multicentre, randomised, open-label trial. Lancet Gastroenterol Hepatol. 2019;4(4):278–86. https://doi.org/10.1016/S2468-1253(19)30016-0.
39. Schultz JK, Yaqub S, Wallon C, Blecic L, Forsmo HM, Folkesson J, Buchwald P, Körner H, Dahl FA, Øresland T, SCANDIV Study Group. Laparoscopic lavage vs primary resection for acute perforated diverticulitis: the SCANDIV randomized clinical trial. JAMA. 2015;314(13):1364–75. https://doi.org/10.1001/jama.2015.12076.
40. Galbraith N, Carter JV, Netz U, Yang D, Fry DE, McCafferty M, Galandiuk S. Laparoscopic lavage in the management of perforated diverticulitis: a contemporary meta-analysis. J Gastrointest Surg. 2017;21(9):1491–9. https://doi.org/10.1007/s11605-017-3462-6.
41. Schultz JK, Wallon C, Blecic L, Forsmo HM, Folkesson J, Buchwald P, Kørner H, Dahl FA, Øresland T, Yaqub S, SCANDIV Study Group. One-year results of the SCANDIV randomized

clinical trial of laparoscopic lavage versus primary resection for acute perforated diverticulitis. Br J Surg. 2017;104(10):1382–92. https://doi.org/10.1002/bjs.10567.

42. Chouillard E, Maggiori L, Ata T, Jarbaoui S, Rivkine E, Benhaim L, et al. Laparoscopic two-stage left colonic resection for patients with peritonitis caused by acute diverticulitis. Dis Colon Rectum. 2007;50(8):1157–63.

43. Coleman C, et al. Incarcerated paraesophageal hernia and gastric volvulus: management options for the acute care surgeon, an Eastern Association for the Surgery of Trauma master class video presentation. J Trauma Acute Care Surg. 2020;88(6):e146–8.

44. Wernick B, Jansen M, Noria S, Stawicki SP, El Chaar M. Essential bariatric emergencies for the acute care surgeon. Eur J Trauma Emerg Surg. 2016;42(5):571–84. https://doi.org/10.1007/s00068-015-0621-x.

45. Yurcisin BM, DeMaria EJ. Management of leak in the bariatric gastric bypass patient: reoperate, drain and feed distally. J Gastrointest Surg. 2009;13(9):1564–6. https://doi.org/10.1007/s11605-009-0861-3.

46. Chang J, Sharma G, Boules M, Brethauer S, Rodriguez J, Kroh MD. Endoscopic stents in the management of anastomotic complications after foregut surgery: new applications and techniques. Surg Obes Relat Dis. 2016;12(7):1373–81. https://doi.org/10.1016/j.soard.2016.02.041. Epub 2016 Mar 2. PMID: 27317605.

47. Scott JW, Olufajo OA, Brat GA, Rose JA, Zogg CK, Haider AH, Salim A, Havens JM. Use of national burden to define operative emergency general surgery. JAMA Surg. 2016;151(6):e160480. https://doi.org/10.1001/jamasurg.2016.0480.

48. Hammer MM, Flagg E, Mellnick VM, Cummings KW, Bhalla S, Raptis CA. Computed tomography of blunt and penetrating diaphragmatic injury: sensitivity and inter-observer agreement of CT signs. Emerg Radiol. 2014;21(2):143–9.

49. Friese RS, Coln CE, Gentilello LM. Laparoscopy is sufficient to exclude occult diaphragm injury after penetrating abdominal trauma. J Trauma Acute Care Surg. 2005;58(4):789–92.

50. D'Souza N, Bruce JL, Clarke DL, Laing GL. Laparoscopy for occult left-sided diaphragm injury following penetrating thoracoabdominal trauma is both diagnostic and therapeutic. Surg Laparosc Endosc Percutan Tech. 2016;26(1):e5–8.

51. Schnüriger B, Lam L, Inaba K, Kobayashi L, Barbarino R, Demetriades D. Negative laparotomy in trauma: are we getting better? Am Surg. 2012;78(11):1219–23.

52. Uranues S, Popa DE, Diaconescu B, Schrittwieser R. Laparoscopy in penetrating abdominal trauma. World J Surg. 2015;39(6):1381–8.

53. Bain K, Meytes V, Chang GC, Timoney MF. Laparoscopy in penetrating abdominal trauma is a safe and effective alternative to laparotomy. Surg Endosc. 2019;33(5):1618–25.

54. Kawahara NT, Alster C, Fujimura I, Poggetti RS, Birolini D. Standard examination system for laparoscopy in penetrating abdominal trauma. J Trauma Acute Care Surg. 2009;67(3):589–95.

55. Berci G, Forde KA. History of endoscopy. Surg Endosc. 2000;14(1):5.

56. Jones CM. Diagnostic and therapeutic considerations of gastrointestinal bleeding. N Engl J Med. 1946;235(22):773–6.

57. Katz D, Friedman E, Selesnick S. Endoscopy in acute upper gastrointestinal bleeding. Am J Dig Dis. 1958;3(10):734–42.

58. Gaisford WD. Endoscopic electrohemostasis of active upper gastrointestinal bleeding. Am J Surg. 1979;137(1):47–53.

59. Tejero E, Mainar A, Fernandez L, Tobío R, De Gregorio MA. New procedure for the treatment of colorectal neoplastic obstructions. Dis Colon Rectum. 1994;37(11):1158–9.

60. Krishnan V, Hutchings K, Godwin A, Wong JT, Teixeira J. Long-term outcomes following endoscopic stenting in the management of leaks after foregut and bariatric surgery. Surg Endosc. 2019;33(8):2691–5.

History of Thoracoscopy in Emergency Surgery and Trauma

Morgan M. Sellers, Fredric M. Pieracci, and Clay Cothren Burlew

The origins of thoracoscopy, as with much of thoracic surgery, are rooted in nineteenth-century attempts to treat tuberculosis. Innovative work in Europe and the United States throughout the 1800s was based on the principle that inducing a pneumothorax caused collapse of the diseased lung, which led to clinical improvement in patients with cavitary pulmonary disease. By the late 1890s, the technique was perfected in Europe and around the time of World War I was widespread within the United States [1].

While the basic technique for inducing pneumothorax required only percutaneous access to the pleural space, it was severely limited in many patients by the pleural adhesions that often developed in diseased lungs, preventing full lobar collapse. Efforts to overcome this limitation drew the attention of Swedish internist Hans Christian Jacobaeus, the same physician noted in the previous chapter, who pioneered laparoscopy. In 1910, he had also published the first recorded description of thoracoscopy in association with the thoracic surgeon Einar Key [2]. This initial report described only two cases of diagnostic thoracoscopy, but over the next few years, Jacobaeus went on to publish reports of nearly 100 cases of thoracoscopy [3].

M. M. Sellers (✉)
Division of Acute Care Surgery, Department of Surgery, University of New Mexico School of Medicine, Albuquerque, NM, USA
e-mail: Mmsellers@salud.unm.edu

F. M. Pieracci
Denver Health Medical Center, Denver, CO, USA

University of Colorado School of Medicine, Aurora, CO, USA
e-mail: fredric.pieracci@dhha.org

C. C. Burlew
Department of Surgery, University of Colorado, Aurora, CO, USA
e-mail: clay.cothren@dhha.org

1913 marked his first thoracoscopic lysis of adhesions to achieve pneumothorax—a procedure which later became known as the "Jacobaeus operation" [4].

Over the next few decades, thoracoscopy spread widely throughout Europe, the United States, and Canada. Performed using local anesthetic with the patient breathing spontaneously, both single and double port techniques were described in two clinical arenas: diagnostic workup of malignancy and lysis of pleural adhesions to allow pneumothorax in patients with tuberculosis. Despite the description of early versions of surgical energy and biopsy forceps, the technical instruments were relatively primitive, and therapeutic uses of thoracoscopy were limited in part by the risk of uncontrolled hemorrhage. A discussant on a paper in a later era described thoracoscopic lysis of adhesions as, "much like patting one's head and rubbing one's abdomen at the same time … The instrument actually made me nervous because of the feeling of inadequate control and the possibility of disaster, such as bronchial leak and hemorrhage" [5]. As medical treatment of tuberculosis advanced in the mid-1900s, the need for lobar collapse therapy evaporated, and the Jacobaeus operation (along with overall familiarity and use of thoracoscopy) was largely abandoned.

Toward the end of this early period, a few individuals did find more varied applications for thoracoscopy, including the first recorded uses in trauma. In 1946, Martins Castello Branco published a paper entitled "Thoracoscopy as a method of exploration in penetrating injuries" [6], describing his practice of inserting a thoracoscope through a penetrating injury "to verify visually, whether the wound bleeds into the thorax, or whether there is a pulmonary lesion, with or without bleeding, as well as lesion of any intrathoracic vein." He went on to describe how "in the absence of hemorrhage, or when it is discovered that the bleeding vein has already been obliterated, this method enables us to avoid thoracotomy, an operation which is much more serious than a thoracoscopy which only requires a simple small pleurotomy. It further enables us to find out whether or not there exists injury to the diaphragm with the possibility of damage to an abdominal organ or vein, requiring laparotomy; and also to discover whether on the left side there exists a wound in the pericardium, with probability of a lesion of the myocardium requiring, in either case, a quick intervention for its suture."

The next few decades marked a period of stagnation and even rejection of thoracoscopy overall [7], particularly in the United States. But individuals in a few centers revived the technique, prompting a resurgence. The use of a double-lumen endotracheal tube to allow single-lung ventilation and increase visibility was introduced in 1970 [8]. In 1978, Miller and Hatcher from Emory University in Atlanta, Georgia [9], described their experience with diagnostic thoracoscopy in 11 patients over a 12-month period as a complement to bronchoscopy, thoracentesis, and pleural biopsy, noting that thoracoscopy was "reinstituted" at their institution in 1976. The 1980s saw a proliferation of diagnostic indications, with many publications noting the revival of the procedure within thoracic surgery, using techniques as varied as a sterilized sigmoidoscope [10], an arthroscopic "needle scope" [11], a laparoscope [12], mediastinoscope [13], and a bronchoscope [14, 15]. Notably, other issues under examination in the literature of this era were whether diagnostic thoracoscopy could be safely performed by pulmonologists [16], and which cases mandated general anesthesia lung isolation.

Thoracoscopy was rediscovered in trauma as well, with the first publications reestablishing the same indications described 30 years prior. In 1976, Jackson and Ferreira published a case series from Johannesburg, South Africa, demonstrating the utility of thoracoscopy in diagnosing occult diaphragmatic injuries [17]. They described the results of thoracoscopy in 11 patients with "penetrating wounds of the left lower chest, who had no definite clinical or radiological indication for operation. In 6 patients the diaphragm was seen clearly, and in 2 of these an unsuspected diaphragmatic injury was found. Both injuries were later confirmed at operation. The other 4 patients had intact diaphragms and were successfully treated conservatively." They went on to suggest that "thoracoscopy is a useful aid in the diagnosis of left-sided, diaphragmatic injury and that the best results are obtained if it is performed within 24 h of injury." A larger case series from the same institution was published in 1982 by Adamthwaite [18].

The introduction of video-based technology to minimally invasive surgery in the early 1990s ushered in a new era for thoracoscopy, with video-assisted thoracoscopic surgery (VATS) allowing a full range of therapeutic as well as diagnostic techniques [19, 20]. While the primary focus for thoracoscopic advances was on oncologic procedures, emergency and trauma procedures began to be more frequently described. A 1993 paper by Smith et al. from Oakland, California [21], examined the use of VATS in 24 patients with ongoing thoracic hemorrhage, clotted hemothorax, and suspected diaphragmatic injury. The report advocated for "wider use of the technique in the trauma setting. It is an accurate, safe, and minimally invasive method for the assessment of diaphragmatic injury … [and] effective in the evacuation of clotted hemothorax." Over the next few decades, evacuation of retained hemothorax became a particularly well-described use of VATS [22] with multiple publications examining idea timing of the procedure and comparing outcomes of VATS to additional chest tubes, the use of fibrinolytics, and other attempted techniques.

These three indications (hemorrhage control, drainage of retained hemothorax, diagnosis, and treatment of diaphragmatic injury) remain the most widely described indications for videothoracoscopy in trauma. However, an increasing range of therapeutic uses have been described including decortication/drainage of posttraumatic thoracic empyema [23, 24], retrieval of foreign bodies [25], stapling of injured lung parenchyma and creation of pericardial window [26], repair of tracheal injury [27], management of posttraumatic persistent pneumothorax [28], treatment of chylothorax [29], and various degrees of thoracoscopic guidance during surgical stabilization of rib fractures [30–32] demonstrating the degree to which videothoracoscopy has become a crucial and versatile tool in the armamentarium of the trauma surgeon.

Additionally, there are clear indications for VATS in nontraumatic emergency surgery. Thoracoscopy as part of minimally invasive treatment of esophageal perforation was described prior to the advent of VATS [33] and continues to undergo refinement and debate [34]. Left-sided VATS has been described to achieve pericardial effusion drainage and relieve tamponade physiology [35]. Slightly less emergent indications include thoracoscopic first rib resection for thoracic outlet syndrome [36] and VATS truncal vagotomy [37].

The current literature shows ongoing efforts to refine these techniques and clarify indications for thoracoscopic procedure while also reexploring currently held assumptions such as the need for general anesthesia and single-lung ventilation [38–40].

References

1. Rosenblatt MB. Pulmonary tuberculosis: evolution of modern therapy. Bull N Y Acad Med. 1973;49:163–96.
2. Jacobaeus. Über die Moglichkeit, die Zystoskopie bei Untersuchung seröser Höhlungen anzuwenden. Munch Med Wochenschr. 1910;57.
3. Jacobaeus HC. The cauterization of adhesions in artificial pneumothorax treatment of pulmonary tuberculosis under thoracoscopic control. Proc R Soc Med. 1923;16:45–62.
4. Pietro MG, Tassi G. Thoracoscopy: an old technique 2 for a modern work-up of the pleural cavity. In: Thoracoscopy for pulmonologists: a didactic approach. Berlin: Springer; 2014. p. 5–16.
5. Oakes DD, Sherck JP, Brodsky JB, Mark JB, Jose Calif S. Therapeutic thoracoscopy. J Thorac Cardiovasc Surg. 1984;87(2):269–73.
6. Martins Castello Branco J. Thoracoscopy as a method of exploration in penetrating injuries of the thorax. Dis Chest. 1946;12:330–5.
7. Braimbridge MV. The history of thoracoscopic surgery. Ann Thorac Surg. 1993;56:610–4.
8. Baumgartner WA, Mark JBD. The use of thoracoscopy in the diagnosis of pleural disease. Arch Surg. 1980;115:420–1.
9. Miller JI, Hatcher CR. Thoracoscopy: a useful tool in the diagnosis of thoracic disease. Ann Thorac Surg. 1978;26:68–72.
10. Radigan LR, Glover JL. Thoracoscopy. Surgery. 1977;82:425–8.
11. Boushy SF, North LB. Thoracoscopy: technique and results in fourteen patients with pleural effusion. Am Rev Respir Dis. 1977;115:89.
12. Sang CTM, Braimbridge MV. Thoracoscopy simplified using the laparoscope. Thorac Cardiovasc Surg. 1981;29:129–30.
13. Lewis RJ, Kunderman PJ, Sisler GE, Mackenzie JW. Direct diagnostic thoracoscopy. Ann Thorac Surg. 1976;21:536–9.
14. Gwin E, Pierce G, Boggan M, Kerby G, Ruth W. Pleuroscopy and pleural biopsy with the flexible fiberoptic bronchoscope. Chest. 1975;67:527–31.
15. Sarkar SK, Purohit SD, Sharma TN, Sharma VK, Ram M, Singh AP. Pleuroscopy in the diagnosis of pleural effusion using a fiberoptic bronchoscope. Tubercle. 1985;66:141–4.
16. Esteva H. Who should perform thoracoscopy? The controversy continues. Chest. 1995;107:1480.
17. Jackson AM, Ferreira AA. Thoracoscopy as an aid to the diagnosis of diaphragmatic injury in penetrating wounds of the left lower chest: a preliminary report. Injury. 1976;7:213–7.
18. Adamthwaite DN. Penetrating injuries of the diaphragm. Injury. 1982;14:151–8.
19. Coltharp WH, Arnold JH, Alford WC, et al. Videothoracoscopy: improved technique and expanded indications. Ann Thorac Surg. 1992;53(5):776–8; discussion 779. https://doi.org/10.1016/0003-4975(92)91434-B.
20. LoCicero J. Video-assisted thoracic surgery study group. Ann Thorac Surg. 1993;56:734–5.
21. Smith RS, Fry WR, Tsoi EKM, Morabito DJ, Koehler RH, Reinganum SJ, Organ CH. Preliminary report on videothoracoscopy in the evaluation and treatment of thoracic injury. Am J Surg. 1993;166:690–5.

22. Villavicencio RT, Aucar JA, Wall MJ. Analysis of thoracoscopy in trauma. Surg Endosc. 1999;13:3–9.
23. Hutter JA, Harari D, Braimbridge M, v. The management of empyema thoracis by thoracoscopy and irrigation. Ann Thorac Surg. 1985;39:517–20.
24. O'Brien J, Cohen M, Solit R, Solit R, Lindenbaum G, Finnegan J, Vernick J. Thoracoscopic drainage and decortication as definitive treatment for empyema thoracis following penetrating chest injury. J Trauma Inj Infect Crit Care. 1994;36:536–40.
25. Bartek JP, Grasch A, Hazelrigg SR. Thoracoscopic retrieval of foreign bodies after penetrating chest trauma. Ann Thorac Surg. 1997;63:1783–5.
26. Pons F, Lang-Lazdunski L, de Kerangal X, Chapuis O, Bonnet PM, Jancovici R. The role of videothoracoscopy in management of precordial thoracic penetrating injuries. Eur J Cardiothorac Surg. 2002;22:7–12.
27. Martínez-Hernández NJ, Sánchez-García F, Váquez-Sánchez A, Galbis-Caravajal JM. Video-assisted thoracic surgical repair of the airway. Ann Thorac Surg. 2019;108:e45–6.
28. Carrillo EH, Schmacht DC, Gable DR, Spain DA, Richardson JD. Thoracoscopy in the management of posttraumatic persistent pneumothorax. J Am Coll Surg. 1998;186:636–9.
29. Shirai T, Amano J, Takabe K. Thoracoscopic diagnosis and treatment of chylothorax after pneumonectomy. Ann Thorac Surg. 1991;52:306–7.
30. Lin HL, Tarng YW, Wu TH, Huang FD, Huang WY, Chou YP. The advantages of adding rib fixations during VATS for retained hemothorax in serious blunt chest trauma—a prospective cohort study. Int J Surg. 2019;65:13–8.
31. Pieracci FM, Johnson JL, Stovall RT, Jurkovich GJ. Completely thoracoscopic, intra-pleural reduction and fixation of severe rib fractures. Trauma Case Rep. 2015;1:39–43.
32. Nowack T, Nonnemacher C, Christie DB. Video-assisted thoracoscopic surgery as an adjunct to rib fixation. Am Surg. 2020;88(6):1338–40.
33. Hutter JA, Fenn A, Braimbridge M, v. The management of spontaneous oesophageal perforation by thoracoscopy and irrigation. Br J Surg. 1985;72:208–9.
34. Aiolfi A, Micheletto G, Guerrazzi G, Bonitta G, Campanelli G, Bona D. Minimally invasive surgical management of Boerhaave's syndrome: a narrative literature review. J Thorac Dis. 2020;12:4411–7.
35. Muhammad MIA. The pericardial window: is a video-assisted thoracoscopy approach better than a surgical approach? Interact Cardiovasc Thorac Surg. 2011;12:174–8.
36. Ohtsuka T, Wolf RK, Dunsker SB. Port-access first-rib resection. Surg Endosc. 1999;13:940–2.
37. Chisholm EM, Chung SCS, Sunderland GT, Leong HT, Li AKC. Surgical workshop. Thoracoscopic vagotomy: a new use for the laparoscope. Br J Surg. 1992;79:254.
38. Gonzalez-Rivas D, Bonome C, Fieira E, Aymerich H, Fernandez R, Delgado M, Mendez L, de la Torre M. Non-intubated video-assisted thoracoscopic lung resections: the future of thoracic surgery? Eur J Cardiothorac Surg. 2016;49:721–31.
39. Pompeo E, Cristino B, Rogliani P, Dauri M. Urgent awake thoracoscopic treatment of retained haemothorax associated with respiratory failure. Ann Transl Med. 2015;3:112.
40. de Jongh R, Koto MZ. Awake emergency department thoracoscopic investigation of penetrating diaphragmatic injuries: a novel minimally invasive technique of diagnosis. J Laparoendosc Adv Surg Tech A. 2020;30:1334–9.

Role and Limitations of Mininvasive Approach in Abdominal Emergencies and Trauma

Marcelo A. F. Ribeiro Jr, Gabriela Karabachian Tebar,
José Lucas Rodrigues Salgueiro,
and Gabriel Franco de Camargo Galindo

1   Introduction

Laparoscopic surgery is stopped being an innovative technology to become standard procedure in many surgical specialties. Its recommendation for trauma patients presenting hemodynamically stable condition has been progressively expanded. Nowadays, improvements observed in the laparoscopic equipment and surgical technique have decreased the rate of lesions that used to go unnoticed during laparoscopic surgeries from 13 to 0.12% [1]. Trauma surgery is traditionally carried out through open procedures; however, the use of laparoscopy in stable patients has been gaining room due to favorable outcomes reported in different studies available in the literature [2].

The hemodynamic stability of trauma patients is the basic condition for video laparoscopic surgery recommendation; this group also includes patients whose condition has stabilized after fluid resuscitation. Computed tomography is often held before laparoscopy in order to increase surgical accuracy and to avoid unnecessary procedures [3].

Nowadays, laparoscopy applied to trauma cases can be divided into screening, diagnosis, and therapeutic applications. Laparoscopic surgery application was initially limited to screening procedure focused on finding peritoneal violations; such a procedure would be followed by exploratory laparotomy. Diagnostic laparoscopy (DL) goes beyond screening, since it is used to fully assess patients' peritoneal

M. A. F. Ribeiro Jr (✉)
Division of Trauma, Critical Care and Acute Care Surgery, Sheikh Shakhbout Medical City, in partnership with Mayo Clinic, Abu Dhabi, UAE

G. K. Tebar · J. L. R. Salgueiro · G. F. de Camargo Galindo
PGY3 of General Surgery at Catholic University of São Paulo, PUCSP-Sorocaba, São Paulo, Brazil

                                                                 23

F. Coccolini et al. (eds.), *Mini-invasive Approach in Acute Care Surgery*,
Hot Topics in Acute Care Surgery and Trauma,
https://doi.org/10.1007/978-3-031-39001-2_3

cavity in a systematic and meticulous way. It can be used as diagnostic tool to rule out intra-abdominal injuries, such as the diaphragmatic ones, which may have gone unnoticed during computed tomography. Therapeutic laparoscopy (TL) application to trauma cases is reported as viable and safe, as long as the hospital provides proper material and experienced surgeon to perform the procedure. Procedures that do not identify injuries, or that the identified injuries do not require repair, are defined as nontherapeutic DL [1].

Laparoscopy has been widely used in the current scenario to treat penetrating trauma, given its sensitivity, specificity, and accuracy close to 100% [3]. However, laparoscopy using to treat blunt abdominal trauma is not yet fully defined. Although several diagnostic methods are available to assess trauma patients, intra-abdominal injury diagnosis remains a challenge in clinical practice, mainly diaphragm, mesentery and small bowel injuries [4].

Noninvasive diagnostic imaging methods can be used at initial penetrating trauma assessment, and computed tomography is among them, although it presents major limitations to assess diaphragmatic injuries. According to estimates, the aforementioned methods can only evidence diaphragmatic injuries in 26% of cases. Patients with gastrointestinal and pancreatic tract injuries, who undergo nontherapeutic laparotomy procedures based on these noninvasive diagnostic imaging methods, may present high morbidity and mortality rates. Laparoscopy can avoid nontherapeutic laparotomy in 63% of cases [5].

2 Indications and Contraindications

The benefits of using laparoscopy in trauma cases as diagnostic tool to rule out intra-abdominal injuries that may have gone unnoticed in computed tomography, such as diaphragmatic injuries, can be easily seen. It can be used to prevent unnecessary laparotomies in patients with penetrating injuries, whose fascial breach cannot be clinically or radiologically ruled out. Furthermore, laparoscopy can play important therapeutic role when the physician in charge of conducting it has the right surgical skills [2].

Among the laparoscopy recommendations in trauma scenarios, one can mention (Table 1) [6]:

Table 1 Laparotomy recommendations for trauma cases

Laparotomy recommendations for trauma cases	Suspected issue
Clinical peritonitis or pneumoperitoneum	It is indicative of gastrointestinal injury
Inconclusive findings in imaging methods	Suspected gastroduodenal, colorectal, or bladder injuries
"Unclear abdomen"	Discrepancy between imaging findings and physical examination
Penetrating abdominal trauma	Doubts about whether there was peritoneal penetration, or not
Penetrating trauma in thoracoabdominal transition:	Suspected diaphragmatic tear

- Hemodynamic stability: grades I and II shock (rapid response to fluid resuscitation) sustaining abdominal trauma.
- Clinical peritonitis or pneumoperitoneum: trauma patients who are clinically stable but present with clinical signs of peritonitis (usually suggests gastrointestinal injury) may benefit from laparoscopy for both, diagnose and also as a therapeutic tool depending on the type of injury and on the surgeon's skill.
- CT findings and diagnostic uncertainty: diagnostic and potentially therapeutic laparoscopy is a valuable diagnostic tool in suspected gastroduodenal, colorectal, or intraperitoneal bladder injuries.
- Trauma of large vessels and retroperitoneal and renal injuries can be laparoscopically investigated or diagnosed, but only highly selected cases should be explored and treated. Open surgery remains the best way to manage retroperitoneal traumas.
- "Unclear abdomen": discrepancy between image finding and physical examination results.
- Unexplained trauma with free fluid in the cavity and no damage to solid organs.
- Suspected or image-confirmed mesenteric injury (free fluid, hematoma, and/or densification of adipose planes).
- Penetrating abdominal trauma with uncertain peritoneal penetration. Digital exploration can be initially performed, but it must be carried out by experienced surgeon based on the appropriate technique. Laparoscopy can be performed in healthcare institutions lacking experience in nonoperative treatments; in case of negative results, patients can be discharged early. However, early diagnosis without sepsis and contamination means better chances of primary repair and better outcome in hollow viscus injury cases.
- Intraperitoneal bladder injury: cases presenting intraperitoneal leakage at cystography or cases with unexplained free fluid may benefit from laparoscopy.
- Penetrating trauma in the thoracoabdominal transition: suspected diaphragmatic tear after penetrating trauma. It comprises cases of splenic trauma eligible for nonoperative treatment used to assess patients' diaphragm, which may be injured in approximately 30% of cases.
- Penetrating trauma presenting evisceration.
- As an exception in splenic trauma in those patients with continuous non-severe venous bleeding and non-compromising hemodynamic status splenectomy can be performed. So far, laparoscopic splenectomy **is not** indicated in upfront treatment in trauma patients.
- High-grade liver trauma can show complications, and the laparoscopic treatment may be indicated for hemoperitoneum or choleperitoneum drainage, infectious perihepatic collection, and biliary peritonitis treatment.
- Pancreatic trauma: exploration, hemostatic agent placement, as well as laparoscopic evacuation and drainage may be alternative approaches to treat this trauma [6].

Table 2 Absolute contraindications and relative contraindications for laparoscopy

Absolute contraindications	Relative contraindications
Hypovolemic shock	Umbilical or diaphragmatic hernia
Impossibility of performing pneumoperitoneum	Severe pulmonary disease with hypercapnia
Septic shock	Previous surgery with significant adhesion
Severe cardiopulmonary dysfunction	Abdominal mass, peritoneal tuberculosis, or obesity
Severe head trauma	Obvious evisceration

Hemodynamic instability is formal contraindication for laparoscopy. Among other absolute contraindications, one finds (Table 2):

- Hypovolemic shock stage II (nonresponsive to fluid resuscitation), III and IV in these cases laparotomy is recommended
- Septic shock
- Severe cardiopulmonary dysfunction
- Severe head trauma
- Impossibility of performing pneumoperitoneum

Most contraindications are relative and exclusively determined based on surgeon's assessment and experience. Among them, one finds [7]:

- Diffuse peritonitis, with severe clinical impairment like septic shock where patients will not tolerate the physiological alterations related to pneumoperitoneum the patient must be managed by laparotomy
- Severe chronic obstructive pulmonary disease with hypercapnia
- Obvious evisceration
- Significant intra-abdominal adhesions
- Previous abdominal surgery
- Abdominal mass
- Cardiorespiratory disease
- Peritoneal tuberculosis
- Insufficient pneumoperitoneum
- Obesity
- Umbilical hernia
- Diaphragmatic hernia

3　Laparoscopic Technique

This technique is applied to patients who must always be in supine position, under general anesthesia, with legs kept together and straight. They must be secured with the aid of belts; however, the health professional applying this technique must be able to change patients' position in all directions to enable adequate laparoscopic exposure of peritoneal organs.

- First access must be performed with the aid of 10/12 mm trocar (Veress needle is not recommended).
- Pneumoperitoneum should be slowly and progressively established (target of 12–14 mmHg); insufflation should be discontinued in case of increased respiratory pressure, hypotension, or tachycardia.
- 0° and 30° optics can be used, but the 30° one is the best.
- If the cavity inventory does not recommend laparotomy, other two trocars (5 or 12 mm) should be inserted in it, preferably without blade and under direct vision, and positioned by taking into consideration the suspected site.
- Patients subjected to supramesocolic region assessment should be placed in reverse Trendelenburg position to enable examining their liver, gallbladder, spleen, diaphragm, pancreas, stomach, and duodenum. Subsequently, the transverse and descending colon, and their mesocolon, should be examined. Finally, patients' position should be changed to Trendelenburg to enable assessing their rectum, Douglas pouch, and pelvic organs, which must be followed by cecum and right colon assessment.
- After cranially moving the omentum, the small intestine should be fully examined with the aid of two atraumatic intestinal clamps, from the ileocecal valve to the Treitz angle.
- Patients' bladder must be fully examined.
- Methylene blue can be applied through transnasal access, via nasogastric tube (NGT) or intravenous route [6].

The assessment should be systematized, and the following steps must be taken to avoid leaving injuries unnoticed:

1. Diaphragm: it is the first region to be examined after the bleeding is controlled, since its communication with the pleural cavity may cause patient instability.
2. Liver and gallbladder.
3. Spleen.
4. Anterior wall of the stomach.
5. Gastrocolic ligament division.
6. Posterior wall of the stomach. It must be lifted with the aid of tweezers to enable assessing underneath it.
7. Pancreas and its associated retroperitoneal area.
8. Duodenum above the mesocolon.
9. Duodenum below the mesocolon.
10. Small intestine—careful inspection of the small intestine is mandatory; if peritoneum violation is confirmed or if pathological contents are identified in the abdominal cavity, it is strongly recommended to reexamine the small intestine twice, from the Treitz angle to the ileocecal junction. Approximately 10 cm of bowel must be spread between two atraumatic forceps, and, subsequently, they

must be rotated to enable full examination. This maneuver should be repeated until the entire bowel is examined. Clots and fibrinous exudate must be carefully removed through suction, and the area must be dried to enable examining the underlying bowel. In case of signs of contusion or suspicious site are identified, blunt atraumatic forceps should be used to assess the bowel wall and to make sure about the absence of partially occluded intestinal injury. Hematomas around the bowel wall should be carefully inspected by using bowel mobilization and dry gauze to carefully remove them and to enable proper bowel wall examination.

11. Right colon (cecum, ascending colon, and hepatic flexure), right kidney, hilum, and ureter. The colon must be mobilized, and the retroperitoneal contents must be examined.
12. Transverse colon.
13. Left colon (splenic flexure, descending and sigmoid colon), left kidney, hilum, and ureter.
14. Pelvic cavity (rectum and urinary bladder).
15. Additional areas of interest and other areas that require extra attention (e.g., inferior vena cava, aorta) [1].

4   Laparoscopy Application in Trauma Cases: When to Convert It?

Laparoscopy application in stable patients with abdominal trauma has been gaining more and more room since its accuracy is close to 100% and because it is a safe approach, as long as the health institution where it is performed in has a high-performance surgical team with advanced laparoscopic skills and appropriate materials [8]. Quality laparoscopic equipment, well-coordinated trauma team with experience in laparoscopic surgery, and strict compliance with steps previously determined for the procedure play essential role in assuring successful laparoscopic procedures.

Assumingly, centers that meet the requirements described above should approach all stable patients through laparoscopy. Systolic blood pressure levels are the criterion most often used to define stable trauma patients, although the numbers significantly differ. SBP values lower than 90, 100, and 110 mmHg were used to indicate hemodynamic instability [9]. On the other hand, our health service considers blood pressure equal to 90 mmHg as minimum hemodynamic parameter to perform imaging or laparoscopic exams.

Laparoscopy recommendations for trauma cases and its conversion into laparotomy significantly differ among health centers. Organ evisceration, multiple intestinal injuries, or even any injury that requires therapeutic procedures have been reported in some centers as indications for laparoscopy conversion into laparotomy; however, these injuries are successfully treated through laparoscopy in other services. Overall, continuous intra-abdominal bleeding that cannot be quickly controlled is the most common reason for conversion; it is followed by multiple highly complex lesions, hemodynamic instability, and intraoperative visualization issues.

However, most patients present more than one reason for laparoscopy conversion into laparotomy. Intra-abdominal bleeding is often associated with multiple complex injuries and with hemodynamic instability [10].

Retroperitoneal injuries are a potentially dangerous site for laparoscopic surgery; thus, several surgeons make the option for adopting laparotomy in these cases. According to Matsevych et al. [11], retroperitoneal lesions in stable patients were approached through laparoscopy, whereas continuous bleeding that could not be readily controlled was the main reason for laparoscopy conversion into laparotomy.

Hemodynamic (HR and SBP) and metabolic (pH, lactate, BE) instability parameters have been correlated to increased trauma patient mortality rates [4]. Increased $PaCO_2$ during pneumoperitoneum resulted in decreased pH, although it went back to normal levels right after deflation. On the other hand, pH decrease after laparotomy was affected by metabolic factors, which persisted for 1 h after surgery. It appears that laparotomy causes more metabolic disorders in trauma patients than laparoscopy. SBP, HR, pH, lactate, and BE were investigated as possible predictors of complications or of conversion into trauma laparoscopy. Although pH was the only parameter presenting statistical significance, differences in values were so small, and they could not be used in practice [10].

Although limited, data comparing laparoscopy to laparotomy in trauma patients have shown statistically significant reduction in the number of operative complications, perioperative mortality rates, earlier recovery of bowel function, lesser postoperative pain, shorter hospitalization time, and lower infection rate in the laparoscopy group [10, 12].

5   Complications

Complications inherent to surgical procedures in trauma patients may be associated with both the laparoscopic and laparotomy approaches; however, Di Saverio et al. have shown lower rate of adhesions, incisional hernias, and surgical site infections. In addition, the best esthetic outcome should be taken into account since younger patients show higher trauma rates. Faster recovery leads to lower costs; besides, cases such as one single affected organ and negative laparoscopies can help reducing hospitalization time. On the other hand, these benefits must be balanced against 16–19% false-negative laparoscopies in trauma cases [5].

The most feared complication associated with laparoscopy application in trauma patients lies on unnoticed injuries during operative exploration. Meta-analysis conducted by Uranues et al. [3] did not find significant difference in the number of unnoticed injuries, although there was significant reduction in surgical wound infection and postoperative pneumonia in the group subjected to the minimally invasive procedure. Reduced number of nontherapeutic laparotomies is another benefit of the laparoscopic therapy [4] (Table 3).

Perioperative complications associated with laparoscopy can result from the technique used to access the abdominal cavity, or they can be secondary to

Table 3 Complications associated with the laparoscopic technique

Complications associated with the laparoscopic technique	
Pneumoperitoneum-related complications	Puncture-related complications
Cardiac arrhythmias and cardiac arrest	Adjacent organ damage
Significant change in pulse and hypotension	Bleeding in solid organs (liver and spleen)
Gas embolism	Puncture, perforation of hollow viscera (stomach, small intestine, and colon)
Barotrauma/pneumothorax	Uterine perforation
Pre-peritoneal fat dissection	Bladder perforation

pneumoperitoneum, due to increased intra-abdominal pressure caused by carbon monoxide insufflation [13] (Table 3).

Postoperative complications deriving from laparoscopic procedures applied to trauma patients after 10-year review performed by Nicolau et al. [14] comprised wall abscess after intestinal and gallbladder perforation. On the other hand, laparoscopic procedures converted into laparotomy procedures presented complications such as surgical site infection and one death due to multiple organ failure. In addition, reduction in the number of negative and nontherapeutic laparotomies can help reducing postoperative complications by 14.5% and 27%, respectively [13].

6 Conclusion

Given the advances in laparoscopic techniques, equipment improvement, and surgeons' training, nowadays, laparoscopy application in trauma patients is a technique to be applied in selected cases, a fact that helps reducing the rates of nontherapeutic laparotomies, as well as their complications.

References

1. Koto MZ, Matsevych OY, Aldous C. Diagnostic laparoscopy for trauma: how not to miss injuries. J Laparoendosc Adv Surg Tech A. 2018;28(5):506–13. https://doi.org/10.1089/lap.2017.0562. Epub 2018 Jan 2. PMID: 29293406.
2. Birindelli A, Podda M, Segalini E, Cripps M, Tonini V, Tugnoli G, Lim RB, Di Saverio S, TraumaLap Study Group. Is the minimally invasive trauma surgeon the next (r)evolution of trauma surgery? Indications and outcomes of diagnostic and therapeutic trauma laparoscopy in a level 1 trauma centre. Updates Surg. 2020;72(2):503–12. https://doi.org/10.1007/s13304-020-00739-0. Epub 2020 Mar 26. PMID: 32219731.
3. Uranues S, Popa DE, Diaconescu B, Schrittwieser R. Laparoscopy in penetrating abdominal trauma. World J Surg. 2015;39(6):1381–8. https://doi.org/10.1007/s00268-014-2904-5. PMID: 25446491.
4. Koto MZ, Matsevych OY, Mosai F, Patel S, Aldous C, Balabyeki M. Laparoscopy for blunt abdominal trauma: a challenging endeavor. Scand J Surg. 2019;108(4):273–9. https://doi.org/10.1177/1457496918816927. Epub 2018 Dec 6. PMID: 30522416.

5. Di Saverio S, Birindelli A, Podda M, Segalini E, Piccinini A, Coniglio C, Frattini C, Tugnoli G. Trauma laparoscopy and the six w's: why, where, who, when, what, and how? J Trauma Acute Care Surg. 2019;86(2):344–67. https://doi.org/10.1097/TA.0000000000002130. PMID: 30489508.

6. Loffer FD, Pent D. Indications, contraindications and complications of laparoscopy. Obstet Gynecol Surv. 1975;30(7):407–27. https://doi.org/10.1097/00006254-197507000-00001. PMID: 124409.

7. Kindel T, Latchana N, Swaroop M, Chaudhry UI, Noria SF, Choron RL, Seamon MJ, Lin MJ, Mao M, Cipolla J, El Chaar M, Scantling D, Martin ND, Evans DC, Papadimos TJ, Stawicki SP. Laparoscopy in trauma: an overview of complications and related topics. Int J Crit Illn Inj Sci. 2015;5:196–205. https://doi.org/10.4103/2229-5151.165004.

8. Clarke DL, Brysiewicz P, Sartorius B, Bruce JL, Laing GL. Hypotension of B110 mmHg is associated with increased mortality in South African patients after trauma. Scand J Surg. 2017;106:261. https://doi.org/10.1177/1457496916680129.

9. Matsevych O, Koto M, Balabyeki M, Aldous C. Trauma laparoscopy: when to start and when to convert? Surg Endosc. 2018;32(3):1344–52. https://doi.org/10.1007/s00464-017-5812-6. Epub 2017 Aug 10. PMID: 28799045.

10. Li Y, Xiang Y, Wu N, Wu L, Yu Z, Zhang M, Wang M, Jiang J, Li Y. A comparison of laparoscopy and laparotomy for the management of abdominal trauma: a systematic review and metaanalysis. World J Surg. 2016;39:2862–71. https://doi.org/10.1007/s00268-015-3212-4.

11. Matsevych OY, Koto MZ, Motilall SR, Kumar N. The role of laparoscopy in management of stable patients with penetrating abdominal trauma and organ evisceration. J Trauma Acute Care Surg. 2016;81(2):307–11. https://doi.org/10.1097/TA.0000000000001064. PMID: 27032004.

12. Hajibandeh S, Hajibandeh S, Gumber AO, Wong CS. Laparoscopy versus laparotomy for the management of penetrating abdominal trauma: a systematic review and meta-analysis. Int J Surg. 2016;34:127–36. https://doi.org/10.1016/j.ijsu.2016.08.524. Epub 2016 Aug 26. PMID: 27575832.

13. Wadlund DL. Laparoscopy: risks, benefits and complications. Nurs Clin North Am. 2006;41(2):219–29. https://doi.org/10.1016/j.cnur.2006.01.003.

14. Nicolau AE, Craciun M, Vasile R, Kitkani A, Beuran M. The role of laparoscopy in abdominal trauma: a 10-year review. Chirurgia (Bucur). 2019;114(3):359–68. https://doi.org/10.21614/chirurgia.114.3.359. PMID: 31264574.

Role of MIS Approaches in Thoracic Emergencies and Trauma

Daniel VanDerPloeg, Clay Cothren Burlew,
and Fredric M. Pieracci

1   Introduction

With the increasing popularity of thoracoscopic techniques, there has been a trend toward using minimally invasive techniques when safe and appropriate to address urgent and emergent thoracic diseases for both acute care and trauma surgery patients. Thoracoscopic surgery is an important minimally invasive technique that significantly decreases postoperative pain and often decreases hospital length of stay when compared to open thoracotomy. It avoids the need for a very painful thoracotomy incision and utilizes port placement through intercostal spaces to gain access to the pleural space. Additionally, studies have demonstrated increased patient satisfaction and decreased pain, decreased pneumonia rates, shorter hospital length of stay, and even a mortality benefit with a thoracoscopic approach. It also allows for the use of laparoscopic energy and stapling devices within the chest to perform a wide selection of operations. There are a variety of indications for the utilization of thoracoscopy within the practice of trauma and acute care surgery.

2   Role 1: Recurrent Spontaneous Pneumothorax

A frequent indication for urgent thoracoscopic intervention is for treatment of a spontaneous pneumothorax. A primary spontaneous pneumothorax is one that presents in the absence of trauma and without underlying lung pathology. A secondary

D. VanDerPloeg (✉)
University of Colorado and Denver Health, Denver, CO, USA
e-mail: daniel.vanderploeg@cuanschutz.edu

C. C. Burlew · F. M. Pieracci
Denver Health, Denver, CO, USA
e-mail: clay.cothren@dhha.org; fredric.pieracci@dhha.org

    33
F. Coccolini et al. (eds.), *Mini-invasive Approach in Acute Care Surgery*,
Hot Topics in Acute Care Surgery and Trauma,
https://doi.org/10.1007/978-3-031-39001-2_4

spontaneous pneumothorax is one that occurs in the presence of underlying lung pathology, most commonly COPD. The incidence of spontaneous pneumothoraces in the United States is thought to exceed 20,000 patients per year [2]. There is a large variability in the management of spontaneous pneumothoraces and a lack of well-accepted, consensus guidelines. Initial management can include simple aspiration, tube thoracostomy, or oxygen supplementation to assist in pneumothorax reabsorption [7, 12]. In emergent situations or in the presence of tension physiology, patient stabilization requires tube thoracostomy for drainage of pneumothorax and re-expansion of the lung. A recent randomized controlled trial demonstrated non-inferiority from a conservative approach that did not include immediate tube decompression [3] for the management of spontaneous pneumothoraces. It prevented the need for 85% invasive procedures and led to a decreased length of hospital stay and decreased adverse events. Finally, computed tomography (CT) is a vital component of the diagnostic workup and should be used to evaluate for pulmonary blebs as they are a major risk factor for recurrent pneumothorax.

Surgical evaluation for primary spontaneous pneumothorax is indicated in patients with a recurrent pneumothorax, persistent air leak after tube thoracostomy more than 4 days, or at first occurrence for patients with occupational risks or for recurrent pneumothorax. A thoracoscopic approach is preferred in these patients as it decreases hospital stay and postoperative pain, with similar recurrence rates when compared to an open surgical approach. There are two main goals of thoracoscopic management [12]. The first involves resection of bullae/blebs or area of persistent air leak with an endoscopic stapler. The second is to induce pleural scarring, or pleurodesis, in order to decrease recurrence. The pleurodesis may be achieved by either mechanical, chemical, or both methods. One commonly used technique is the instillation of talcum powder into the pleural space to create a chemical pleurodesis. However, with the recall of talcum powder, other sclerosing agents are used, such as betadine, tetracycline, doxycycline, or gentamicin. Mechanical pleurodesis may be performed by formal parietal pleurectomy or by disrupting the pleura with direct contact with Bovie scratch pad or gauze. Although chemical pleurodesis may be performed at bedside via chest tube, without the need for operative intervention, it is often poorly tolerated by the patient due to pain, and sometimes this requires conscious sedation.

Patient positioning is one of the important first steps in any thoracoscopic operation. Lateral decubitus with appropriate padding and arm rests is the position of choice for thoracoscopic pleurodesis. Additionally, the break of the operating room table should be positioned at the level of the xiphoid process in order to open the rib spaces to increase working space during the operation. Attention to port placement is also important in order to allow for working space and maneuverability within the chest. See Fig. 1.

Below is the preferred technique for thoracoscopic pleurodesis and bleb resection at our institution. After confirmation of appropriate lung isolation with either double-lumen endotracheal tube or endobronchial blocker, the authors favor entering the chest using the optical viewing technique (with an endoscope inserted into a 12 mm port) in the anterior-axillary line at the fourth or fifth intercostal space. The

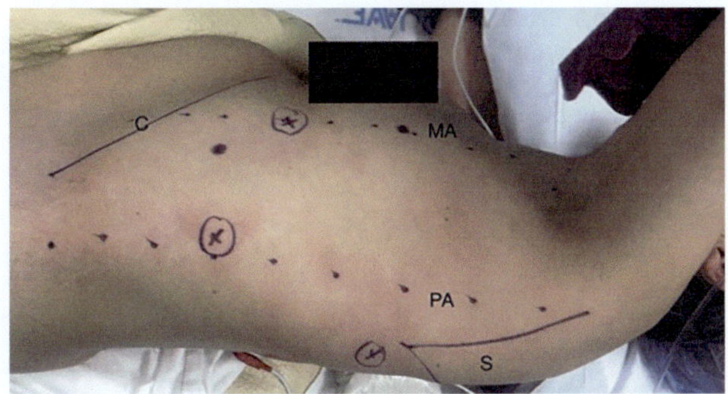

Fig. 1 Patient positioning in the right lateral decubitus position with circled X marking proposed port sites placement. Costal margin (C), scapular tip (S), midaxillary line (MA), and posterior axillary line (PA)

chest is entered at the planned site of the chest tube placement after the operation, directing the scope toward the scapular tip. The open technique is also acceptable for initial entry into the chest. This involves an incision at the upper border of the fourth or fifth intercostal space and using surgical energy to dissect through the intercostal muscle until the pleural space is entered. This may be the preferred approach as it is similar to that for chest tube insertion. An additional 12 mm port, to accommodate a stapler, is placed under direct visualization in the posterior-axillary line. Our final 5 mm port is placed in the eighth or ninth intercostal space along the midaxillary line and under direct visualization. The pleural space is evaluated, and any blebs are resected with endoscopic stapler using medium staple height loads (2.5–3.5 mm). See Figs. 2 and 3.

Sometimes there may be adhesions already present at the site of ruptured blebs. Careful lysis of adhesions may be required to free the bleb off of the chest wall in order to perform a resection. Next, attention is turned to performing the chemical pleurodesis. The preferred sclerosing agent at our institution is betadine. See Fig. 4. It is used to coat the entire parietal and visceral pleural surfaces by instilling it into the chest via red rubber catheter and Toomey syringe or via suction irrigator.

Once all the pleural surfaces are covered, the lung is then reinflated under direct visualization in order to assess for air leaks. Once satisfied with the pleurodesis, a chest tube is introduced through the anterior axillary port site and directed posterior and apically. The chest tube is placed to continuous suction at 20 cm H_2O for 48 h to ensure pleural apposition.

A mechanical pleurodesis, using a Bovie scratch pad, requires the open technique for the anterior axillary site in order to use a working port rather than performing the pleurodesis via ports. The rest of the ports are placed per the above technique under direct visualization. To perform the mechanical pleurodesis, a Bovie scratch pad is folded in half and clasped with an empty ringed forceps. This is then used to scratch the parietal pleura in order to induce scarring.

Recurrent pneumothorax still remains an area of concern, even after thoracoscopic bleb resection and pleurodesis. Recurrence after surgery is cited to occur in between 5 and 19% of patients [1]. There have been a number of studies done to identify risk factors for recurrence. Smoking increases the risk of recurrence by up to four times when compared to nonsmokers [4]. One retrospective study identified

Figs. 2 and 3 Thoracoscopic stapled blebectomy after identifying source of air leak by submerging lung in saline (top) and resected blebectomy specimen (bottom)

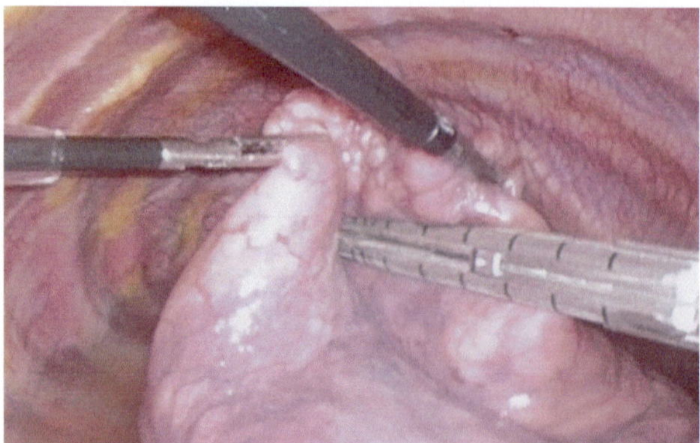

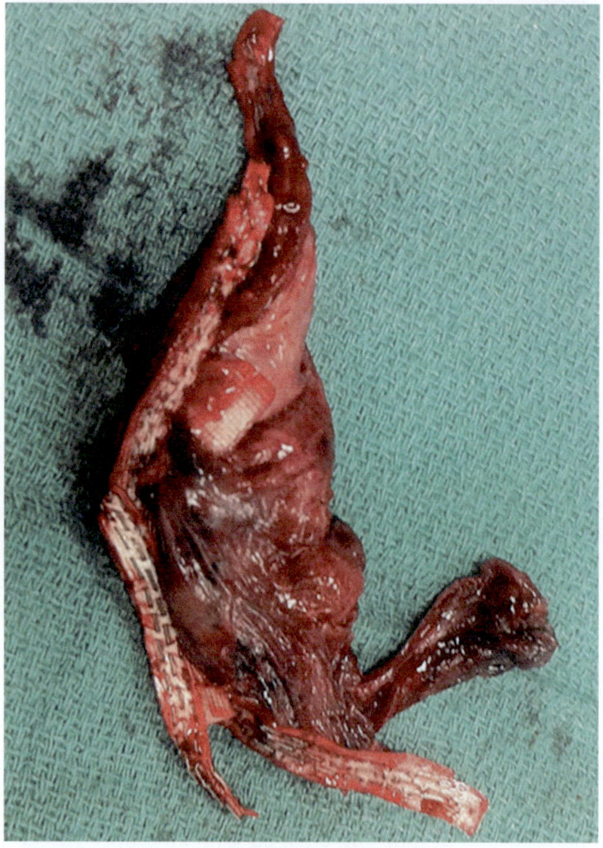

risk factors for recurrence that included age <20, inability to identify bleb on preoperative CT imaging, and history of ipsilateral pneumothorax [1]. Another retrospective study identified female gender and prolonged air leak as risk factors for recurrence after thoracoscopic surgery [9].

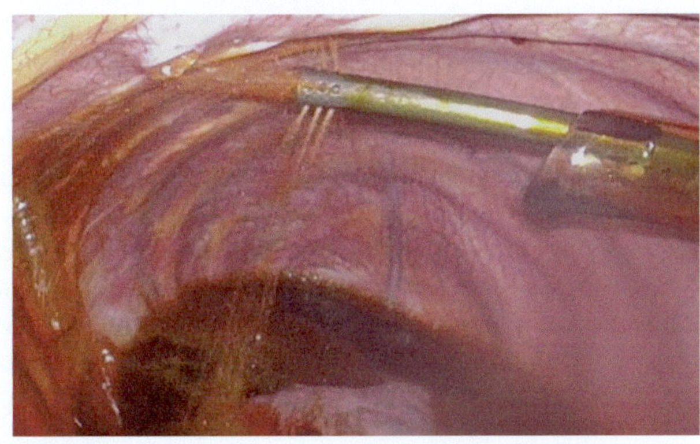

Fig. 4 Betadine pleurodesis being used to cover the pleural spaces via suction irrigator. Betadine was injected into a bag of saline and connected to irrigator port and used to coat the pleural space

3   Role 2: Pericardial Window for Pericardial Effusion

A pericardial window can be done using thoracoscopy. This technique is preferred for loculated, posterior effusions, or recurrent effusions as echocardiogram-guided pericardial drain or pericardiocentesis are best for addressing more anterior effusions. One main advantage is that it offers access to different areas of the pericardium that can be difficult to access with a subxiphoid approach. The thoracoscopic technique is also advocated for evaluation for pericardial injury in the setting of penetrating chest trauma. In select patients, it is a safe and effective approach to rule out injury to the heart for patients with penetrating trauma. However, a thoracoscopic approach should not be used in hemodynamically unstable patients or patients with clear tamponade physiology as median sternotomy needs to be used in these patients for immediate decompression.

Retrospective studies have been done that demonstrate comparable morbidity and mortality between a thoracoscopic and a classical open subxiphoid approach. Both techniques are effective at addressing and draining pericardial effusions. One advantage of a thoracoscopic approach is the added potential to address concomitant pleural or pulmonary issues at the time of pericardial window [8].

Techniques to perform thoracoscopic pericardial drainage often utilize a left-sided approach as it allows access to most areas of the pericardium. A right-sided approach may be indicated for a loculated right-sided effusion, but this can often still be addressed via left-sided drainage. The surgical approach requires single-lung ventilation and often requires slightly lower port placement compared to the previously described lung parenchymal procedure to allow better manipulation of the pericardium. Three ports are usually sufficient for performing the procedure with a camera port, grasping instrument, and working instrument. The camera port is placed in the eighth or ninth intercostal space in the midaxillary line. The port for the grasper is along the posterior axillary line, and the working instrument is along the anterior axillary line. The working instrument is typically a laparoscopic scissors or energy device that are used to incise the pericardium. The grasping instrument is used to grab the pericardium and elevate it away from the heart to prevent injury when incising the pericardium. The scissors are used to incise the pericardium and then remove a square 2 cm portion of the pericardium. This can be sent for pathological analysis but also ensures a communication between the pericardial and pleural spaces. This communication allows for both rapid and continued drainage of the pericardial effusion.

A thoracoscopic technique is sufficient to treat pericardial effusions. It allows for treatment of concomitant pleural or pulmonary issues at the same time. It does require entry into two anatomical spaces but often provides better visualization when compared to the classical subxiphoid, preperitoneal approach. It allows for the same pathological and cytological fluid analyses. Studies have been done that demonstrate safety and efficacy of a thoracoscopic approach, even in the setting of early echocardiographic signs of pericardial tamponade.

4   Role 3: Retained Hemothorax

A retained hemothorax is a complication often seen after thoracic trauma. It is defined as hemothorax persisting after tube thoracostomy as demonstrated on chest radiograph or chest CT. See Figs. 5 and 6. Some practice patterns advocate for the

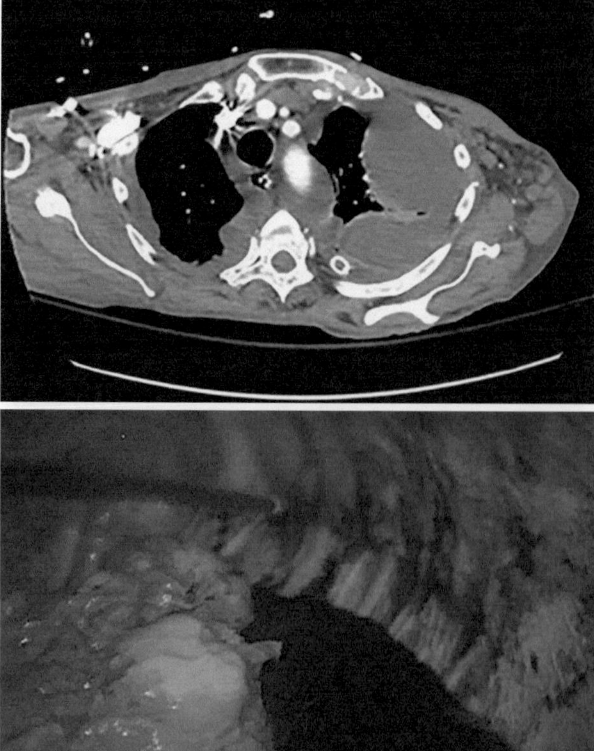

Figs. 5 and 6 CT scan demonstrating retained hemothorax after chest tube placement (top). Thoracoscopic visualization of early moderate volume retained hemothorax (bottom)

placement of an additional chest tubes after a persistent hemothorax is identified on imaging. A retained hemothorax is an important diagnostic distinction as it may occur in up to one third of trauma patients that initially present with hemothorax [5]. Additionally, it is a risk factor for increased morbidity such as empyema or a fibrothorax, also known as a trapped lung. It leads to such complications due to the remodeling of retained blood products in the pleural space that can serve as a nidus for infection or scarring. Surgical intervention becomes a point of discussion to decrease these risks when imaging reveals a retained hemothorax. When utilized appropriately, early thoracoscopic evacuation can lead to decrease length of hospital stay, decreased length of chest tube duration, and decreased hospital cost [13]. One additional benefit of intervention is the ability to address causes of retained hemothoraces, such as lung lacerations or chest wall injury, that would have been otherwise untreated if undergoing tube thoracostomy alone. Therefore, early thoracoscopic evacuation is an important tool in the acute care surgeon's armamentarium for the management of thoracic trauma.

Tissue plasminogen activator (tPA) and DNase is described for the treatment of empyema and parapneumonic effusions. While intrapleural lytics have demonstrated some efficacy for treating empyemas, there is hesitancy to use these agents in the acute setting of traumatic hemothorax due to the risk of rebleeding. A large randomized control trial demonstrated improved pleural effusions at 7 days, decreased hospital stay, decreased surgical referral, and no increase in adverse events for pleural infections [16]. There have been a lack of prospective randomized controlled trials to evaluate thoracoscopic evacuation versus tPA for retained hemothoraces. There have been some retrospective studies evaluating thoracoscopic evacuation compared to streptokinase that demonstrated the superiority of surgery [14]. Additionally, a large majority of trauma patients have multisystem injuries that often prohibit thrombolytic use in this population. There is also a lack of trials done to determine appropriate dosing for intrapleural thrombolytics and DNase. Although some studies have advocated that intrapleural thrombolytics and DNase is safe in the trauma population, it is often associated with an increased hospital stay and cost that could potentially be avoided with early thoracoscopic evacuation [5, 13].

Operative intervention requires similar positioning in the lateral decubitus position. Here, a 12 mm port is placed in the midaxillary line at the fourth or fifth intercostal space. An additional 5 mm port is placed along the anterior axillary line in the sixth or seventh intercostal space to allow direct evacuation of the retained hemothorax most commonly located along the diaphragm at the base of the lung. A suction irrigator system is used to evacuate the retained hemothorax, and the pleural space is irrigated until clear. If necessary to achieve adequate hemostasis or evacuation of hemothorax, an additional port may be placed along the posterior axillary line. Evaluation of the entire pleural space is performed in order to identify and treat any reversible cause of retained hemothorax such as pulmonary laceration or chest wall bleeding. This may require upsizing the anterior axillary port to 12 mm in order to accommodate an endoscopic stapler. Once the hemothorax is completely evacuated, a posterior and apical chest tube can be placed under direct visualization via previously placed port incision to allow for improved drainage postoperatively. A

24–28 French chest tube is used as there is no better drainage with a larger bore chest tube [10]. Additionally, the option to place a right-angled chest tube can be utilized if increased basilar drainage along the diaphragm is desired.

An area of ongoing, particular interest is whether a retained hemothorax can be prevented with sterile pleural irrigation at time of initial chest tube placement [11]. Current multicenter trials are underway to examine whether sterile pleural irrigation with normal saline or sterile water is effective at preventing retained hemothorax. The hypothesis behind pleural irrigation is that it breaks down the clotted blood within the hemothorax, allowing for better evacuation and avoidance of need for surgical evacuation.

5 Role 4: Diaphragm Evaluation for Thoracoabdominal Penetrating Trauma

Thoracoabdominal penetrating trauma is an important injury pattern to consider thoracoscopic intervention. It is defined as an injury that occurs within the zone delineated between the nipple, costal margin, and scapula. Organs with the chest and abdomen are at risk of injury, including peritoneal and retroperitoneal structures as well as the diaphragm. There is high incidence of diaphragmatic injury in thoracoabdominal wounds, up to approximately 20% [15]. Radiographic studies are very poor at the evaluation of the diaphragm and have a wide range of sensitivity from 8 to 63% [18]. One reason is that the diaphragm laceration may be very small in penetrating trauma. A retrospective single institution study compared the newer 256-slice CT scanners to the older 64-slice scanners to evaluate whether the newer scanners improved the diagnostic capabilities [18]. The study failed to diagnose traumatic diaphragm injuries in over 40% of patients. The study also found that CT scanners result in a higher incidence of false negatives, confirming that intraoperative analysis should still be the gold standard. Thus, a high level of suspicion is warranted and should drive the surgeon to operatively evaluate patients with thoracoabdominal penetrating trauma for a diaphragmatic injury.

Although many institutions prefer laparoscopy to evaluate for a diaphragmatic injury, thoracoscopic evaluation is an important alternative approach. One advantage of a thoracoscopic approach is in the setting of other thoracic injuries, most commonly a pneumothorax or hemothorax that requires chest tube placement. In this situation, two thoracoscopic ports should be placed, one in the midaxillary line and one in the anterior axillary line. This can also be done with the patient in the supine position for conversion to exploratory laparotomy or laparoscopy if thoracoscopic exploration mandates further abdominal exploration. It allows for the insertion of an endoscope through a port for visual inspection of the pleural space and diaphragm. It also allows for directed and more complete drainage of the pleural space and chest tube placement under direct vision. There are studies that compare thoracoscopy to exploratory laparotomy for the identification of diaphragmatic injuries [17, 19]. They demonstrate that thoracoscopy is a safe and reliable method for the evaluation of diaphragmatic injuries in the setting of thoracoabdominal trauma. There has, however, not been a comparison of a thoracoscopic to a laparoscopic approach for the diagnosis of diaphragmatic injury. With the lack of randomized control trials or direct comparison, the recommendation is to use the approach that the operating trauma surgeon is the most comfortable performing or would best evaluate the concern for other injuries. Some patients may require both approaches.

Some institutions advocate for the use of a thoracoscope in the emergency department to determine the need for further surgical evaluation and intervention. Following bedside tube thoracostomy, a thoracoscope is introduced under sterile conditions to survey the pleural space. This technique is promoted as a novel minimally invasive technique to evaluate the pleural space for diaphragm injury or ongoing bleeding that will require operative intervention [6]. It removes the requirement for general anesthesia as it can be performed under local anesthesia and conscious sedation. The technique is also thought to allow for better determination of the need for chest exploration for a hemothorax. It allows for immediate evacuation of hemothorax and removes the need to wait for repeated chest X-rays. Most of the reports describing this technique are small cohorts, and they demonstrated no increased morbidity and a trend of decreased nontherapeutic operations. In order to validate this technique, prospective clinical trials are needed to compare it to the classically accepted diagnostic laparoscopic or thoracoscopic evaluation of thoracoabdominal penetrating trauma.

6 Role 5: Foreign Body Removal

Foreign bodies may enter the pleural space as a result of penetrating trauma or iatrogenic injury. Provided the patient is clinically stable, these objects may be readily retrieved via thoracoscopic exploration. Depending upon the nature of the foreign body and associated injury, additional chest wall debridement and/or reconstruction may be necessary on an individual basis. Additionally, standard thoracoscopic port sites may need to be enlarged to facilitate safe object retrieval.

7 Conclusions

VATS can be very helpful for a variety of acute pathologies including trauma. It requires single-lung ventilation, proper positioning, and hemodynamic stability. Acute patients who are unstable should undergo a thoracotomy if chest pathology is suspected. The minimally invasive approach to the chest has several advantages including decreased postoperative pain, decreased length of hospital stay, earlier recovery of pulmonary function, and decreased narcotic requirements, decreased incidence of postoperative complications, and lower overall cost. With increasing popularity and training in minimally invasive techniques, VATS is a great tool for the modern trauma and acute care surgeon.

References

1. Asano H, Ohtsuka T, Noda Y, et al. Risk factors for recurrence of primary spontaneous pneumothorax after thoracoscopic surgery. J Thorac Dis. 2019;11(5):1940–4. https://doi.org/10.21037/jtd.2019.04.105.
2. Baumann MH, Strange C, Heffner JE, et al. Management of spontaneous pneumothorax: an American College of Chest Physicians Delphi consensus statement. Chest. 2001;119(2):590–602. https://doi.org/10.1378/chest.119.2.590.
3. Brown SGA, Ball EL, Perrin K, Asha SE, Braithwaite I, Egerton-Warburton D, Jones PG, Keijzers G, Kinnear FB, Kwan BCH, Lam KV, Lee YCG, Nowitz M, Read CA, Simpson G, Smith JA, Summers QA, Weatherall M, Beasley R, et al. Conservative versus interventional treatment for spontaneous pneumothorax. N Engl J Med. 2020;382:405–15. https://doi.org/10.1056/NEJMoa19107.
4. Cardillo G, Bintcliffe OJ, Carleo F, et al. Primary spontaneous pneumothorax: a cohort study of VATS with talc poudrage. Thorax. 2016;71(9):847–53. https://doi.org/10.1136/thoraxjnl-2015-207976.
5. Chou YP, Lin HL, Wu TC. Video-assisted thoracoscopic surgery for retained hemothorax in blunt chest trauma. Curr Opin Pulm Med. 2015;21(4):393–8. https://doi.org/10.1097/MCP.0000000000000173.
6. de Jongh R, Koto MZ. Awake emergency department thoracoscopic investigation of penetrating diaphragmatic injuries: a novel minimally invasive technique of diagnosis. J Laparoendosc Adv Surg Tech A. 2020;30(12):1334–9. https://doi.org/10.1089/lap.2020.0232.
7. Devanand A, Koh MS, Ong TH, Low SY, Phua GC, Tan KL, Philip Eng CT, Samuel M. Simple aspiration versus chest-tube insertion in the management of primary spontaneous pneumothorax: a systematic review. Respir Med. 2004;98(7):579–90. https://doi.org/10.1016/j.rmed.2004.04.006.
8. Georghiou GP, Stamler A, Sharoni E, et al. Video-assisted thoracoscopic pericardial window for diagnosis and management of pericardial effusions. Ann Thorac Surg. 2005;80(2):607–10. https://doi.org/10.1016/j.athoracsur.2005.02.068.
9. Imperatori A, Rotolo N, Spagnoletti M, et al. Risk factors for postoperative recurrence of spontaneous pneumothorax treated by video-assisted thoracoscopic surgery†. Interact Cardiovasc Thorac Surg. 2015;20(5):647–52. https://doi.org/10.1093/icvts/ivv022.
10. Inaba K, Lustenberger T, Recinos G, et al. Does size matter? A prospective analysis of 28-32 versus 36-40 French chest tube size in trauma. J Trauma Acute Care Surg. 2012;72(2):422–7. https://doi.org/10.1097/TA.0b013e3182452444.
11. Kugler NW, Carver TW, Milia D, Paul JS. Thoracic irrigation prevents retained hemothorax: a prospective propensity scored analysis. J Trauma Acute Care Surg. 2017;83(6):1136–41. https://doi.org/10.1097/TA.0000000000001700.
12. Luh SP. Review: diagnosis and treatment of primary spontaneous pneumothorax. J Zhejiang Univ Sci B. 2010;11(10):735–44. https://doi.org/10.1631/jzus.B1000131.
13. Meyer DM, Jessen ME, Wait MA, Estrera AS. Early evacuation of traumatic retained hemothoraces using thoracoscopy: a prospective, randomized trial. Ann Thorac Surg. 1997;64(5):1396–401. https://doi.org/10.1016/S0003-4975(97)00899-0.
14. Oğuzkaya F, Akçali Y, Bilgin M. Videothoracoscopy versus intrapleural streptokinase for management of post traumatic retained haemothorax: a retrospective study of 65 cases. Injury. 2005;36(4):526–9. https://doi.org/10.1016/j.injury.2004.10.008.
15. Parreira JG, Rasslan S, Utiyama EM. Controversies in the management of asymptomatic patients sustaining penetrating thoracoabdominal wounds. Clinics (Sao Paulo). 2008;63(5):695–700. https://doi.org/10.1590/s1807-59322008000500020.
16. Rahman NM, Maskell NA, West A, et al. Intrapleural use of tissue plasminogen activator and DNase in pleural infection. N Engl J Med. 2011;365(6):518–26. https://doi.org/10.1056/NEJMoa1012740.

17. Spann JC, Nwariaku FE, Wait M. Evaluation of video-assisted thoracoscopic surgery in the diagnosis of diaphragmatic injuries. Am J Surg. 1995;170(6):628–31. https://doi.org/10.1016/s0002-9610(99)80030-0.

18. Uhlich R, Kerby JD, Bosarge P, Hu P. Diagnosis of diaphragm injuries using modern 256-slice CT scanners: too early to abandon operative exploration. Trauma Surg Acute Care Open. 2018;3(1):e000251. https://doi.org/10.1136/tsaco-2018-000251.

19. Uribe RA, Pachon CE, Frame SB, Enderson BL, Escobar F, Garcia GA. A prospective evaluation of thoracoscopy for the diagnosis of penetrating thoracoabdominal trauma. J Trauma. 1994;37(4):650–4. https://doi.org/10.1097/00005373-199410000-00020.

Acute Appendicitis

Andrea Pakula and Ruby Skinner

1 Introduction

Appendectomy for acute appendicitis is one of the most commonly performed surgical procedures for acute care surgeons. The estimated lifetime risk for acute appendicitis is 7–8%, and there are approximately 300,000 patients diagnosed with acute appendicitis in the United States. Luminal obstruction of the appendix is commonly causative of appendicitis, and this obstruction can be related to a fecalith, impacted stool, or lymphoid hyperplasia [1, 2].

Surgical approaches to appendectomy have evolved from open surgery to minimally invasive approaches. Kurt Semm performed the first laparoscopic appendectomy in September 1980, and with the subsequent evolution of the minimally invasive technology, an open appendectomy is not frequently done in the adult populations [3].

In a 2010 meta-analysis of randomized controlled trials comparing minimally invasive to open appendectomy, it was determined that laparoscopy offers significant advantages over open appendectomy to include less pain, a lower incidence of surgical site infection, a decreased length of hospital stay, an earlier return to work, a lower overall cost, and better quality of life scores. This was an early study documenting the superiority of the minimally invasive approach based on high strength studies that allowed for the strong recommendation of the laparoscopic approach for both uncomplicated and complicated acute appendicitis [4].

Similarly, in a more recent 2017 meta-analysis comparing laparoscopic versus open appendectomy in cases of complicated appendicitis, laparoscopy

A. Pakula (✉)
Adventist Health Simi Valley Hospital, Simi Valley, CA, USA
e-mail: pakulaam@ah.org

R. Skinner
St. Bernadine's Medical Center, San Bernadino, CA, USA
e-mail: ruby.skinner@commonspirit.org

© The Author(s), under exclusive license to Springer Nature Switzerland AG 2023
F. Coccolini et al. (eds.), *Mini-invasive Approach in Acute Care Surgery*,
Hot Topics in Acute Care Surgery and Trauma,
https://doi.org/10.1007/978-3-031-39001-2_5

demonstrated less surgical site infections, reduced time to oral intake, and length of hospitalization. There was no significant difference in intra-abdominal abscess rates. Operative time was longer for laparoscopy but did not reach statistical significance in the RCT subgroup analysis [5]. Overall, laparoscopy for appendectomy is safe and can be applied in traditionally high-risk populations. Laparoscopy is safe for patients with obesity, the elderly population with medical comorbid conditions, and pregnant patients in all trimesters [6–9].

The adoption of robotic-assisted laparoscopic techniques has become more prevalent in general surgery, and approaches to acute care cases are evolving [10, 11]. The adoption of robotic-assisted laparoscopic appendectomy into the surgical armamentarium of the acute care surgeon is also feasible.

2 Preoperative Diagnosis and Indications for Surgery

Patient presentation can vary from minimal symptoms with vague lower abdominal pain to more localized pain with or without peritoneal inflammation. The classic physical exam findings and patient complaints are described as periumbilical pain that radiates and ultimately localizes to the right lower quadrant. If the appendix is more anterior and adjacent to the parietal peritoneum, patients will have focal tenderness on palpation. If the appendix is located in the retrocecal position, physical exam findings may not be as clear. Common laboratory findings include leukocytosis and an elevated c-reactive protein. Though imaging is not always necessary, ultrasound is recommended in pregnant or pediatric patients, and computed tomography (CT) of the abdomen and pelvis is the preferred diagnostic study in adults. In the 2016 ACS NSQIP database, CT scan was shown to have higher positive predictive values compared to ultrasound (US) and MRI [12]. CT is specifically useful in identifying a periappendiceal phlegmon or abscess if the duration of symptoms is questionable. The utilization of imaging or modality selected is based on physician preference and confidence in the diagnosis.

3 Operative Technique for Laparoscopic and Robotic Appendectomy

Prior to making skin incisions, local anesthesia can be injected into the skin. The first step is to then gain access to the peritoneal cavity. This can be done using a Veress needle, open/Hassan, or optical view entry technique. Port placement for laparoscopic appendectomy relies on triangulation of instruments to the right lower quadrant. Selection of port size is surgeon preference, but at least one 12 mm port is needed if an endoscopic stapler is to be used. For the robotic-assisted approach, either three 8 mm or two 8 mm and a 12 mm cannula are used. Again, the 12 mm port is necessary to accommodate the stapler if this is the chosen technique. There are some variations to port placement utilizing the robotic approach which are shown in (see Figs. 1 and 2) Fig. 2a, b. Once ports have been placed and

Fig. 1 Laparoscopic port placement

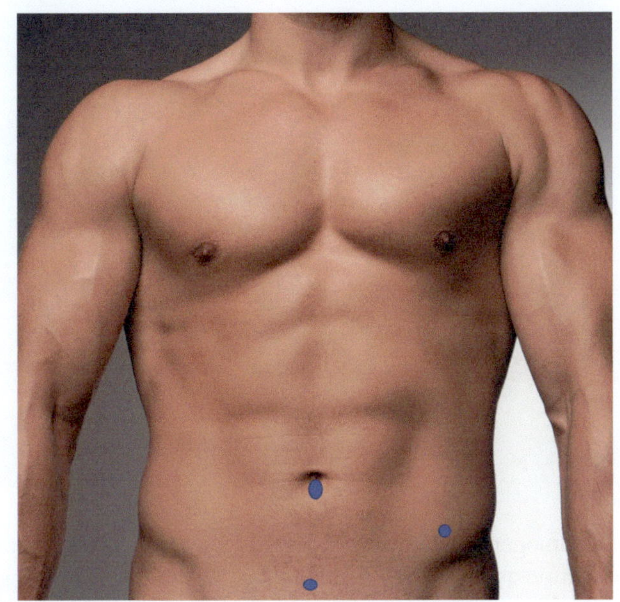

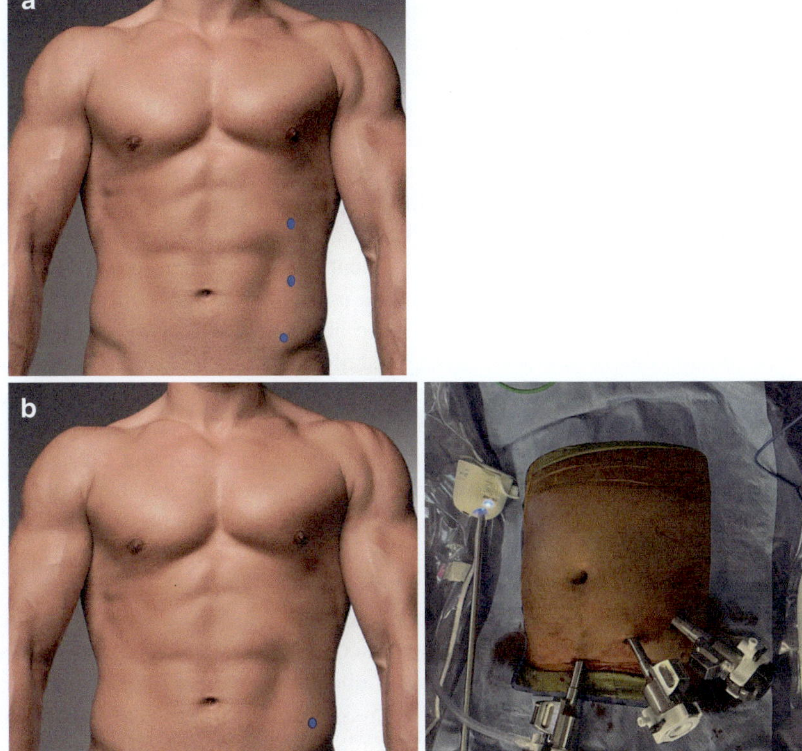

Fig. 2 Robotic assisted port placement

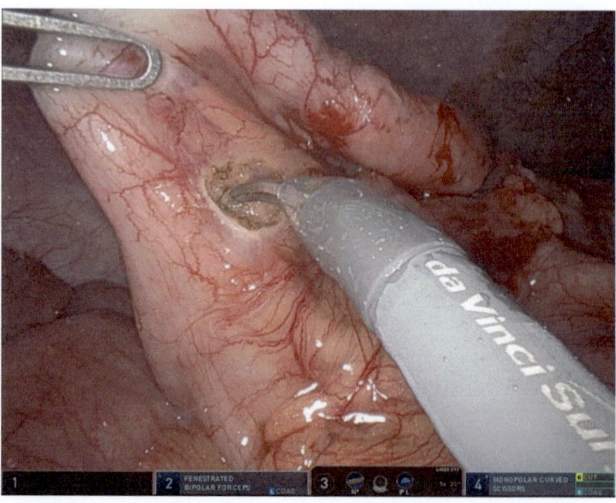

Fig. 3 Creation of mesenteric window

pneumoperitoneum is achieved to 15 mmHg, the patient is placed in Trendelenburg position and rotated left side down. The operation begins with initial exploration to identify any unexpected pathology. Atraumatic graspers are then inserted, and the first step is to identify the appendix. This can sometimes be difficult so identifying the cecum can help to facilitate this step. The ligament of Treves located on the distal ileum near the ileocecal valve can also be used to locate the appendix. During acute appendicitis, it is often adherent to the mesoappendix or the appendix itself. The omentum and small bowel are gently swept away from the right lower quadrant. The appendix can be found lateral to the ileal cecal valve at the base of the taenia. If the appendix is in the retrocecal position, the cecum will need to be mobilized medially by dividing the white line of Toldt in order to expose the appendix. The principles of mesenteric division as well as division of the appendix are similar regardless of the minimally invasive approach. Once identified, the appendix can be gently grasped taking care not to cause rupture. The mesoappendix should be identified, and either a window can be created at the base of the appendix using a dissector or the mesoappendix can be divided moving distally to proximally (Fig. 3). The window would allow for hemoclips, a suture, or an endoscopic stapler to be used to control the mesoappendix vessels. Alternatively, an energy device such as the ultrasonic scalpel, advanced bipolar energy, simple bipolar, or monopolar energy can be used to divide the mesoappendix which contains the appendiceal artery.

There are several different techniques for dividing the appendix itself, and this depends on surgeon preference as well as the characteristics of the appendiceal tissue. These include stapled division, suture ligation, or placement of an Endoloop with or without dunking of the appendiceal stump. The robotic technology facilitates suturing, though this can be done laparoscopically as well. If a stapler is used, a short-height load (2.0–3.0 mm) is typically chosen to seal the mesoappendix and artery, and a medium height staple load (2.5–3.5 mm) is often used to divide the appendix itself (Fig. 4). Once divided, the staple lines are inspected to assure there

Fig. 4 Division of base of
appendix with stapler

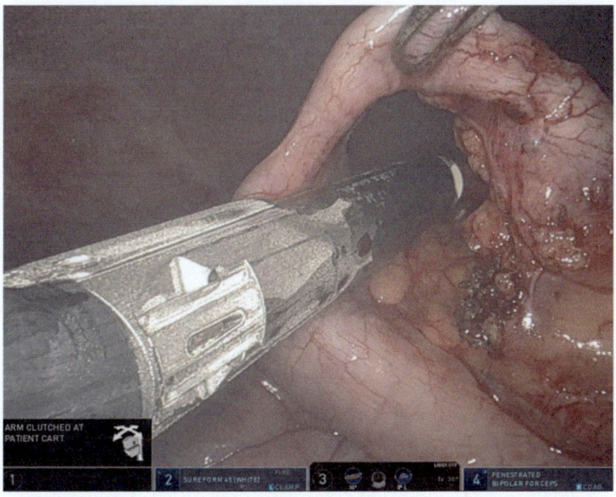

is no bleeding or leakage of stool. Next the appendix can be placed in a retrieval bag
and removed through the larger port. If there is evidence of contamination, this can
be judiciously irrigated and suctioned. Once the procedure is complete, the ports are
removed, and the fascial incision at any port site larger than 5 mm is closed to prevent hernia formation. This is usually done with a 0-vicryl suture. Skin incisions are
then closed, and sterile dressing or skin glue is applied.

4　　Complicated Appendicitis

In patients who present with signs and symptoms consistent with appendicitis and
demonstrate evidence of perforation with phlegmon or abscess on preoperative
imaging, immediate surgical intervention is not always recommended. If the patient
is not septic requiring immediate surgical exploration, they are admitted to the hospital, started on IV antibiotics, and treated nonoperatively, which may or may not
include radiology-guided drain placement to control the infection depending on the
location and size of the phlegmon or abscess. These patients can then go on to
undergo appendectomy in 6–8 weeks after resolution of acute inflammatory changes
and drainage of the abscess. 25% of appendectomies performed each year are due
to complicated appendicitis [13].

5　　Conclusion

Appendectomy for acute appendicitis is one of the most common procedures performed by acute care surgeons, and minimally invasive approaches are standard.
Laparoscopy in general is associated with significant clinical benefits and overall
cost benefits for patient care, and patients with acute appendicitis are afforded with

those benefits. High-risk populations including elderly patient, those with obesity, and pregnant patients, all can safely be managed with laparoscopy for acute appendicitis. Finally, robotic-assisted appendectomies are being performed; although the literature is sparse for this application, there are evolving benefits reported of applying robotic surgery for common acute care surgical emergencies.

References

1. Stewart B, Khanduri P, McCord C, et al. Global disease burden of conditions requiring emergency surgery. Br J Surg. 2014;101:e9–e22.
2. Bhangu A, Soreide K, Di Saverio S, et al. Acute appendicitis: modern understanding of pathogenesis, diagnosis , and management. Lancet. 2015;383:1278–87.
3. Meljnikov I, Radojcic B, Grebeldinger S, Radojcic N. History of surgical treatment of appendicitis. Med Pregl. 2009;62(9–10):489–92.
4. Li X, Zhang J, Sang L, et al. Laparoscopic versus conventional appendectomy—a meta-analysis of randomized controlled trials. BMC Gastroenterol. 2010;10:129.
5. Athanasiou C, Lockwood S, Markides GA. Systematic review and meta-analysis of laparoscopic versus open appendicectomy in adults with complicated appendicitis: an update of the literature. World J Surg. 2017;41(12):3083–99. https://doi.org/10.1007/s00268-017-4123-3.
6. Werkgartner G, Cerwenka H, El Shabrawi A, et al. Laparoscopic versus open appendectomy for complicated appendicitis in high risk patients. Int J Color Dis. 2015;30:397–401.
7. Wang D, Dong T, Shao Y, et al. Laparoscopy versus open appendectomy for elderly patients, a meta-analysis and systematic review. BMC Surg. 2019;19:54.
8. Michailidou M, Sacco Casamassima MG, Goldstein SD, et al. The impact of obesity on laparoscopic appendectomy: results from the ACS National Surgical Quality Improvement Program pediatric database. J Pediatric Surg. 2015;50:1880–4.
9. Lee SH, Lee JY, Choi YY, et al. Laparoscopic appendectomy versus open appendectomy for suspected appendicitis during pregnancy: a systematic review and updated meta-analysis. BMC Surg. 2019;19:41.
10. Certulo LN, Harmon K, Ortiz J, et al. Case report of a robotic-assisted laparoscopic repair of a giant incarcerated recurrent inguinal hernia containing bladder and ureters. Int J Med Robot. 2015;1:15–7.
11. Cengiz TB, Aghayeva A, Atasoy D, et al. Robotic TAPP repair of incarcerated femoral hernia with utilization of indocyanine green dye—a video vignette. Color Dis. 2017;19(8):186.
12. Agathis AZ, Miller M, Divino CM. National trends in diagnostic imaging for appendicitis: a cross-sectional analysis using NSQIP. Am Surg. 2019;85(6):625–30.
13. Perez KS, Allen SR. Complicated appendicitis and considerations for interval appendectomy. JAAPA. 2018;31(9):35–41.

Acute Cholecystitis and Emergency Common Bile Duct Exploration

Simone Frassini, Paola Fugazzola, Matteo Tomasoni, and Luca Ansaloni

1 Background

1.1 Anatomy and Physiology

The gallbladder is a small hollow organ attached to the inferior surface of the liver, and it is divided into four components: neck, infundibulum, body, and fundus [1] (Fig. 1).

The gallbladder function is to store and concentrate the bile synthesized by the liver—from 30 to 60 mL per day—as an extrahepatic reservoir. Vagal stimulation and release of cholecystokinin from neuroendocrine cells in the duodenum, in response to the presence of the fat in the diet, cause gallbladder contraction and the transport of the bile down along the cystic duct [2].

The cystic duct drains into the common bile duct forming typically an acute angle and can range from 1 to 5 cm in length: there are several uncommon anatomic variations in cystic duct anatomy, and knowledge of these variations is important to avoid possible injury to the biliary tree during surgery.

Above the cystic duct lies the common hepatic duct, draining the left and the right hepatic duct system: after the conjunction with the gallbladder, the common bile duct descends behind the first part of the duodenum and passes through the

S. Frassini (✉) · L. Ansaloni
General Surgery I Unit, Fondazione IRCCS Policlinico San Matteo, University of Pavia, Pavia, Italy

Department of Clinical, Surgical, Diagnostic and Pediatric Sciences, Università degli Studi di Pavia, Pavia, Italy
e-mail: simone.frassini01@universitadipavia.it; l.ansaloni@smatteo.pv.it

P. Fugazzola · M. Tomasoni
General Surgery I Unit, Fondazione IRCCS Policlinico San Matteo, University of Pavia, Pavia, Italy
e-mail: p.fugazzola@smatteo.pv.it; m.tomasoni@smatteo.pv.it

F. Coccolini et al. (eds.), *Mini-invasive Approach in Acute Care Surgery*,
Hot Topics in Acute Care Surgery and Trauma,
https://doi.org/10.1007/978-3-031-39001-2_6

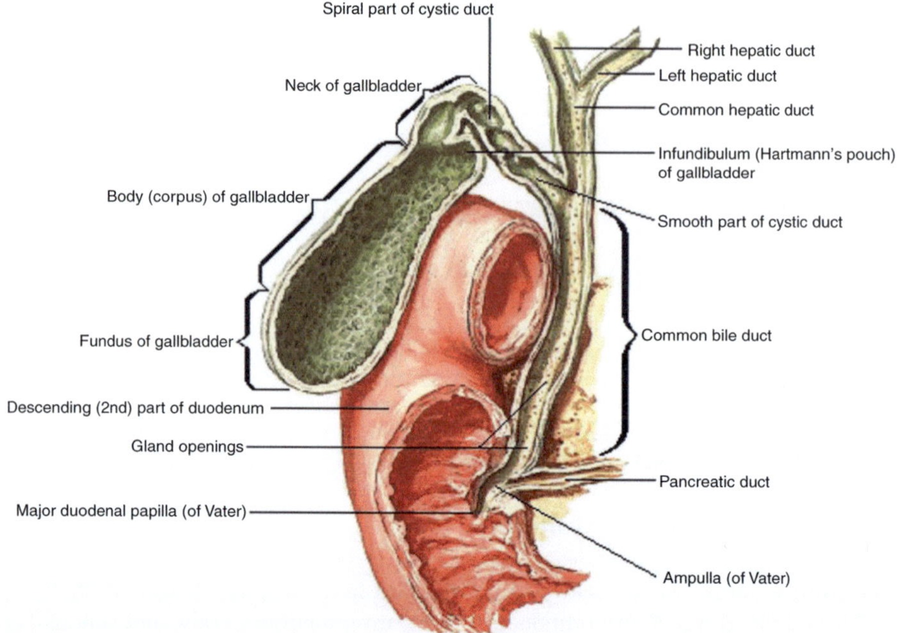

Fig. 1 Anatomy of gallbladder and the biliary tract

pancreas head forming the intrapancreatic portion of the biliary tree. The pancreatic duct also joins the common bile duct on its distal part, composing the ampulla of Vater and finally going within the wall of the third part of the duodenum to release its content. Rarely, the common bile duct and the pancreatic duct may have a separate course encompassed by the head of the pancreas with two separate orifices in the duodenum (Figs. 2 and 3).

1.2　Pathogenesis

Acute cholecystitis is an acute inflammatory process involving the gallbladder, mainly attributable to the presence of gallstones but also due to other factors such as ischemia, motility disorders, direct chemical injury, infections, collagen disorders, and allergic reactions. In a recent survey in the United States, over 10% of patients with gallstone-related complications have a first clinical presentation with acute calculous cholecystitis (ACC) [3, 4]. The pathological process of acute cholecystitis is an obstruction of the neck or in the cystic duct by a gallstone with two factors determining the progression and the severity of the disease: the degree of obstruction and the duration of obstruction. When the obstruction is of short duration and partial, the patients can experience biliary colic; otherwise, when the obstruction is complete and of long duration, the patients can develop acute cholecystitis, and more serious septic complications can occur. Possible complications when gallstone-related ACC is ignored or misdiagnosed are acute cholangitis, acute biliary

Figs. 2 and 3 Possible anatomic variations of biliary tract tree

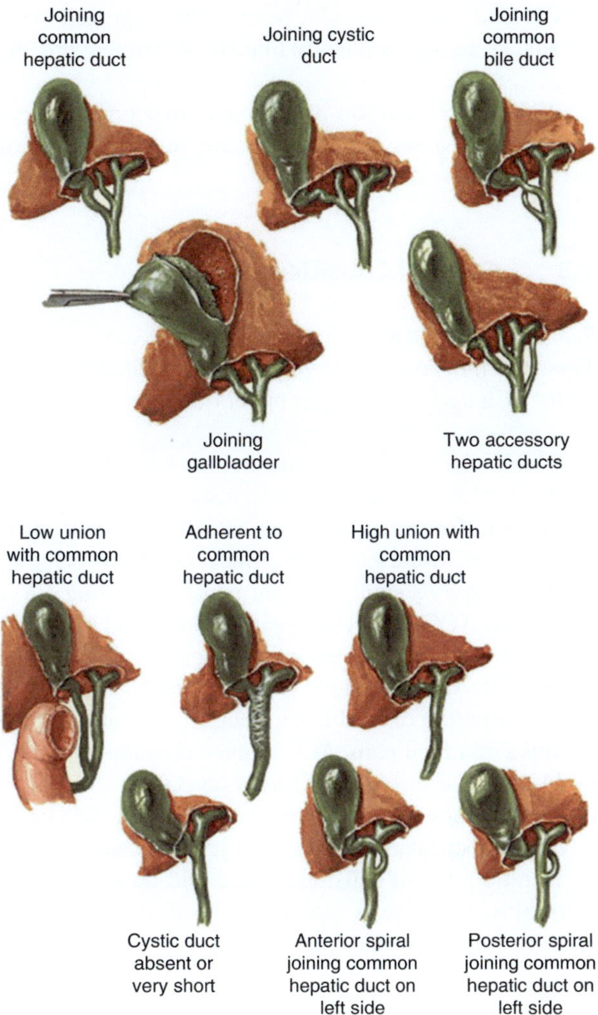

pancreatitis, gallstone ileus, Mirizzi syndrome, gallbladder carcinoma, and porcelain gallbladder [5]. According to the most recent evidence, the pathogenesis of ACC goes through a four-step classification:

1. Edematous cholecystitis (0–4 days): first reactive pathological phase, with interstitial fluid and parietal edema but tissues are intact without deeper layer involvement.
2. Necrotizing cholecystitis (3–5 days): gallbladder has edematous changes with areas of necrosis and local hemorrhage. There are portions of scattered necrosis, but they are superficial and do not involve the full thickness of the wall.
3. Suppurative cholecystitis (7–10 days): the active repairing process of inflammation is evident. The gallbladder wall is thickened by fibrous proliferation, and pericholecystic abscesses are present.

4. Chronic cholecystitis: it occurs after repeated occurrence of mild cholecystitis attacks and consequently fibrotic or atrophic process in the gallbladder wall.

With the obstruction of a tubular structure as the cystic duct, pain may come from increased intraluminal pressure, and it precedes infectious complications due to the biliary stasis.

1.3 General Consideration

1.3.1 Symptoms

The three most common symptoms associated with the biliary disease are resumed by the "Charcot triad": right upper quadrant pain, fever, and jaundice.

- PAIN: when the gallbladder lumen cannot fully empty due to obstruction by a stone, pain fibers are activated resulting in a typical abdominal pain in the epigastrium or the right upper quadrant. From a weak and occasional postprandial pain, in case of severe ACC, the clinical condition can evolve to abdominal tenderness and Murphy's sign. A recent paper, including 17 studies about clinical assessment of ACC, showed a positive likelihood ratio for right upper quadrant tenderness and Murphy's sign in the diagnosis of acute cholecystitis [6].
- FEVER: this symptom is a common systemic manifestation of infection or inflammation of the biliary tract. In case of fever associated with common right upper quadrant pain, ACC or even cholangitis must be immediately suspected.
- JAUNDICE: a serum bilirubin level of 2.5 mg/dL or even more is necessary to detect scleral icterus; levels above 5 mg/dL will cause cutaneous jaundice. Fever, right upper quadrant pain, and jaundice suggest generally a blockage of biliary secretion due to gallstones but could be also secondarily to other less common origins. Jaundice is typically related to surgical, from obstruction, or medical, from hepatocellular disease, cause.

1.3.2 Laboratory Test

When a biliary alteration is suspected, the routine hepatic panel of blood test is mandatory as a first-level diagnostic tool. Determination of the conjugated or unconjugated level of bilirubin, alkaline phosphatase, and serum transaminases is useful to detect and discriminate a hepatic or cholestatic source of the pathological process.

In addition, in the case of ACC, also phlogistic signals in the blood exams must be checked out: white blood cells count (WBC), C-reactive protein (CRP), and procalcitonin (PCT) increase when infection or inflammation are evolving, and they represent also a key component of all the existing diagnostic score.

1.3.3 Imaging

- Ultrasound (US): Transabdominal ultrasound is an inexpensive, sensitive, accurate, and reproducible test—when in expert hands—to evaluate the gallbladder and the biliary tree; this diagnostic tool is the first-choice technique to separate a possible medical cause of jaundice from a surgical obstructive one. Gallstones, gallbladder diseases, and common bile duct dilatations are commonly diagnosed via US assessment. Pathologic signs for gallbladder are wall thickening, pericholecystic fluid, calcified gallbladder wall, and intraluminal stones.

- Computed tomography (CT): Although the US is worldwide identified as the first choice in the diagnostic path of biliary disease, CT scan provides a more accurate anatomical delineation and could be necessary when US findings are ambiguous. In some clusters of patients not fit for an ultrasound diagnosis—elderly people, obese—CT could be chosen as the first step in diagnostic evaluation.
- Magnetic resonance (MR): MR delineates a superior anatomic definition of the intrahepatic and extrahepatic biliary tree and pancreas. This diagnostic tool, compared to CT scan, avoids radiation exposure and, as a second-step imaging exam, could be very useful to detect any alteration along the cystic duct and common bile duct; on the other hand, it's expensive and not always available even in the major specialistic centers.

2 Acute Calculus Cholecystitis (ACC)

As abovementioned, ACC is the first clinical presentation with a prevalence of 10–15% in patients with gallstone-related complications.

Due to the importance of this topic, a lot of studies have been published aiming to define parameters for the diagnosis, classification, and management of ACC. The Tokyo Guidelines (TG) first edition—produced based on the results of expert consensus at the Tokyo Consensus Meeting in 2007—was published in 2007 (TG07) and then revised in 2013 (TG13) and more recently in 2018 (TG18): consecutive versions provided an up-to-date point of view on diagnosis, classification, and management of ACC [7–9]. These guidelines have become widely adopted in recent years, but in 2016, also the World Society of Emergency Surgery (WSES) published the first edition of its guidelines for ACC [10]. In 2018, the scientific board of the sixth World Congress of WSES evaluated the TG18 on ACC and found how this last edition concluded closer to the recommendations of the 2016 WSES guidelines. Furthermore, this was the occasion for a revision and update of the guideline, along with the availability of new evidence. The final product was the "2020 World Society of Emergency Surgery update guidelines for the diagnosis and treatment of acute calculus cholecystitis," with still some difference from TG18 on important topics [11].

2.1 Diagnosis of ACC

According to the Tokyo Guidelines of 2013, and confirmed by TG18 [8, 9], diagnosis of ACC can be made when are satisfied at least one item from each criteria they proposed (Table 1).

Table 1 TG18/TG13 diagnostic criteria for acute cholecystitis

(a)	Local signs of inflammation	– Murphy's sign
		– RUQ mass/pain/tenderness
(b)	Systemic signs of inflammation	– Fever
		– Elevated PCR
		– Elevated WBC count
(c)	Imaging findings	Findings of acute cholecystitis
Suspected diagnosis		One item A + One item B
Definitive diagnosis		One item A + One item B + C

An ACC can be suspected when the patient presents one item from the local signs of inflammation criteria (Criteria A) and one item from the systemic signs of inflammation criteria (Criteria B). These diagnostic criteria have been judged from numerous validation studies as indicators in daily clinical practice, without any addition in the last edition from 2018; for example, some studies tried to evaluate additional lab tests—such as procalcitonin (PCT)—as a useful diagnostic tool for ACC but without statistical significance. Studies have found that diagnostic accuracy of TG13/TG18 criteria ranges from 60.4 to 94.0% if pathological samples are used as the gold standard [12].

However, WSES in 2020 [11] affirms that the TG criteria appear to be limited for the diagnosis of ACC. For the diagnosis of ACC, they suggest using a combination of anamnesis and clinical examination—fever, right upper quadrant pain, abdominal tenderness, Murphy's sign, vomiting, etc., —laboratory features, CRP, PCT, WBC, and imaging analysis with suggestive findings for the gallbladder inflammation. The best combination of these criteria is not known, but WSES guidelines suggest not to rely on a single or few findings but to extend the point of view.

2.2   Imaging for ACC

Abdominal ultrasound (US) is recommended as the first-choice initial imaging method for the diagnosis of acute calculus cholecystitis: in a recent review and meta-analysis, the US has a sensitivity of 81% and a specificity of 83% [13]. TG13/TG18 and WSES guidelines agree with this statement because of its low invasiveness, cost-effectiveness balance, wide-spread availability, easy-to-use, and good accuracy for gallstones diagnosis. The typical US signs of ACC are the presence of gallstones, thickened walls of more than 5 mm, pericholecystic fluid, debris echo, and US Murphy's sign [14].

When abdominal US does not provide a definitive diagnosis about ACC and a clear definition of the biliary tract anatomy, without an indication about a possible associated common bile duct stones presence, a further imaging technique is suggested. The presence of stones along with the biliary tract results in evidence of common bile duct enlargement due to obstruction and associated signs of inflammation: this condition makes mandatory a definitive diagnostic assessment and eventually a treatment before or associated with the surgical treatment.

Magnetic resonance cholangiopancreatography (MRI) has a diagnostic accuracy better than the abdominal US and enables the visualization of the biliary tract anatomy without contrast-agent use [15]. The diagnostic yield of MRI for ACC provides 85% sensitivity and 81% specificity [16]. On the other hand, it must be taken into account how MRI is expensive, not routinely applicable, not commonly used in the emergency setting, and roughly comparable to US accuracy [17]. Diagnostic accuracy of CT scan is poor, with the lowest sensitivity compared with every other imaging technique in the field (59.8%) [18]. Advantages of the CT scan performance are a relatively low cost and that it is easy to perform and rapid even in the emergency setting. CT scan is recommended when a gangrenous ACC is suspected: specific findings are irregular thickening of the gallbladder wall, poor contrast enhancement of gallbladder wall, increased density of fatty tissue around the gallbladder, gas in the gallbladder lumen or wall, membranous structures within the lumen, and peri-gallbladder abscess. Finally, cholescintigraphy with hepatobiliary iminodiacetic acid (HIDA scan) has the highest sensitivity and specificity for the diagnosis of ACC [18]: in the clinical practice, HIDA scan utilization is limited due to its scarce availability, long time required to perform the exam, and the important exposure to radiation.

2.3   Grading and Classification of ACC

TG 13/18 suggests a classification for ACC, structured in three different levels of severity, based on the characteristic of the acute inflammatory process [8, 9]:

1. Grade III, *Severe ACC*: an ACC associated with organ dysfunction
    (a) Cardiovascular dysfunction: hypotension with dopamine >5 µg/kg per min, or norepinephrine
    (b) Neurological dysfunction: decreased level of consciousness
    (c) Respiratory dysfunction: PaO_2/FiO_2 ratio < 300
    (d) Renal dysfunction: oliguria, creatinine>2.0 mg/dL
    (e) Hepatic dysfunction: PT-INR > 1.5
    (f) Hematological dysfunction: platelet count <100,000/mm^3
2. Grade II, *Moderate ACC*, associated with any one of the following conditions:
    (a) Elevated white blood cell count (>18,000/mm^3)
    (b) Palpable tender mass in the right upper abdominal quadrant
    (c) Duration of complaints >72 h
    (d) Marked local inflammation (gangrenous cholecystitis, pericholecystic abscess, hepatic abscess, biliary peritonitis, emphysematous cholecystitis)
3. Grade I, *Mild ACC* does not meet the criteria of "Grade III" or "Grade II" ACC: grade I can also be defined as AC in a healthy patient with no organ dysfunction and mild inflammatory changes in the gallbladder, making cholecystectomy a safe and low-risk operative procedure.

The criteria used in the Tokyo guidelines to assess a severity grading for ACC have been validated in numerous studies, and they are significantly related to prognosis, length of hospital stay, conversion to open surgery, and medical costs [19, 20]. A grade III ACC is well regarded as a factor predicting patients' prognosis and, in some circumstances, may require treatment in intensive care unit: nevertheless, the mortality rate for ACC remains around 1% [21]. In particular, a recent work by Endo et al. identified factors such as jaundice, neurological dysfunction, and respiratory dysfunction that were significantly associated with prognosis [22]. An analysis from the US in 2015 showed that severe ACC according to TG13 guidelines was an independent predictor for conversion from laparoscopic to open surgery, and complications after surgery are also more common for patients with higher severity grade [19, 23]: however, recent data state TG13 cannot be used as an unquestionable assessment for surgical treatment difficulties, and cholecystectomy is feasible even in case of severe ACC with conversion or subtotal cholecystectomy also a possible rescue procedure [24, 25].

3 Common Bile Duct Associated to ACC

3.1 Initial Evaluation

A subset of patients with the condition of gallstones also has choledocholithiasis—i.e., the presence of common bile duct stones (CBDS)—ranging from 10 to 20% and from 5 to 10% in the case of ACC [26, 27]. Approach to patients with suspected choledocholithiasis must be careful because a missed diagnosis and proper treatment of CBDS means a risk of recurrent symptoms, pancreatitis, and cholangitis: the main issue is to identify patients with a high likelihood of CBDS for further diagnostic tests and treatment.

The initial evaluation of suspected CBDS associated with ACC should include:

- *Serum liver biochemical test*
  - Alanine aminotransferase (ALT)
  - Aspartate aminotransferase (AST)
  - Alkaline phosphatase (ALP)
  - Bilirubin
  - Gamma-glutamyl transferase (GGT)
  - GGT has been validated by recent studies as the most reliable liver function test for CBDS with a sensitivity of 80.6% and a specificity of 75.3% using a cutoff level of 224 U/L [28].
- *Transabdominal US*
  - As above mentioned, the US is the first-line technique for ACC diagnosis, but the biliary tract can be visualized at the same time. This imaging tool has relatively poor sensitivity for detecting CBDS; however, US reliable detects are an increased diameter of the common bile duct and the direct visualization of a stone in the biliary tract [29, 30].
  - Anyhow, scientific literature and specifically WSES 2020 guidelines recommend against the use of laboratory tests or US findings as the only method to identify CBDS in patients with ACC, but a complete risk assessment and consequently decisions are suggested by experts as mandatory [11].

Table 2 Risk factors and classification of risk for CBDS according to WSES 2020 guidelines

CBDS risk factors	
Very strong	Evidence of CBDS at the abdominal US
	Ascending cholangitis
Strong	Common bile duct diameter > 6 mm
	Total serum bilirubin level > 1.8 mg/dL
Moderate	Abnormal liver biochemical test
	Age > 55 years
	Clinical gallstone pancreatitis
Risk class for choledocolithiasis	
High	Presence of any very strong
Low	No predictors present
Intermediate	All other patients

3.2 Risk Assessment of CBDS Associated with ACC

The American Society of Gastrointestinal Endoscopy (ASGE) and the Society of American Gastrointestinal Endoscopic Surgery (SAGES) proposed a strategy in 2010 to assign risk of choledocholithiasis looking at some clinical and imaging predictors (Table 2) [31]. ASGE and SAGES identified very strong predictors of choledocholithiasis, CBDS at US imaging, evidence of clinical ascending cholangitis, bilirubin level > 4 mg/dL; strong predictors of CBDS, common bile duct dilatation on the US (>6 mm) or a bilirubin level from 1.8 to 4 mg/dL; and moderate predictors of choledocholithiasis, abnormal liver biochemical tests other than bilirubin, age older than 55 years old, and clinical pancreatitis. These clinical predictors build a stratification of risk for CBDS: in case any very strong predictor or both strong predictors are present, CBDS likelihood is >50% (high-risk patients); when no predictors are present, probability of CBDS is <10% (low-risk patients); and finally, all other patients with predictors have a risk from 10 to 50% (moderate-risk patients) [32–35].

WSES 2020 guidelines suggest stratifying the risk of CBDS associated with ACC with a modified classification from the previous ASGE and SAGES' one: only patients with evidence of CBDS at US imaging should be considered at high risk, meanwhile patients with no imaging evidence of CBDS but indirect US signs and laboratory alterations should be considered as moderate-risk population [11].

Up-to-date risk stratification of CBDS associated with ACC is a key point to establish planning for further second diagnostic level investigations or treatment decisions.

3.3 Clinical Implications of CBDS Risk Stratification

The appropriate treatment of CBDS associated with ACC is the biliary system drainage either preoperatively, intraoperatively, or postoperatively according to the local resources and experience [36].

Approaches are different according to risk stratification:

- *Low risk of CBDS associated with ACC*

  When patients are a candidate for surgery, they should undergo cholecystectomy without any other kind of diagnostic investigation.

- *Moderate risk of CBDS associated with ACC*

  Patients with an intermediate probability of CBDS associated with ACC should benefit from additional second-level imaging exams. The diagnostic examinations options are endoscopic ultrasound (EU) and magnetic resonance cholangiopancreatography (MRCP) before any kind of surgical approach, laparoscopic US, and intraoperative cholangiography during cholecystectomy. ASGE and WSES guidelines agree that patients with moderate risk of CBDS associated with ACC are recommended to undergo one of the previous imaging techniques of biliary tract obstruction detection [11, 31].

- *High risk if CBDS associated with ACC*

  In case of high risk of choledocholithiasis associated with ACC, due to the frequent necessity of operative management, the first-line treatment choice is a preoperative endoscopic retrograde cholangiopancreatography (ERCP). With this approach, a second-level diagnostic examination is avoided, and patients have a faster way from endoscopy directly to surgery. ERCP has both a diagnostic and a therapeutic role in the management of CBDS, but it is also an invasive procedure with the risk of a complication from 1 to 10% when associated with sphincterotomy [37]. The endoscopic approach is widespread in Western countries, when available, also because it can be performed postoperatively when CBDS are misdiagnosed. Other possible approaches to CBDS are intraoperative cholangiography (IOC) followed by laparoscopic or open common bile duct exploration at the time of surgery, or even an ERCP performed directly in the operating room. IOC and intraoperative ERCP significantly increase the length of surgery and require a dedicated staff in the operating room, but ERCP performed with associated sphincterotomy need a careful posttreatment observation to detect any sign of complication—including pancreatitis, cholangitis, biliary system bleeding, or perforation.

  A meta-analysis comparing procedures of biliary duct treatments before or during surgery (ERCP versus IOC and common bile duct exploration) states the two approaches are equivalent in terms of safety and efficacy; on the other hand, intraoperative management of CBDS has lauded of major cost [38]. No differences in morbidity, mortality, and success rate were reported; therefore, all these techniques can be considered suitable options depending on local facilities [11].

4   Treatment of ACC

Literature evidence over the years reported how different data and changes in the clinical management of ACC succeeded, but the surgical approach to ACC with cholecystectomy is still the gold standard for symptomatic cholelithiasis [39].

During these years, a lot of reports, case series, and randomized clinical trials have been published discussing the better surgical technique and the better timing for cholecystectomy in ACC, early (ELC) or delayed (DLC).

Conservative management with pharmacological therapy—fluids, analgesia, and antibiotics—has been proposed as an alternative for patients with symptomatic ACC, but 30% of them develop recurrent gallstone-related complications and 60% undergo a subsequent cholecystectomy [40]. According to TG18, an optimal treatment strategy for acute cholecystitis should consider the assessment of ACC severity: in case of grade I (mild) ACC, cholecystectomy should ideally be performed soon after the patient's admission to the hospital, and a conservative approach should be considered only if patients cannot withstand surgery. For moderate (grade II) ACC, the surgical treatment remains the gold standard but in the case of patients fit for surgery and in the advanced surgical center. If patients cannot withstand surgery, conservative medical treatment should be considered as an alternative to surgery with the indication to urgent biliary drainage if the clinical status is not getting better. Grade III (severe) ACC is a condition accompanied by organ dysfunction with the necessity of organ support in addition to a standard initial medical treatment: if the patient can withstand surgery and an experience in intensive care management is allowed, cholecystectomy remains the first-line treatment considering pharmacological support and biliary drainage as a second-line option for patients unfit for surgery [9]. Typical methods used by intensive care personnel and anesthesiologists to stratify patients' risk at the moment of surgical evaluation are the Charlson Comorbidity Index (CCI) and the American Society of Anesthesiologists' physical status classification (ASA-Score). Patients that are candidates to cholecystectomy with CCI $\geq$ 4 and ASA-Score $\geq$ 3 are considered at high risk [41–43]. Furthermore, TG18 defined neurological and respiratory dysfunction and jaundice as negative predictive factors in the case of grade III ACC because they are associated with higher mortality [9].

WSES 2020 guidelines, as previously stated and reported in Fig. 4, recommend the surgical approach as the preferred first-line treatment choice in patient with ACC, considering as contraindications for cholecystectomy only an ongoing septic shock and anesthesiologic inadvisability [11]. After this initial agreement with TG18 indications, the experts' panel of WSES focused on surgical indications in the case of ACC, going deep inside technical advice and stating the optimal timing of treatment.

4.1 Surgical Management of ACC

Surgical removal of the gallbladder is generally considered the standard treatment for ACC, and the laparoscopic cholecystectomy has been supported as the gold-standard approach: local inflammation is a risk factor for bile duct injuries, bleeding, longer operative time, morbidity, and mortality rates but recently has been demonstrated how laparoscopy is safe and feasible in case of ACC [44, 45]. When anatomic identification of structures is difficult and the risk of biliary tract injuries

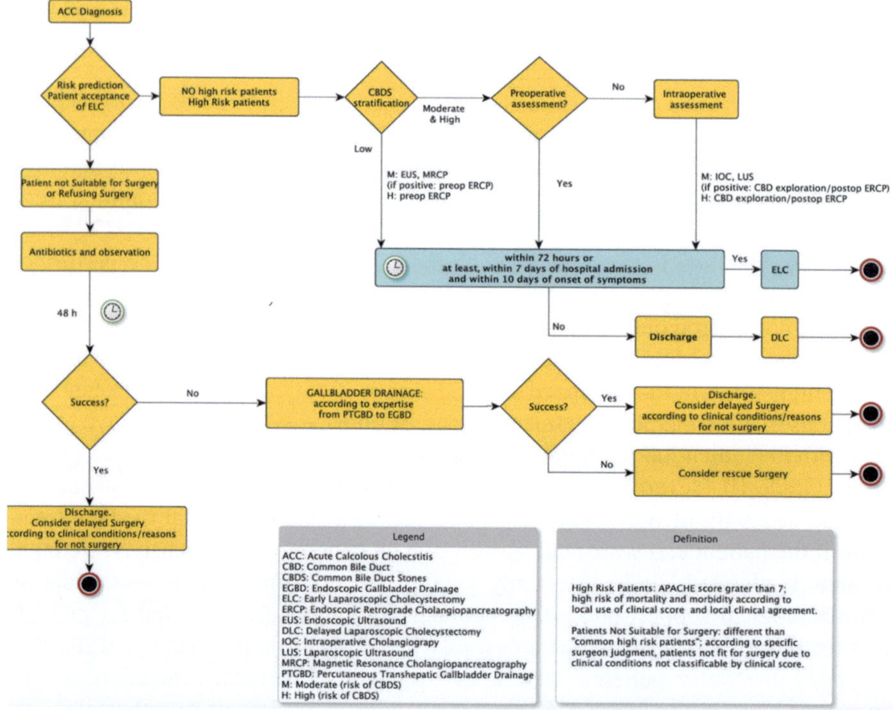

Fig. 4 WSES 2020 Flowchart for the management of patients with ACC

is high, open surgical conversion or bailout procedures, e.g., laparoscopic subtotal cholecystectomy or fundus first technique, are valid alternative procedures [46]. The reasons that must be considered for a change of approach with an open cholecystectomy conversion from laparoscopic treatment are severe local inflammation, strong adhesions, major bleeding from Calot's triangle, and suspicion of bile duct injury. The review of relevant recent literature confirmed strong support for the recommendation that the laparoscopic approach should be attempted in the case of ACC because it is associated with a lower complication rate, shorter length of hospital stay, and operative time becoming progressively faster [47]. WSES 2020 guidelines suggest even performing laparoscopic cholecystectomy for ACC in patients with liver cirrhosis, in the elderly, and in cases of pregnancy [48].

Another key point to be addressed talking about cholecystectomy for ACC is timing: WSES 2020 guidelines state ELC—performed as soon as possible, when associated CBDS risk is assessed, within 7 days from hospital admission and 10 days from the onset of symptoms—is the preferable approach compared to intermediate laparoscopic cholecystectomy (ILC), performed between 7 days from hospital admission and 6 weeks, or DLC, performed between 6 weeks and 3 months. DLC should be considered as a second-line treatment option only when an early approach is not considered feasible and safe. Also in TG18, an early surgical approach within 72 h or even a week from hospital admission for ACC is considered the optimal strategy with a shorter length of hospital stay, reduction of recurrence and complications, and a reduction of costs too [49, 50].

4.2 Alternative Treatment for ACC

As previously cited, recent data from a long/medium follow-up time study confirm that about 30% of patients with symptomatic acute cholecystitis who did not undergo surgery developed recurrent gallstone-related complications—compared with 3% of patients treated with cholecystectomy—and 60% had the following necessity of surgical approach [43]. According to this evidence, nonoperative management (NOM) with medical treatments (i.e., antibiotics, fluids, analgesia, and observation) is to consider as a second-line therapy only when patients are refusing surgery or are not fit for surgical intervention. Observation and medical therapy are safe with a typically low incidence of adverse outcomes, but this latter approach has a high incidence of recurrence.

In patients who are not suitable for surgery but with an increasing septic condition due to biliary infection, gallbladder drainage is an alternative when the NOM approach failed in the first 24–48 h [51]. Gallbladder drainage decompresses the infected bile or pus, removes the infected collection, reduces inflammation condition, and improves clinical condition without removing the gallbladder [52]. A recent multicentric randomized trial (CHOCOLATE trial) compared ELC to percutaneous transhepatic gallbladder drainage (PTGBD) and showed how surgical approach must be considered the gold standard technique also in high-risk patients. Recently, endoscopic biliary drainage, e.g., endoscopic transpapillary gallbladder drainage (ETGBD), with or without positioning of nasogastric drainage and a gallbladder stent, or endoscopic ultrasound-guided transmural gallbladder drainage (EUS-GBD) with a lumen-apposing self-expandable metal stent to be removed within 4 weeks, have taken hold [52]. DRAC 1 trial by Teoh AYB et al. compared endoscopic procedures with PTGBD in high-risk patients with ACC, and it evidenced improved outcomes in ETGBD and EUS-GBD in terms of adverse events, reintervention rate, unplanned readmissions, recurrence of ACC, and analgesic requirements [53].

4.3 Antibiotics for ACC

The use of antibiotics for ACC remains a mainstay in the treatment choice, and it has been defined how a deep selection of antimicrobial agents, targeted organism, pharmacokinetics and pharmacodynamics, and actual patient's condition must be a key point for antibiotic selection. Organisms most often involved in biliary infections are the Gram-negative aerobes—*E. coli* and *K. pneumoniae*—and anaerobes, especially *Bacteroides fragilis*; antimicrobial regimen, when indicated, should be based on the presumed pathogens involved and the risk factors for major resistance

Table 3 Antimicrobial regimens suggested for acute calculous cholecystitis

Good penetration efficiency antibiotics	Low penetration efficiency antibiotics
Bile/serum (≥5)	Bile/serum (<1)
Piperacillin/tazobactam	Cefotaxime
Tigecycline	Meropenem
Amoxicillin/clavulanate	Ceftazidime
Ciprofloxacin	Vancomycin
Ampicillin/sulbactam	Amikacin
Ceftriaxone	Gentamicin
Levofloxacin	Cefepime
Penicillin G	Imipenem

patterns [54]. Microbiological analyses help design targeted therapeutic strategies for individual patients, mostly if patients are at high risk for antimicrobial resistance: on the other hand, an antibiotic regimen has been demonstrated not to be routinely necessary after the source control (Table 3). WSES 2020 recommended against the use of postoperative antibiotics when the infection focus is controlled by surgery in uncomplicated ACC while in case of complicated ACC is recommended to prescribe the pharmacological regimen based on the presumed pathogens involved [11]. Similarly, TG18 suggests the use of antimicrobial therapy only before and at the time of surgery for patients with mild or moderate ACC, and for the duration of 4–7 days after surgery for grade III ACC [9].

References

1. Towsend CM, et al. Sabiston textbook of surgery, 20th ed. Elsevier.
2. Hansen JT, Koeppen BM. Netter's atlas of human physiology.
3. Kimura Y, Takada T, Strasberg SM, Pitt HA, Gouma DJ, Garden OJ, Büchler MW, Windsor JA, Mayumi T, Yoshida M, Miura F, Higuchi R, Gabata T, Hata J, Gomi H, Dervenis C, Lau WY, Belli G, Kim MH, Hilvano SC, Yamashita Y. TG13 current terminology, etiology, and epidemiology of acute cholangitis and cholecystitis. J Hepatobiliary Pancreat Sci. 2013;20(1):8–23. https://doi.org/10.1007/s00534-012-0564-0.
4. Stinton LM, Shaffer EA. Epidemiology of gallbladder disease: cholelithiasis and cancer. Gut Liver. 2012;6(2):172–87. https://doi.org/10.5009/gnl.2012.6.2.172.
5. Portincasa P, Di Ciaula A, de Bari O, Garruti G, Palmieri VO, Wang DQ. Management of gallstones and its related complications. Expert Rev Gastroenterol Hepatol. 2016;10(1):93–112. https://doi.org/10.1586/17474124.2016.1109445.
6. Trowbridge RL, Rutkowski NK, Shojania KG. Does this patient have acute cholecystitis? JAMA. 2003;289(1):80–6. https://doi.org/10.1001/jama.289.1.80.
7. Kimura Y, Takada T, Kawarada Y, Nimura Y, Hirata K, Sekimoto M, Yoshida M, Mayumi T, Wada K, Miura F, Yasuda H, Yamashita Y, Nagino M, Hirota M, Tanaka A, Tsuyuguchi T, Strasberg SM, Gadacz TR. Definitions, pathophysiology, and epidemiology of acute cholangitis and cholecystitis: Tokyo guidelines. J Hepatobiliary Pancreat Surg. 2007;14(1):15–26. https://doi.org/10.1007/s00534-006-1152-y.
8. Takada T, Strasberg SM, Solomkin JS, Pitt HA, Gomi H, Yoshida M, Mayumi T, Miura F, Gouma DJ, Garden OJ, Büchler MW, Kiriyama S, Yokoe M, Kimura Y, Tsuyuguchi T, Itoi T, Gabata T, Higuchi R, Okamoto K, Hata J, Murata A, Kusachi S, Windsor JA, Supe AN, Lee S, Chen XP, Yamashita Y, Hirata K, Inui K, Sumiyama Y. Tokyo guidelines revision committee.

TG13: updated Tokyo guidelines for the management of acute cholangitis and cholecystitis. J Hepatobiliary Pancreat Sci. 2013;20(1):1–7. https://doi.org/10.1007/s00534-012-0566-y.

9. Yokoe M, Hata J, Takada T, Strasberg SM, Asbun HJ, Wakabayashi G, Kozaka K, Endo I, Deziel DJ, Miura F, Okamoto K, Hwang TL, Huang WS, Ker CG, Chen MF, Han HS, Yoon YS, Choi IS, Yoon DS, Noguchi Y, Shikata S, Ukai T, Higuchi R, Gabata T, Mori Y, Iwashita Y, Hibi T, Jagannath P, Jonas E, Liau KH, Dervenis C, Gouma DJ, Cherqui D, Belli G, Garden OJ, Giménez ME, de Santibañes E, Suzuki K, Umezawa A, Supe AN, Pitt HA, Singh H, Chan ACW, Lau WY, Teoh AYB, Honda G, Sugioka A, Asai K, Gomi H, Itoi T, Kiriyama S, Yoshida M, Mayumi T, Matsumura N, Tokumura H, Kitano S, Hirata K, Inui K, Sumiyama Y, Yamamoto M. Tokyo guidelines 2018: diagnostic criteria and severity grading of acute cholecystitis (with videos). J Hepatobiliary Pancreat Sci. 2018;25(1):41–54. https://doi.org/10.1002/jhbp.515.

10. Ansaloni L, Pisano M, Coccolini F, Peitzmann AB, Fingerhut A, Catena F, Agresta F, Allegri A, Bailey I, Balogh ZJ, Bendinelli C, Biffl W, Bonavina L, Borzellino G, Brunetti F, Burlew CC, Camapanelli G, Campanile FC, Ceresoli M, Chiara O, Civil I, Coimbra R, De Moya M, Di Saverio S, Fraga GP, Gupta S, Kashuk J, Kelly MD, Koka V, Jeekel H, Latifi R, Leppaniemi A, Maier RV, Marzi I, Moore F, Piazzalunga D, Sakakushev B, Sartelli M, Scalea T, Stahel PF, Taviloglu K, Tugnoli G, Uraneus S, Velmahos GC, Wani I, Weber DG, Viale P, Sugrue M, Ivatury R, Kluger Y, Gurusamy KS, Moore EE. 2016 WSES guidelines on acute calculous cholecystitis. World J Emerg Surg. 2016;11:25. https://doi.org/10.1186/s13017-016-0082-5.

11. Pisano M, Allievi N, Gurusamy K, Borzellino G, Cimbanassi S, Boerna D, Coccolini F, Tufo A, Di Martino M, Leung J, Sartelli M, Ceresoli M, Maier RV, Poiasina E, De Angelis N, Magnone S, Fugazzola P, Paolillo C, Coimbra R, Di Saverio S, De Simone B, Weber DG, Sakakushev BE, Lucianetti A, Kirkpatrick AW, Fraga GP, Wani I, Biffl WL, Chiara O, Abu-Zidan F, Moore EE, Leppäniemi A, Kluger Y, Catena F, Ansaloni L. 2020 World Society of Emergency Surgery updated guidelines for the diagnosis and treatment of acute calculus cholecystitis. World J Emerg Surg. 2020;15(1):61. https://doi.org/10.1186/s13017-020-00336-x.

12. Naidu K, Beenen E, Gananadha S, Mosse C. The yield of fever, inflammatory markers and ultrasound in the diagnosis of acute cholecystitis: a validation of the 2013 Tokyo guidelines. World J Surg. 2016;40(12):2892–7. https://doi.org/10.1007/s00268-016-3660-5.

13. Kiewiet JJ, Leeuwenburgh MM, Bipat S, Bossuyt PM, Stoker J, Boermeester MA. A systematic review and meta-analysis of diagnostic performance of imaging in acute cholecystitis. Radiology. 2012;264(3):708–20. https://doi.org/10.1148/radiol.12111561.

14. Fuks D, Mouly C, Robert B, Hajji H, Yzet T, Regimbeau JM. Acute cholecystitis: preoperative CT can help the surgeon consider conversion from laparoscopic to open cholecystectomy. Radiology. 2012;263(1):128–38. https://doi.org/10.1148/radiol.12110460.

15. Bates DD, LeBedis CA, Soto JA, Gupta A. Use of magnetic resonance in pancreaticobiliary emergencies. Magn Reson Imaging Clin N Am. 2016;24(2):433–48. https://doi.org/10.1016/j.mric.2015.11.010.

16. Watanabe Y, Nagayama M, Okumura A, Amoh Y, Katsube T, Suga T, Koyama S, Nakatani K, Dodo Y. MR imaging of acute biliary disorders. Radiographics. 2007;27(2):477–95. https://doi.org/10.1148/rg.272055148.

17. Pinto A, Reginelli A, Cagini L, Coppolino F, Stabile Ianora AA, Bracale R, Giganti M, Romano L. Accuracy of ultrasonography in the diagnosis of acute calculous cholecystitis: review of the literature. Crit Ultrasound J. 2013;5 Suppl 1(Suppl 1):S11. https://doi.org/10.1186/2036-7902-5-S1-S11.

18. Changphaisarnkul P, Saengruang-Orn S, Boonya-Asadorn T. The diagnosis of acute cholecystitis: sensitivity of sonography, cholescintigraphy and computed tomography. J Med Assoc Thail. 2015;98(8):812–9.

19. Paul Wright G, Stilwell K, Johnson J, Hefty MT, Chung MH. Predicting length of stay and conversion to open cholecystectomy for acute cholecystitis using the 2013 Tokyo guidelines in a US population. J Hepatobiliary Pancreat Sci. 2015;22(11):795–801. https://doi.org/10.1002/jhbp.284.

20. Ambe PC, Christ H, Wassenberg D. Does the Tokyo guidelines predict the extent of gallbladder inflammation in patients with acute cholecystitis? A single center retrospective analysis. BMC Gastroenterol. 2015;15:142. https://doi.org/10.1186/s12876-015-0365-4.

21. Yokoe M, Takada T, Hwang TL, Endo I, Akazawa K, Miura F, Mayumi T, Mori R, Chen MF, Jan YY, Ker CG, Wang HP, Itoi T, Gomi H, Kiriyama S, Wada K, Yamaue H, Miyazaki M, Yamamoto M. Descriptive review of acute cholecystitis: Japan-Taiwan collaborative epidemiological study. J Hepatobiliary Pancreat Sci. 2017;24(6):319–28. https://doi.org/10.1002/jhbp.450.

22. Endo I, Takada T, Hwang TL, Akazawa K, Mori R, Miura F, Yokoe M, Itoi T, Gomi H, Chen MF, Jan YY, Ker CG, Wang HP, Kiriyama S, Wada K, Yamaue H, Miyazaki M, Yamamoto M. Optimal treatment strategy for acute cholecystitis based on predictive factors: Japan-Taiwan multicenter cohort study. J Hepatobiliary Pancreat Sci. 2017;24(6):346–61. https://doi.org/10.1002/jhbp.456.

23. Cheng WC, Chiu YC, Chuang CH, Chen CY. Assessing clinical outcomes of patients with acute calculous cholecystitis in addition to the Tokyo grading: a retrospective study. Kaohsiung J Med Sci. 2014;30(9):459–65. https://doi.org/10.1016/j.kjms.2014.05.005.

24. Kamalapurkar D, Pang TC, Siriwardhane M, Hollands M, Johnston E, Pleass H, Richardson A, Lam VW. Index cholecystectomy in grade II and III acute calculous cholecystitis is feasible and safe. ANZ J Surg. 2015;85(11):854–9. https://doi.org/10.1111/ans.12986.

25. Amirthalingam V, Low JK, Woon W, Shelat V. Tokyo guidelines 2013 may be too restrictive and patients with moderate and severe acute cholecystitis can be managed by early cholecystectomy too. Surg Endosc. 2017;31(7):2892–900. https://doi.org/10.1007/s00464-016-5300-4.

26. Csendes A, Burdiles P, Diaz JC, Maluenda F, Korn O, Vallejo E, Csendes P. Prevalence of common bile duct stones according to the increasing number of risk factors present. A prospective study employing routinely intraoperative cholangiography in 477 cases. Hepatogastroenterology. 1998;45(23):1415–21.

27. Ko CW, Lee SP. Epidemiology and natural history of common bile duct stones and prediction of disease. Gastrointest Endosc. 2002;56(6 Suppl):S165–9. https://doi.org/10.1067/mge.2002.129005.

28. Ahn KS, Yoon YS, Han HS, Cho JY. Use of liver function tests as first-line diagnostic tools for predicting common bile duct stones in acute cholecystitis patients. World J Surg. 2016;40(8):1925–31. https://doi.org/10.1007/s00268-016-3517-y.

29. Gurusamy KS, Giljaca V, Takwoingi Y, Higgie D, Poropat G, Štimac D, Davidson BR. Ultrasound versus liver function tests for diagnosis of common bile duct stones. Cochrane Database Syst Rev. 2015;2015(2):CD011548. https://doi.org/10.1002/14651858.CD011548.

30. Boys JA, Doorly MG, Zehetner J, Dhanireddy KK, Senagore AJ. Can ultrasound common bile duct diameter predict common bile duct stones in the setting of acute cholecystitis? Am J Surg. 2014;207(3):432–5; discussion 435. https://doi.org/10.1016/j.amjsurg.2013.10.014.

31. ASGE Standards of Practice Committee, Maple JT, Ben-Menachem T, Anderson MA, Appalaneni V, Banerjee S, Cash BD, Fisher L, Harrison ME, Fanelli RD, Fukami N, Ikenberry SO, Jain R, Khan K, Krinsky ML, Strohmeyer L, Dominitz JA. The role of endoscopy in the evaluation of suspected choledocholithiasis. Gastrointest Endosc. 2010;71(1):1–9. https://doi.org/10.1016/j.gie.2009.09.041.

32. Barkun AN, Barkun JS, Fried GM, Ghitulescu G, Steinmetz O, Pham C, Meakins JL, Goresky CA. Useful predictors of bile duct stones in patients undergoing laparoscopic cholecystectomy. McGill Gallstone Treatment Group. Ann Surg. 1994;220(1):32–9. https://doi.org/10.1097/00000658-199407000-00006.

33. Cronan JJ. US diagnosis of choledocholithiasis: a reappraisal. Radiology. 1986;161(1):133–4. https://doi.org/10.1148/radiology.161.1.3532178.

34. Bose SM, Mazumdar A, Prakash VS, Kocher R, Katariya S, Pathak CM. Evaluation of the predictors of choledocholithiasis: comparative analysis of clinical, biochemical, radiological, radionuclear, and intraoperative parameters. Surg Today. 2001;31(2):117–22. https://doi.org/10.1007/s005950170194.

35. Abboud PA, Malet PF, Berlin JA, Staroscik R, Cabana MD, Clarke JR, Shea JA, Schwartz JS, Williams SV. Predictors of common bile duct stones prior to cholecystectomy: a meta-analysis. Gastrointest Endosc. 1996;44(4):450–5. https://doi.org/10.1016/s0016-5107(96)70098-6.

36. Dasari BV, Tan CJ, Gurusamy KS, Martin DJ, Kirk G, McKie L, Diamond T, Taylor MA. Surgical versus endoscopic treatment of bile duct stones. Cochrane Database Syst Rev. 2013;2013(12):CD003327. https://doi.org/10.1002/14651858.CD003327.pub4.

37. Christensen M, Matzen P, Schulze S, Rosenberg J. Complications of ERCP: a prospective study. Gastrointest Endosc. 2004;60(5):721–31. https://doi.org/10.1016/s0016-5107(04)02169-8.

38. Wang B, Liu Z, Lü Y, Zhao S, Chen L. A meta-analysis of preoperative versus intraoperative endoscopic sphincterotomy in patients with gallbladder and suspected common bile duct stones. Zhonghua Yi Xue Za Zhi. 2015;95(18):1425–9.

39. De U. Evolution of cholecystectomy: a tribute to Carl August Langenbuch. Indian J Surg. 2004;66:97–100.

40. Schmidt M, Søndenaa K, Vetrhus M, Berhane T, Eide GE. Long-term follow-up of a randomized controlled trial of observation versus surgery for acute cholecystitis: non-operative management is an option in some patients. Scand J Gastroenterol. 2011;46(10):1257–62. https://doi.org/10.3109/00365521.2011.598548.

41. Charlson ME, Carrozzino D, Guidi J, Patierno C. Charlson comorbidity index: a critical review of clinimetric properties. Psychother Psychosom. 2022;91(1):8–35. https://doi.org/10.1159/000521288.

42. Sundararajan V, Henderson T, Perry C, Muggivan A, Quan H, Ghali WA. New ICD-10 version of the Charlson comorbidity index predicted in-hospital mortality. J Clin Epidemiol. 2004;57(12):1288–94. https://doi.org/10.1016/j.jclinepi.2004.03.012.

43. https://www.asahq.org/standards-and-guidelines/asa-physical-status-classification-system

44. Catena F, Ansaloni L, Bianchi E, Di Saverio S, Coccolini F, Vallicelli C, Lazzareschi D, Sartelli M, Amaduzzi A, Amaduzz A, Pinna AD. The ACTIVE (acute cholecystitis trial invasive versus endoscopic) study: multicenter randomized, double-blind, controlled trial of laparoscopic versus open surgery for acute cholecystitis. Hepatogastroenterology. 2013;60(127):1552–6.

45. Johansson M, Thune A, Nelvin L, Stiernstam M, Westman B, Lundell L. Randomized clinical trial of open versus laparoscopic cholecystectomy in the treatment of acute cholecystitis. Br J Surg. 2005;92(1):44–9. https://doi.org/10.1002/bjs.4836.

46. Hussain A. Difficult laparoscopic cholecystectomy: current evidence and strategies of management. Surg Laparosc Endosc Percutan Tech. 2011;21(4):211–7. https://doi.org/10.1097/SLE.0b013e318220f1b1.

47. Coccolini F, Catena F, Pisano M, Gheza F, Fagiuoli S, Di Saverio S, Leandro G, Montori G, Ceresoli M, Corbella D, Sartelli M, Sugrue M, Ansaloni L. Open versus laparoscopic cholecystectomy in acute cholecystitis. Systematic review and meta-analysis. Int J Surg. 2015;18:196–204. https://doi.org/10.1016/j.ijsu.2015.04.083.

48. Pisano M, Ceresoli M, Cimbanassi S, Gurusamy K, Coccolini F, Borzellino G, Costa G, Allievi N, Amato B, Boerma D, Calcagno P, Campanati L, Campanile FC, Casati A, Chiara O, Crucitti A, di Saverio S, Filauro M, Gabrielli F, Guttadauro A, Kluger Y, Magnone S, Merli C, Poiasina E, Puzziello A, Sartelli M, Catena F, Ansaloni L. 2017 WSES and SICG guidelines on acute calculous cholecystitis in elderly population. World J Emerg Surg. 2019;14:10. https://doi.org/10.1186/s13017-019-0224-7.

49. Gutt CN, Encke J, Köninger J, Harnoss JC, Weigand K, Kipfmüller K, Schunter O, Götze T, Golling MT, Menges M, Klar E, Feilhauer K, Zoller WG, Ridwelski K, Ackmann S, Baron A, Schön MR, Seitz HK, Daniel D, Stremmel W, Büchler MW. Acute cholecystitis: early versus delayed cholecystectomy, a multicenter randomized trial (ACDC study, NCT00447304). Ann Surg. 2013;258(3):385–93. https://doi.org/10.1097/SLA.0b013e3182a1599b.

50. Pucher PH, Brunt LM, Davies N, Linsk A, Munshi A, Rodriguez HA, Fingerhut A, Fanelli RD, Asbun H, Aggarwal R, SAGES Safe Cholecystectomy Task Force. Outcome trends and safety measures after 30 years of laparoscopic cholecystectomy: a systematic review and pooled data analysis. Surg Endosc. 2018;32(5):2175–83. https://doi.org/10.1007/s00464-017-5974-2.

51. van Dijk AH, de Reuver PR, Tasma TN, van Dieren S, Hugh TJ, Boermeester MA. Systematic review of antibiotic treatment for acute calculous cholecystitis. Br J Surg. 2016;103(7):797–811. https://doi.org/10.1002/bjs.10146.
52. Loozen CS, van Santvoort HC, van Duijvendijk P, Besselink MG, Gouma DJ, Nieuwenhuijzen GA, Kelder JC, Donkervoort SC, van Geloven AA, Kruyt PM, Roos D, Kortram K, Kornmann VN, Pronk A, van der Peet DL, Crolla RM, van Ramshorst B, Bollen TL, Boerma D. Laparoscopic cholecystectomy versus percutaneous catheter drainage for acute cholecystitis in high risk patients (CHOCOLATE): multicentre randomised clinical trial. BMJ. 2018;363:k3965. https://doi.org/10.1136/bmj.k3965.
53. Teoh AYB, Kitano M, Itoi T, Pérez-Miranda M, Ogura T, Chan SM, Serna-Higuera C, Omoto S, Torres-Yuste R, Tsuichiya T, Wong KT, Leung CH, Chiu PWY, Ng EKW, Lau JYW. Endosonography-guided gallbladder drainage versus percutaneous cholecystostomy in very high-risk surgical patients with acute cholecystitis: an international randomised multicentre controlled superiority trial (DRAC 1). Gut. 2020;69(6):1085–91. https://doi.org/10.1136/gutjnl-2019-319996.
54. Sartelli M, Catena F, Ansaloni L, Coccolini F, Corbella D, Moore EE, Malangoni M, Velmahos G, Coimbra R, Koike K, Leppaniemi A, Biffl W, Balogh Z, Bendinelli C, Gupta S, Kluger Y, Agresta F, Di Saverio S, Tugnoli G, Jovine E, Ordonez CA, Whelan JF, Fraga GP, Gomes CA, Pereira GA, Yuan KC, Bala M, Peev MP, Ben-Ishay O, Cui Y, Marwah S, Zachariah S, Wani I, Rangarajan M, Sakakushev B, Kong V, Ahmed A, Abbas A, Gonsaga RA, Guercioni G, Vettoretto N, Poiasina E, Díaz-Nieto R, Massalou D, Skrovina M, Gerych I, Augustin G, Kenig J, Khokha V, Tranà C, Kok KY, Mefire AC, Lee JG, Hong SK, Lohse HA, Ghnnam W, Verni A, Lohsiriwat V, Siribumrungwong B, El Zalabany T, Tavares A, Baiocchi G, Das K, Jarry J, Zida M, Sato N, Murata K, Shoko T, Irahara T, Hamedelneel AO, Naidoo N, Adesunkanmi AR, Kobe Y, Ishii W, Oka K, Izawa Y, Hamid H, Khan I, Attri A, Sharma R, Sanjuan J, Badiel M, Barnabé R. Complicated intra-abdominal infections worldwide: the definitive data of the CIAOW study. World J Emerg Surg. 2014;9:37. https://doi.org/10.1186/1749-7922-9-37.

Acute Colonic Diverticulitis

Dario Tartaglia, Federico Coccolini, Alessio Mazzoni, Valerio Genovese, Camilla Cremonini, Enrico Cicuttin, and Massimo Chiarugi

1   Percutaneous Drainage

Diverticulitis may occur with a pericolic or distant abscess in the pelvis: pericolic in 1B and pelvic distant from the colon in grade 2 according to Wasvary's modified Hinchey's classification [1]. The size of the abscess is the mainstream for proper treatment. The intravenous administration of large-spectrum antibiotics could be associated with the need to place percutaneous drainage, mainly in case of larger abscesses. The exact size cutoff in which one should apply for percutaneous drainage has been a topic of debate for a long time, and nowadays, we still do not have a definitive answer. Since the early 2000s, the cutoff value diameter for amenability of the percutaneous abscess has progressively been reduced from 5 to 3 cm [2, 3]. Abscesses under 3 cm can be treated with IV, broad-spectrum antibiotics that cover Gram-negative and anaerobic bacteria. This medical approach could lead to a resolution in more than 80% of cases.

On the other hand, larger abscesses might be evacuated with US- or CT-guided percutaneous drainage (Figs. 1 and 2). The choice to use US or CT as guidance depends on the abscess location: for instance, superficial ones could be easily chased by ultrasound. Therefore, CT scan represents the preferred method of evacuation [4]. However, this procedure is not free of risks: it has been shown that it is

D. Tartaglia (✉)
Emergency Surgery Unit and Trauma Center, University Hospital of Pisa, Pisa, Italy

Emergency Surgery Unit and Trauma Center, Cisanello Hospital, University of Pisa, Pisa, Italy
e-mail: dario.tartaglia@unipi.it

F. Coccolini · A. Mazzoni · V. Genovese · C. Cremonini · E. Cicuttin · M. Chiarugi
Emergency Surgery Unit and Trauma Center, University Hospital of Pisa, Pisa, Italy
e-mail: federico.coccolini@unipi.it; massimo.chiarugi@unipi.it

F. Coccolini et al. (eds.), *Mini-invasive Approach in Acute Care Surgery*,
Hot Topics in Acute Care Surgery and Trauma,
https://doi.org/10.1007/978-3-031-39001-2_7

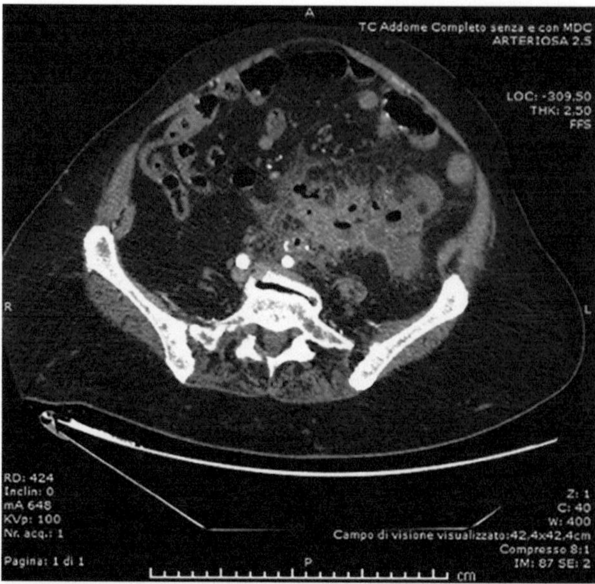

Fig. 1 A CT scan with contrast showing a large pelvic collections along the left paracolic gutter

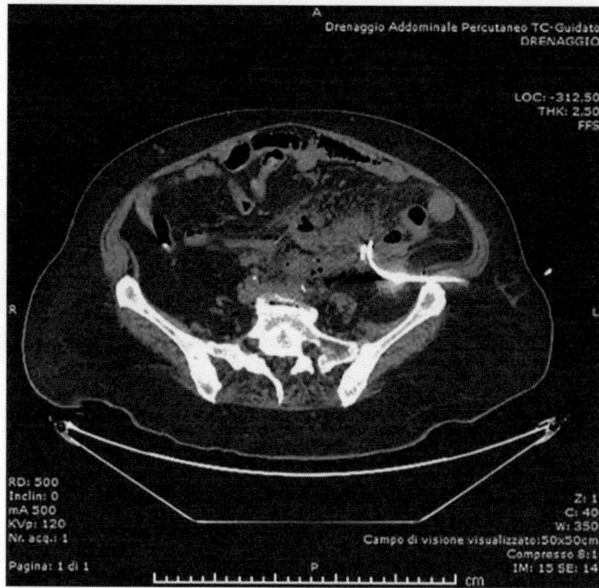

Fig. 2 The pericolic abscess treated with a percutaneous "pig-tail" drain

related to 3% of complications, mainly constituted by visceral injuries rather than vascular ones.

Furthermore, it has been established that 57% of patients develop a fistulous communication to the colon, subsequently to drain placement. Moreover, these patients had longer procedure times and larger abscess sizes. Conversely, female sex

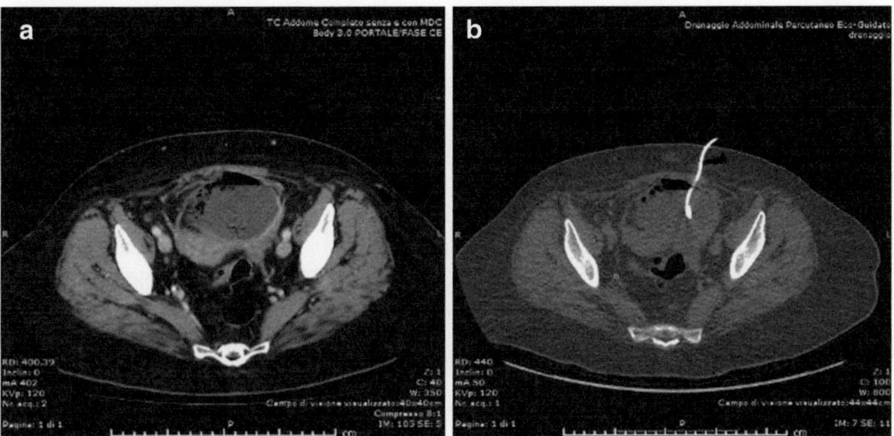

Fig. 3 A 10 cm pelvic abscess with an air level inside. (**a**, **b**) The abscess treated with a percutaneous drain. For the presence of enteric material from the drain and the worsening of the patient's clinical condition, a sigmoid resection was performed

and higher BMI may represent protective factors against the development of intestinal fistulous communications [5].

The more the diameter increases, the higher is the risk of failure to control source infection in the percutaneous draining [6]. The presence of significant comorbidities, ASA (American Society of Anesthesiologists) score 4, elevated values of Charlson Comorbidity Index, and immunosuppression state represent other factors of risk of PCD failure [7, 8].

The recurrence rate after percutaneous drainage is about 25% [3]. Also, in these cases, abscesses larger than 5 cm have an increased risk of recurrence [9].

Although the best treatment for larger abscesses is still not defined, we can assume that PCD must be almost always considered as the first choice in non-peritonitis patients. In fact, acute surgery is related to a high rate of postoperative complications, permanent stoma, and short-term mortality (up to 12%).

Surgery is mandatory in case of PCD failure, a patient's clinical worsening, and hemodynamical instability. A cutoff size of 5 cm is predictive for the need for emergency surgery within 30 days from the presentation (Fig. 3) [10].

In their retrospective study on 105 patients undergoing CT-guided abscess drainage, Raman et al. showed that 57% of patients presented a post-procedural fistula. An 85% required surgical intervention, 83% of them with minimally invasive surgery. Interestingly, they found that men's gender, lower BMIs, current tobacco users, higher ASA class, and larger abscess on initial presentation were related to fistulous communication [11].

In conclusion, PCD could be a valuable tool in patients with diverticular abscess without signs of peritonitis. However, it might not be resolutive in larger abscesses and clinically compromised cases. Therefore, if the procedure fails, surgery must be advocated.

2   Laparoscopic Peritoneal Lavage

It has been widely described that laparoscopic peritoneal lavage has represented a potentially viable option for patients with purulent diverticulitis. By itself, the procedure presents quite simple steps: placement of three ports, complete evacuation of the purulent collection, accurate visualization of the descending colon and sigma, execution of a hydropneumatic or methylene bleu test to rule out eventual visceral discontinuity, and finally putting some drains in situ. In the 1990s, several retrospective studies showed very promising results that started a "hot" debate about the efficacy of this procedure in the treatment of peritonitis due to acute perforated diverticulitis. The discussion is heavily still going on [12–14]. These first studies reported very low rates of morbidity (0–4%), mortality (<2%), reoperation (2–7%), and diverticulitis recurrence (0–5%) during 12- to 48-month follow-up. As a result, the conclusions were very optimistic: the laparoscopic peritoneal lavage was considered a safe and effective alternative to traditional surgical resection allowing to avoid elective colon resection in most cases [14]. However, during the second decade of this century, the scientific community raised a need to clarify the real benefit deriving from laparoscopic peritoneal lavage. Thus, three randomized studies from northern Europe were conducted: LADIEs, SCANDIV, and DILALA trials [15–17]. The first one in chronological order, the LADIEs with the LOLA arm, was prematurely interrupted because of an exceedingly high rate of complications in laparoscopic lavage [15]. The Scandinavian SCANDIV study reported a higher complication rate, short-term morbidity, and mortality in laparoscopic lavage, even though long-term follow-up showed no differences in severe complications [18]. Furthermore, the authors identified that recurrence of diverticulitis after laparoscopic lavage was more common (21% vs. 4%), often leading to sigmoid resection (30%). The authors agreed that a higher resection rate must be weighed against the lower stoma prevalence in laparoscopic lavage, encouraging to take "shared" decisions, considering both short-term and long-term consequences. On the other hand, the DILALA trial reported better results for laparoscopic lavage, identifying shorter operative time, and hospital stay with no differences in terms of morbidity and mortality [17]. At the 2-year follow-up, the laparoscopic lavage was associated with a 45% reduced risk of undergoing operations than Hartmann's. In the study by Kohl et al., the authors considered the laparoscopic lavage a *better* option for perforated diverticulitis with purulent peritonitis than open resection and colostomy [19]. However, an important criticism merging from the literature versus these encouraging results was represented by the very limited number of patients *per arm* enrolled in the DILALA: 39 in the lavage group and 36 in Hartmann's procedure [20]. A multicentric prospective international study was conducted in 2018: the LLO Study, which included 231 patients affected by purulent peritonitis caused by acute diverticulitis. Among 212 patients who underwent lavage, the postoperative morbidity rate was 33%, the mortality rate was 2%, and the readmission rate was 10%. Overall, the technique was successful in 172 patients (81%): there were no signs of sepsis and no need for further surgery during the hospital stay and 60 days after discharge.

Nevertheless, 46 episodes (26.7%) of acute diverticulitis were recorded during the 11-month follow-up [21].

Several meta-analyses have been performed with different results [22–33]. The difference in the results was due to the variability of the considered studies, the type of the analysis, and the focused outcomes analyzed. Some reviews concluded that laparoscopic lavage does not represent a safe approach for purulent diverticular peritonitis because of the high rate of reoperations (up to 30%), higher rate of post-operative intra-abdominal abscesses, and the relevant risk of not recognizing a carcinoma in almost 10% of patients [24, 25, 27, 29, 34, 35]. Other reviews gave more prudent conclusions, reporting that laparoscopic lavage can be comparable to sigmoid resection in terms of mortality. At the same time, it is related to a significantly higher rate of reoperations and intra-abdominal abscesses [23, 26, 33]. Conversely, other meta-analyses supported the use of laparoscopic lavage, stating that the procedure may be an effective and safe option for the treatment of patients with purulent diverticular peritonitis; in fact, the lavage is associated with a lower risk of reoperations within the first 12 months after index surgery, lower hospital costs, and comparable morbidity and mortality than resections [22, 30, 31].

An important point in favor of the laparoscopic lavage is the reduced risk of colostomy at 1- and 2-year follow-up, when the procedure is *effective* [19, 36]. Schultz et al. described a significantly lower stoma rate in the lavage group than resection (14% vs. 42%) at the 1-year follow-up of the SCANDIV study. However, the quality of life did not differ between groups, as laparoscopic lavage was associated with deeper surgical-site infections (32% vs.13%) and more unplanned reoperations (27% vs. 10%) [36]. Kohl et al., instead, reported better results in their 2-year results of the randomized clinical trial DILALA. The lavage group had a 45% reduced risk of undergoing one or more operations, fewer operation rates than Hartmann's group, and a more reduced stoma rate (7% vs. 23%). In addition, the authors did not find significant differences in the mean number of readmissions and mortality [19].

Very few studies focused on comparing laparoscopic peritoneal lavage versus laparoscopic sigmoidectomy in complicated acute diverticulitis. A multicentric study by Catry et al. enrolled 40 patients with purulent diverticular peritonitis and compared 15 laparoscopic peritoneal lavages versus 25 sigmoidectomies. In the latter group, only four were treated with a laparoscopic approach. 40% of laparoscopic lavage patients required reoperation for peritonitis (26.6%), intra-abdominal bleeding (13.3%), intra-abdominal abscess (7%), ileus (7%), and wound infections (7%). For these reasons, the authors concluded that laparoscopic lavage is associated with a high risk of failure in daily practice. Consequently, laparoscopic sigmoidectomy should be the primary option for treating purulent diverticular peritonitis [37]. In a multicenter study led by our Institution, 66 patients with a pelvic abscess not amenable to conservative management or with purulent diverticular peritonitis were enrolled: 28 (42%) underwent laparoscopic lavage and 38 (58%) underwent laparoscopic sigmoidectomy. The authors found that the failure to achieve source control and the need to return to the operating room were more frequent in laparoscopic lavage (29.6% vs. 2.6% and 18.5% vs. 0, respectively). Furthermore, diverticular recurrence was significantly higher in the lavage group (27.3% vs. 0%). As a result, the authors concluded that laparoscopic lavage for perforated diverticulitis carries a high risk of failure in daily practice [38].

Laparoscopic lavage is cheaper than colonic resection. In the Swedish DILALA trial, clinical effectiveness and resource use were derived from the 43 patients randomized in the laparoscopic lavage group and the remaining 40 treated with Hartmann's procedure. In the laparoscopic lavage group, the authors found a mean discount per patient of almost €9000 at the short-term analysis (first 12 months) and almost €19,794 at the long-term analysis. So far, they concluded that the significant cost reduction, the safeness, and the efficacy of laparoscopic lavage make the procedure eligible for a *routinary* use for the treatment of complicated diverticular peritonitis [39]. Quite similar results were obtained by Vennixet al. in their economic evaluation of the randomized LOLA (LaparOscopicLAvage) arm of the Ladies trial. They demonstrated that total medical costs for lavage were lower (almost €3500) at 12 months, although surgical interventions may increase costs. The same was for the long-term results, where lavage was associated with a reduced cost of almost €6377. It must be said that stoma reversal operations can also get costs increased in the Hartmann's procedure group. However, considering the failure in carrying on the LOLA arm in the LADIES study due to an unacceptable too much high rate of postoperative complications, the authors were more prudent in exalting the lavage.

The positions about laparoscopic lavage from the major international surgical societies' guidelines are very different. The recent guidelines from the World Society of Emergency Surgery state: *We suggest performing laparoscopic peritoneal lavage and drainage only in very selected patients with generalized peritonitis. It is not considered as the first line treatment in patients with peritonitis from acute colonic diverticulitis*, notwithstanding weak recommendation [40]. The European Association for Endoscopic Surgery (EAES) and Society of American Gastrointestinal and Endoscopic Surgeons (SAGES) guidelines on acute diverticulitis management recommend that: *Lavage should be considered in selected Hinchey III patients by surgeons with appropriate expertise and the ability to closely watch for and manage complications; the lower stoma rate should be weighed against the higher risk of complications and re-intervention.* Also, in this case, recommendations were weak [41]. Recently, the European Society of Coloproctology guidelines stated more straightforwardly: *Laparoscopic lavage is feasible in selected patients with Hinchey III peritonitis. Alternatively, resection is recommended* [42]. The 2020 American Society of Colon and Rectal Surgeons Guidelines for the management of left-sided colonic diverticulitis recommends colectomy for both feculent and purulent peritonitis, stating that *In patients with purulent peritonitis, colectomy is preferred over laparoscopic lavage. Laparoscopic lavage is associated with higher rates of secondary intervention in comparison with colectomy* [43]. Interestingly, the Japanese guidelines for diverticular disease management did neither consider the laparoscopic lavage [44].

Briefly, we could conclude that laparoscopic peritoneal lavage is feasible in patients with purulent diverticulitis. Still, it should be reserved only in very selected patients with satisfactory immunological competency, without comorbidities, and evident parietal discontinuities of the involved colonic tract.

3   Laparoscopic Sigmoidectomy

After 30 years from the first laparoscopic colectomy, this technique has progressively gained a prominent role in the surgical management of diverticular disease, mainly, thanks to reducing postoperative complications with equal effectiveness compared to the open approach. However, the evidence of the laparoscopic sigmoidectomy is well defined in elective settings. Conversely, its role in the context of complicated acute diverticulitis is still unclear and remains a topic of discussion.

A minimally invasive approach is associated with a lower rate of respiratory complications. The less postoperative pain allows a greater thoracic excursion and, consequently, improved alveolar ventilation. Furthermore, laparoscopy determines a lower intensive inflammatory response that facilitates regenerative processes, such as faster healing and lower ileus. All these factors lower the duration of hospitalization than open surgery [45–47].

Like in elective settings, it has been demonstrated that the laparoscopic colonic resection is associated with lower surgical and medical postoperative complications, also in complicated diverticulitis [48]. In a recent study by Lee et al., 3756 cases undergoing emergent sigmoidectomy for perforated diverticulitis were analyzed. Of them, 282 were laparoscopic-completed, 175 laparoscopic-converted-to-open, and 3299 open. They found that the laparoscopic-completed approach had significantly better outcomes than open and laparoscopic-converted cases. In the intention-to-treat analysis, the laparoscopic-completed approach had significantly fewer complications, less unplanned intubation, and acute renal failure than the open group. Furthermore, laparoscopic groups presented shorter hospital lengths of stay although with longer operating times. Interestingly, when comparing laparoscopic and open colonic resections, the laparoscopic group showed favorable outcomes. So far, the authors have promoted minimally invasive surgery in perforated diverticulitis, suggesting the need for randomized studies to define an optimal operative approach in patients requiring emergency surgery for diverticular perforation [48].

There is no doubt that laparoscopic resections must be considered when patient's clinical conditions are permissive (hemodynamical stability), and there is no severe and diffuse peritoneal contamination, such as Hinchey's IV fecal peritonitis [40, 49–51]. Abraha et al. conducted a meta-analysis from three randomized studies comparing open vs. laparoscopic colonic resections with an overall population of 392 patients. The authors showed no significant differences in mean hospitalization, 30-day mortality, surgical complications, early and late morbidity, major and minor complications, intraoperative blood loss, time for reintroducing liquid and solid diet, and recurrence of diverticulitis. On the other hand, the postoperative pain and the perceived quality of life in patients undergoing laparoscopic resection were significantly better than the open approach, albeit with a very low level of evidence.

However, important risks of attrition, detection, and performance bias were highlighted among studies, which were inhomogeneous in discriminating open and laparoscopic sigmoidectomies, both in the emergency and elective regimes. As a result, the authors were unable to support or reject the safety and efficacy of laparoscopic surgery over traditional surgery in acute diverticulitis [46]. Elgawki et al. highlighted the importance of a minimally invasive approach to the surgical management of acute diverticulitis, reporting the outcomes on 260 patients undergoing laparoscopic sigmoid colectomy in emergency. Hinchey's I diverticulitis (88%) was the most relevant percentage, while only 9% of the overall cohort of patients presented purulent peritonitis. The authors reported a very low rate of intraoperative complications (1%), constituted by anastomotic failure attributable to stapler defect, small bowel, and urinary bladder injuries. Furthermore, they identified a conversion rate of 6%, an anastomotic leak rate of 1.9%, overall 30-day morbidity of 3.8%, and 30-day mortality of 0.7%. Considering these encouraging results, the authors concluded that, in the hands of experienced surgeons, laparoscopic colonic resection for sigmoid diverticulitis might be considered the "gold-standard" treatment for patients with Hinchey's grades I–II. At the same time, for Hinchey III, further studies are necessary to prove its efficacy. However, no comparison was made. The study was limited to a simple cas series report [52]. Similarly, in their meta-analysis of 14 studies for a total population of 918 patients, Lin et al. supported the superiority of the laparoscopic approach over open surgery in acute complicated diverticulitis due to a reduction in morbidity and mortality [53].

A keypoint for a successful outcome of a laparoscopic sigmoidectomy is the surgeon's expertise and the high specialization of the hospital [54]. In a survey conducted by De Simone et al., it emerges that the therapeutic strategies of acute diverticulitis are often subordinated to the surgeon's experience. The authors suggest using the laparoscopic approach in Hinchey's grades 3 and 4 acute diverticulitis in hemodynamically stable patients, whereas adequate materials and personnel are present [55]. A laparoscopic resection requires more expensive equipment and longer operative time than the laparotomic approach [56]. However, a shorter hospital stay, reduced consumption of painkillers, and a faster return to normal activities may balance the overall costs between the two approaches. Klarenbeek et al. conducted an economic evaluation of the randomized control "SIGMAtrial," comparing elective laparoscopic sigmoid resection to open ones in patients with symptomatic diverticulitis, identifying a not statistically significant difference (total healthcare costs: 9969 euro vs. 9366 euro). Thus, the authors stated that, as clinical outcomes favored laparoscopic resection, elective sigmoidectomy should be preferably approached laparoscopically [57]. Unfortunately, no studies have been published about cost-effectiveness in emergency settings, where many other factors can influence the decision-making process, and healthcare costs might have limited importance.

Primary anastomosis with or without proximal diversion should be considered in the settings of an appropriate patient's physiology and tissue quality, as it is associated with reduced morbidity and mortality [58]. Several randomized studies have by now demonstrated that resection with primary anastomosis is a safe alternative to non-restorative colon resection in selected patients with purulent or fecal diverticular peritonitis [59–62]. In a retrospective study on 415 patients undergoing laparoscopic sigmoid resection without diversion, Dreifuss et al. identified 73 cases (20.8%) of perforated diverticulitis. In these settings, laparoscopic sigmoidectomy for perforated diverticulitis has morbidity, anastomotic leak, and mortality rates similar to elective ones [63]. Furthermore, recent evidence has shown that laparoscopic colonic resection may be more difficult in Hinchey grade II and III. The longer exposition to inflammation may determine a more edematous, friable, and thicker mesentery rather than Hinchey grade IV. In a recent study by Pellinoet al., it has been described that laparoscopic sigmoidectomy could be easier than open surgery also in hemodynamically stable patients suffering from Hinchey grade 3 and 4 diverticulitis, when performed by expert surgeons. Interestingly, the authors report a recanalization rate of 88% in patients undergoing laparoscopic Hartmann's compared to 62% of patients undergoing traditional surgery, probably due to the lower presence of adhesions and easier execution of the operation. Consequently, the authors stated that colonic resection with primary laparoscopic anastomosis in perforated diverticulitis is technically feasible in hemodynamically stable patients. However, patient selection and additional factors, including surgeon expertise and hospital resources, are crucial and require careful consideration [47].

If the primary anastomosis is unsafe for the treatment of complicated diverticulitis, a laparoscopic Hartmann's procedure has been described [64]. Agaba et al. reported seven patients with an average operative time of 154 min and an average length of stay of 6 days. All patients were reversed approximately 2–3 months later through a laparoscopic approach [65]. Although little has been published, some studies have compared laparoscopic and open approaches for the reversal of the Hartmann's procedure [66]. Overall, these small series support laparoscopy during Hartmann's reversal to be technically feasible and safe with outcomes like those seen with open surgery. In a multicenter retrospective study on 2937 patients with diverticular perforation undergoing emergent sigmoid colon resection with a colostomy, Moghadamyeghaneh et al. identified a rate of minimally invasive surgery of 11.4% with a 38.6% conversion rate to open. Interestingly, the authors demonstrated that the open approach to sigmoidectomy was associated with higher morbidity compared to the laparoscopic approach (67.2% vs. 56.8%), although no significant differences in risk of reoperation (8.5% vs. 3.9%) or intra-abdominal abscess (11.6% vs. 10.2%). Furthermore, patients who had an open Hartmann's procedure presented significantly higher respiratory complications and unplanned intubations rates, with longer hospitalization length than the mini-invasive approach. Even though important limitations, the authors were able to conclude that a mini-invasive approach to emergent Hartmann's procedure for perforated diverticulitis is feasible and is associated with decreased morbidity and hospitalization length [45].

Although the literature seems to be favorable to laparoscopic surgery also in the emergency settings, we should be aware of the important limits of the considered studies, mainly deriving from patients' selection bias, the absence of a clinical stratification of the acute diverticulitis, the small number of population-based registries analyzed, and the frequent retrospective nature. In most cases, laparoscopic groups included elective sigmoidectomy with patients who are undoubtedly more fit for surgery than the open group. Only in 2018, it has been launched a multicentric randomized study called "LaCeS feasibility trial" (Laparoscopic versus Open Colorectal Surgery in the Acute Setting) from England; the first one aimed to assess the feasibility, safety, and acceptability of performing a large-scale definitive phase III randomized controlled trial with a comparison of emergency laparoscopic with open surgery for acute colorectal pathology [67].

In conclusion, even though the laparoscopic sigmoidectomy for acute complicated diverticulitis is technically feasible in stable hemodynamic patients with adequate clinical reserves, this procedure should be preferably performed by experienced surgeons in specialized centers. Furthermore, a primary anastomosis could be considered if the patient's conditions allow it.

4 Robotic Colonic Resection

The mini-invasive treatment of diverticulitis could be arduous due to the chronically inflamed tissues, distorted anatomic planes, and increased tendency to bleeding, which increases the risk of injury on other organs. In these difficult conditions, the disadvantages of laparoscopy are represented by lower ergonomics in confined spaces, rigid instrumentation, decreased freedom of motion, tremor effect, 2-D visualization, and reduced depth perception. These factors may limit a proper dissection and, consequently, its use. The robotic approach has several advantages and disadvantages than the conventional laparoscopy [68, 69] (Table 1).

The robotic technique has constantly been gaining popularity in colorectal surgery. Unfortunately, only a few studies focusing on robotic colonic resection in patients with diverticulitis have been published.

Robotic surgery can be safe and feasible for noncomplicated and complicated diverticulitis. XIa et al. compared robotic-assisted surgery for complicated and noncomplicated diverticulitis: they demonstrated that the complicated group was

Table 1 Advantages and disadvantages of the robotic surgery

Advantages	Disadvantages
1. Surgeon-controlled camera and stable camera platform	1. Reduced haptic feedback
2. High definition and 3D vision with tenfold magnification	2. Use of larger ports
3. Conversion of surgeon's coarse movements to accurate movements of the robot	3. Greater number of ports
4. Filter to eliminate tremor	4. Repeating the docking
5. Improved strength of action	5. Costs
6. Articulating instruments improving maneuverability and facilitate fine dissection	
7. Extended length of instrumentation (helpful in obese patients and close pelvis)	
8. A third operating arm controlled by the surgeon	
9. Improved operative comfort with more ergonomic position of the surgeon	

related to a higher conversion rate (3.1% vs. 22.2%), a longer mean operative time (171 min vs. 196 min), and a higher ostomy rate (9.4% vs. 33.3%). Instead, no significant differences were identified regarding estimated blood loss, length of postoperative stay, complication rate, time to return normal bowel function, and readmission rate [68].

Among studies comparing robotic and laparoscopic colectomy for diverticulitis, data are very heterogeneous, mainly in conversion rate, complications rate, length of postoperative stay, and operative time. Al-Temimi et al. compared robotic and laparoscopic elective colectomy for diverticulitis in a multivariate analysis [70]. They observed that the robotic approach was associated with a better overall morbidity, shortened length of stay, and lower conversion rate. Instead, the operation time resulted longer. These findings were similar in other reports [71–74].

A longer operative time associated with robotic surgery probably has multifactorial reasons. The most important one may be represented by the limited experience of the attending surgeons. It has been demonstrated that the presence of a dedicated team is associated with decreased operative times [71, 72, 75, 76]. Another important aspect that must be considered is the type of the used robot. Most of the studies show results referring to the *Da Vinci Si*, the oldest one. With the new version, the *Da Vinci Xi*, many limits have been overcome. The *Da Vinci Xi* is enriched with the Integrated Table Motion®: this device allows to change the patient positioning during the different phases of the procedure without moving the robotic trocars. So far, it could be possible to perform the splenic flexure takedown without recurring to the "hybrid" "technique or redocking. That requires undoubtedly less time [75, 77].

As far as the conversion rate is concerned, the literature gives us opposite results. Beltzer et al. compared robotic ($n = 60$) and laparoscopic ($n = 46$) sigmoid resections for uncomplicated, complicated, or recurrent diverticular disease. The authors did not find significant differences in terms of operative time (130 versus 118 min), anastomotic leakage (6.7% versus 6.5%), need for a stoma (6.7% versus 4.3%), conversion (1.7% versus 0%), reoperation (8.3% versus 15.2%), overall complications (30.0% versus 30.4%), and mortality (1.7% versus 0%) rates [76]. Conversely, Al-Temimi et al. and Maciel et al. identified lower conversion rates: 7.5% vs. 14.3% and 0 vs.14.55%, respectively [70, 73, 74]. On the contrary, Elliott et al. and Ogilvie JW et al. found lower conversion rates for the laparoscopic resections than robotic ones [71, 78].

There is no clear superiority from robotic surgery over laparoscopy regarding morbidity and major complication rates. In their small cohort of patients, Elliott et al. found that robotic resection for colonic diverticulitis with fistula had operative time, complication, and readmission rates very similar to laparoscopy [78]. Comparably, in a matched cohort of elective sigmoid resection for diverticular diseases, Ogilvie et al. had demonstrated that laparoscopic and robotic-assisted surgery resulted in a clinically equivalent return to bowel function, length of stay, postoperative pain, and morbidity [71]. Cassini et al. analyzed 156 consecutive patients with a history of complicated diverticulitis undergoing elective mini-invasive colonic resections: 92 fully laparoscopic (FL) and 64 robotic hybrid approaches (RHA). They found that overall postoperative morbidity and major postoperative morbidity rates were higher in FL (21.6% vs. 12.3% and 13% vs. 4.6%, respectively). Interestingly, no significant differences were recognized in mean operative time, mean intraoperative blood loss, mean hospital stay, and mortality. Conversely, the surgeon's compliance was notably increased in the robotic arm [79]. In a retrospective propensity score-matched analysis on a multicentric database performed by Raskin et al., more than 12,000 sigmoidectomies, split in 9.9% robotic, 28.9% open, and 61.2% laparoscopic approaches, were analyzed. The authors found that robotic surgery was associated with significantly lower postoperative complication rates and postoperative ileus than the LS group. However, no other significant differences were identified between robotic and laparoscopic groups [72]. The postoperative length of hospital stay (LOS) is closely related to the conversion and complication rates. In this case, the results are extremely heterogeneous [80].

Robotic colorectal surgery is related to increased costs compared to laparoscopy. The very high cost of the robotic equipment, its maintenance, and each upgrade/addition undoubtedly represents the main obstacle to the full spread of the robotic technique. Furthermore, the presence of a single globally employed company in the field of robotic surgery might determine a barrier to the decrease in costs. Probably, increased competition among companies will be able to reduce overall costs. Some authors have speculated that a shorter hospital stay, a lower complication rate, and a reduced need for intensive care unit support associated with the robotic surgery may limit the expensiveness of the robot. However, that must still be demonstrated [70, 74, 81]. More recent studies have shown similar costs between total hospitalization of robotic colorectal surgery compared with laparoscopy [82].

In short, robotic colonic resection is feasible and safe in the elective management of diverticular disease and is related to similar short-term outcomes compared with laparoscopic technique. However, additional studies are needed to evaluate the role of robotic surgery over laparoscopic surgery for the management of left-sided diverticulitis, mainly in the context of emergency.

References

1. Wasvary H, Turfah F, Kadro O, Beauregard W. Same hospitalization resection for acute diverticulitis. Am Surg. 1999;65(7):632–6.
2. Benoist S, et al. Can failure of percutaneous drainage of postoperative abdominal abscess be predicted? Am J Surg. 2002;184:148–53.
3. Gregersen R, et al. Treatment of patients with acute colonic diverticulitis complicated by abscess formation: a systematic review. Int J Surg. 2016;35:201.
4. Hall J, Hardiman K, Lee S, et al. The American Society of Colon and Rectal Surgeons clinical practice guidelines for the treatment of left-sided colonic diverticulitis. Dis Colon Rectum. 2020;63(6):728–47.
5. Raman S, Gorvet M, Lange K, et al. Outcomes after CT guided drainage of diverticular abscesses and predictive factors for fistulous communication to the colon. Am J Surg. 2021;222(1):193–7. https://doi.org/10.1016/j.amjsurg.2020.10.010.
6. Elagili F, Stocchi L, Ozuner G, Kiran RP. Antibiotics alone instead of percutaneous drainage as initial treatment of large diverticular abscess. Tech Coloproctol. 2015;19(2):97–103.
7. Stabile BE, Puccio E, van Sonnenberg E, Neff CC. Preoperative percutaneous drainage of diverticular abscesses. Am J Surg. 1990;159(1):99–104.

8. Felder SI, Barmparas G, Lynn J, Murrell Z, Margulies DR, Fleshner P. Can the need for colectomy after computed tomography-guided percutaneous drainage for diverticular abscess be predicted? Am Surg. 2013;79(10):1013–6.

9. Gaertner WB, Willis DJ, Madoff RD, Rothenberger DA, Kwaan MR, Belzer GE, et al. Percutaneous drainage of colonic diverticular abscess: is colon resection necessary? Dis Colon Rectum. 2013;56(5):622–6.

10. Lambrichts DPV, Bolkenstein HE, van der Does DCHE, et al. Multicentre study of non-surgical management of diverticulitis with abscess formation. Br J Surg. 2019;106:458–66. https://doi.org/10.1002/bjs.11129.

11. Raman S, Gorvet M, Lange K, Rettenmaier N. Outcomes after CT guided drainage of diverticular abscesses and predictive factors for fistulous communication to the colon. Am J Surg. 2020;222:193.

12. O'Sullivan GC, Murphy D, O'Brien MG, Ireland A. Laparoscopic management of generalized peritonitis due to perforated colonic diverticula. Am J Surg. 1996;171(4):432–4.

13. Myers E, Hurley M, O'Sullivan GC, et al. Laparoscopic peritoneal lavage for generalized peritonitis due to perforated diverticulitis. Br J Surg. 2008;95(1):97–101.

14. Sorrentino M, Brizzolari M, Scarpa E, Malisan D, Bruschi F, Bertozzi S, Bernardi S, Petri R. Laparoscopic peritoneal lavage for perforated colonic diverticulitis: a definitive treatment? Retrospective analysis of 63 cases. Tech Coloproctol. 2015;19(2):105–10. https://doi.org/10.1007/s10151-014-1258-1. Epub 2014 Dec 31. PMID: 25550116.

15. Vennix S, Musters GD, Mulder IM, et al. Laparoscopic peritoneal lavage or sigmoidectomy for perforated diverticulitis with purulent peritonitis: a multicentre, parallel-group, randomized open-label trial. Lancet. 2015;386(10000):1269–77.

16. Schultz JK, Yaqub S, Wallon C, et al. Laparoscopic lavage vs primary resection for acute perforated diverticulitis: the SCANDIV randomized clinical trial. JAMA. 2015;314(13):1364–75.

17. Angenete E, Thornell A, Burcharth J, et al. Laparoscopic lavage is feasible and safe for the treatment of perforated diverticulitis with purulent peritonitis: the first results from the randomized controlled trial DILALA. Ann Surg. 2016;263(1):117–22.

18. Azhar N, Johanssen A, Sundström T, Folkesson J, Wallon C, Kørner H, Blecic L, Forsmo HM, Øresland T, Yaqub S, Buchwald P, Schultz JK, SCANDIV Study Group. Laparoscopic lavage vs primary resection for acute perforated diverticulitis: long-term outcomes from the Scandinavian diverticulitis (SCANDIV) randomized clinical trial. JAMA Surg. 2021;156(2):121–7. https://doi.org/10.1001/jamasurg.2020.5618. PMID: 33355658; PMCID: PMC7758831.

19. Kohl A, Rosenberg J, Bock D, Bisgaard T, Skullman S, Thornell A, Gehrman J, Angenete E, Haglind E. Two-year results of the randomized clinical trial DILALA comparing laparoscopic lavage with resection as treatment for perforated diverticulitis. Br J Surg. 2018;105(9):1128–34. https://doi.org/10.1002/bjs.10839. Epub 2018 Apr 16. PMID: 29663316; PMCID: PMC6055876.

20. Guimarães M, Barbosa L. Safety and effectiveness of laparoscopic peritoneal lavage in Hinchey III diverticulitis. J Coloproctol. 2020;40(3):300–8.

21. Binda GA, Bonino MA, Siri G, Di Saverio S, Rossi G, Nascimbeni R, et al. Multicentre international trial oflaparoscopic lavage for Hinchey III acute diverticulitis (LLOStudy). Br J Surg. 2018;105:1835–43.

22. Angenete E, Bock D, Rosenberg J, Haglind E. Laparoscopic lavage is superior to colon resection for perforated purulent diverticulitis—a meta-analysis. Int J Color Dis. 2017;32:163–9.

23. Ceresoli M, Coccolini F, Montori G, Catena F, Sartelli M, Ansaloni L. Laparoscopic lavage versus resection in perforated diverticulitis with purulent peritonitis: a meta-analysis of randomized controlled trials. World J Emerg Surg. 2016;11:42.

24. Gervaz P, Ambrosetti P. Critical appraisal of laparoscopic lavage for Hinchey III diverticulitis. World J Gastrointest Surg. 2016;8(5):371–5.

25. Cirocchi R, Di Saverio S, Weber DG, et al. Laparoscopic lavage versus surgical resection for acute diverticulitis with generalised peritonitis: a systematic review and meta-analysis. Tech Coloproctol. 2017;21:93–110.

26. Daher R, Barouki E, Chouillard E. Laparoscopic treatment of complicated colonic diverticular disease: a review. World J Gastrointest Surg. 2016;8(2):134–42.
27. Galbraith N, Carter JV, Netz U, et al. Laparoscopic lavage in the management of perforated diverticulitis: a contemporary meta-analysis. J Gastrointest Surg. 2017;21:1491–9.
28. Marshall JR, Buchwald PL, Gandhi J, et al. Laparoscopic lavage in the management of Hinchey grade III diverticulitis: a systematic review. Ann Surg. 2017;265:670–6.
29. Penna M, Markar SR, Mackenzie H, Hompes R, Cunningham C. Laparoscopic lavage versus primary resection for acute perforated diverticulitis: review and metanalysis. Ann Surg. 2018;267:252–8.
30. Cirocchi R, Trastulli S, Vettoretto N, Milani D, Cavaliere D, Renzi C, Adamenko O, Desiderio J, Burattini MF, Parisi A, Arezzo A, Fingerhut A. Laparoscopic peritoneal lavage. Medicine. 2015;94(1):e334.
31. Shaikh FM, Stewart PM, Walsh SR, Davies RJ. Laparoscopic peritoneal lavage or surgical resection for acute perforated sigmoid diverticulitis: a systematic review and meta-analysis. Int J Surg. 2017;38:130–7.
32. Acuna SA, Wood T, Chesney TR, et al. Operative strategies for perforated diverticulitis: a systematic review and meta-analysis. Dis Colon Rectum. 2018;61:1442–53.
33. Schmidt S, Ismail T, Puhan MA, Soll C, Breitenstein S. Meta-analysis of surgical strategies in perforated left colonic diverticulitis with generalized peritonitis. Langenbecks Arch Surg. 2018;403:425–33.
34. Acuna S, Wood T, Chesney T, Dossa F, Wexner SD, Quereshy FA, Chadi SA, Baxter NN. Operative strategies for perforated diverticulitis. Dis Colon Rectum. 2018;61(12):1442–53.
35. Marshall J, Buchwald P, Gandhi J, Schultz JK, Hider PN, Frizelle FA, Eglinton TW. Laparoscopic lavage in the management of Hinchey grade III diverticulitis. Ann Surg. 2017;265(4):670–6.
36. Schultz JK, Wallon C, Blecic L, et al. One-year results of the SCANDIV randomized clinical trial of laparoscopic lavage versus primary resection for acute perforated diverticulitis. Br J Surg. 2017;104:1382–92.
37. Catry J, Brouquet A, Peschaud F, et al. Sigmoid resectionwith primary anastomosis and ileostomy versus laparoscopic lavagein purulent peritonitis from perforated diverticulitis: outcome analysisin a prospective cohort of 40 consecutive patients. Int J Color Dis. 2016;31(10):1693–9.
38. Tartaglia D, Di Saverio S, Stupalkowska W, Giannessi S, Robustelli V, Coccolini F, Ioannidis O, Nita GE, Muñoz-Cruzado VMD, Ciuró FP, Chiarugi M. Laparoscopic peritoneal lavage versus laparoscopic sigmoidectomy in complicated acute diverticulitis: a multicenter prospective observational study. Int J Color Dis. 2019;34(12):2111–20.
39. Gehrman J, Angenete E, Björholt I, Bock D, Rosenberg J, Haglind E. Health economic analysis of laparoscopic lavage versus Hartmann's procedure for diverticulitis in the randomized DILALA trial. Br J Surg. 2016;103(11):1539–47. https://doi.org/10.1002/bjs.10230.
40. Sartelli M, Weber DG, Kluger Y, Ansaloni L, Coccolini F, Abu-Zidan F, Augustin G, Ben-Ishay O, Biffl WL, Bouliaris K, Catena R, Ceresoli M, Chiara O, Chiarugi M, Coimbra R, Cortese F, Cui Y, Damaskos D, De'Angelis GL, Delibegovic S, Demetrashvili Z, De Simone B, Di Marzo F, Di Saverio S, Duane TM, Faro MP, Fraga GP, Gkiokas G, Gomes CA, Hardcastle TC, Hecker A, Karamarkovic A, Kashuk J, Khokha V, Kirkpatrick AW, Kok KYY, Inaba K, Isik A, Labricciosa FM, Latifi R, Leppäniemi A, Litvin A, Mazuski JE, Maier RV, Marwah S, McFarlane M, Moore EE, Moore FA, Negoi I, Pagani L, Rasa K, Rubio-Perez I, Sakakushev B, Sato N, Sganga G, Siquini W, Tarasconi A, Tolonen M, Ulrych J, Zachariah SK, Catena F. 2020 update of the WSES guidelines for the management of acute colonic diverticulitis in the emergency setting. World J Emerg Surg. 2020;15(1):32. https://doi.org/10.1186/s13017-020-00313-4.
41. Francis NK, Sylla P, Abou-Khalil M, Arolfo S, Berler D, Curtis NJ, Dolejs SC, Garfinkle R, Gorter-Stam M, Hashimoto DA, Hassinger TE, Molenaar CJL, Pucher PH, Schuermans V, Arezzo A, Agresta F, Antoniou SA, Arulampalam T, Boutros M, Bouvy N, Campbell K, Francone T, Haggerty SP, Hedrick TL, Stefanidis D, Truitt MS, Kelly J, Ket H, Dunkin BJ, Pietrabissa A. EAES and SAGES 2018 consensus conference on acute diverticulitis management: evidence-based recommendations for clinical practice. Surg Endosc. 2019;33(9):2726–41. https://doi.org/10.1007/s00464-019-06882-z.

42. Schultz JK, Azhar N, Binda GA, Barbara G, Biondo S, Boermeester MA, Chabok A, Consten ECJ, van Dijk ST, Johanssen A, Kruis W, Lambrichts D, Post S, Ris F, Rockall TA, Samuelsson A, Di Saverio S, Tartaglia D, Thorisson A, Winter DC, Bemelman W, Angenete E. European Society of Coloproctology: guidelines for the management of diverticular disease of the colon. Color Dis. 2020;22(Suppl 2):5–28. https://doi.org/10.1111/codi.15140.

43. Hall J, Hardiman K, Lee S, Lightner A, Stocchi L, Paquette IM, Steele SR, Feingold DL, Prepared on behalf of the Clinical Practice Guidelines Committee of the American Society of Colon and Rectal Surgeons. The American Society of Colon and Rectal Surgeons clinical practice guidelines for the treatment of left-sided colonic diverticulitis. Dis Colon Rectum. 2020;63(6):728–47.

44. Nagata N, Ishii N, Manabe N, Tomizawa K, Urita Y, Funabiki T, Fujimori S, Kaise M. Guidelines for colonic diverticular bleeding and colonic diverticulitis: Japan Gastroenterological Association. Digestion. 2019;99(Suppl 1):1–26. https://doi.org/10.1159/000495282. Epub 2019 Jan 9. PMID: 30625484.

45. Moghadamyeghaneh Z, Talus H, Fitzgerald S, Muthusamy M, Stamos MJ, Roudnitsky V. Outcomes of minimally invasive colectomy for perforated diverticulitis. Am Surg. 2021;87(4):561–7. https://doi.org/10.1177/0003134820950295. Epub ahead of print. PMID: 33118383.

46. Abraha I, Binda GA, Montedori A, Arezzo A, Cirocchi R. Laparoscopic versus open resection for sigmoid diverticulitis. Cochrane Database Syst Rev. 2017;11(11):CD009277. Published 2017 Nov 25. https://doi.org/10.1002/14651858.CD009277.pub2.

47. Pellino G, Podda M, Wheeler J, Davies J, Di Saverio S. Laparoscopy and resection with primary anastomosis for perforated diverticulitis: challenging old dogmas. Updates Surg. 2020;72(1):21–8. https://doi.org/10.1007/s13304-020-00708-7. Epub 2020 Jan 28. PMID: 31993993.

48. Klarenbeek BR, Veenhof AA, Bergamaschi R, van der Peet DL, van den Broek WT, de Lange ES, Bemelman WA, Heres P, Lacy AM, Engel AF, Cuesta MA. Laparoscopic sigmoid resection for diverticulitis decreases major morbidity rates: a randomized control trial: short-term results of the Sigma trial. Ann Surg. 2009;249:39–44.

49. Lee YF, Brown RF, Battaglia M, Cleary RK. Laparoscopic versus open emergent sigmoid resection for perforated diverticulitis. J Gastrointest Surg. 2020;24(5):1173–82. https://doi.org/10.1007/s11605-019-04490-9. Epub 2019 Dec 16. PMID: 31845141.

50. Kockerling F, Schneider C, Reymond MA, et al. Laparoscopic resection of sigmoid diverticulitis: results of a multicenter study. Laparoscopic Colorectal Surgery Study Group. Surg Endosc. 1999;13:567–71.

51. Trebuchet G, Lechaux D, Lecalve JL. Laparoscopic left colon resection for diverticular disease: results from 170 consecutive cases. Surg Endosc. 2002;16:18–21.

52. El ZarrokElgazwi K, Baca I, Grzybowski L, Jaacks A. Laparoscopic sigmoidectomy for diverticulitis: a prospective study. JSLS. 2010;14(4):469–75. https://doi.org/10.4293/108680810X12924466008088. PMID: 21605507; PMCID: PMC3083034.

53. Lin H, Zhuang Z, Huang X, Li Y. The role of emergency laparoscopic surgery for complicated diverticular disease: a systematic review and meta-analysis. Medicine (Baltimore). 2020;99(40):e22421. https://doi.org/10.1097/MD.0000000000022421.

54. Nascimbeni R, Amato A, Cirocchi R, Serventi A, Laghi A, Bellini M, Tellan G, Zago M, Scarpignato C, Binda GA. Management of perforated diverticulitis with generalized peritonitis. A multidisciplinary review and position paper. Tech Coloproctol. 2021;25(2):153–65. https://doi.org/10.1007/s10151-020-02346-y. Epub 2020 Nov 5. PMID: 33155148; PMCID: PMC7884367.

55. De Simone B, Chouillard E, Sartelli M, Ansaloni L, Di Saverio S, Chiara O, Coccolini F, Marini P, IPOD Survey Collaborative Group, Catena F. Current management of acute left colon diverticulitis: what have Italian surgeons learned after the IPOD study? Updates Surg. 2021;73(1):139–48. https://doi.org/10.1007/s13304-020-00891-7. Epub 2020 Oct 3. PMID: 33010025.

56. National Guideline Centre (UK). Evidence review for laparoscopic versus open sigmoid resection for acute diverticulitis: diverticular disease: diagnosis and management: evidence review. London: National Institute for Health and Care Excellence (UK); 2019. PMID: 32525635. Excellence (UK).

57. Klarenbeek BR, Coupé VM, van der Peet DL, Cuesta MA. The cost effectiveness of elective laparoscopic sigmoid resection for symptomatic diverticular disease: financial outcome of the randomized control Sigma trial. Surg Endosc. 2011;25(3):776–83.

58. Constantinides VA, et al. Primary resection with anastomosis vs. Hartmann's procedure in nonelective surgery for acute colonic diverticulitis: a systematic review. Dis Colon Rectum. 2006;49(7):966–81.

59. Oberkofler CE, Rickenbacher A, Raptis DA, Lehmann K, Villiger P, Buchli C, Grieder F, Gelpke H, Decurtins M, Tempia-Caliera AA, Demartines N, Hahnloser D, Clavien PA, Breitenstein S. A multicenter randomized clinical trial of primary anastomosis or Hartmann's procedure for perforated left colonic diverticulitis with purulent or fecal peritonitis. Ann Surg. 2012;256:819–26.

60. Binda GA, Karas JR, Serventi A, Sokmen S, Amato A, Hydo L, Bergamaschi R, Study Group on Diverticulitis. Primary anastomosis vs nonrestorative resection for perforated diverticulitis with peritonitis: a prematurely terminated randomized controlled trial. Color Dis. 2012;14:1403–10.

61. Bridoux V, Regimbeau JM, Ouaissi M, Mathonnet M, Mauvais F, Houivet E, Schwarz L, Mege D, Sielezneff I, Sabbagh C, Tuech JJ. Hartmann's procedure or primary anastomosis for generalized peritonitis due to perforated diverticulitis: a prospective multicenter randomized trial (DIVERTI). J Am Coll Surg. 2017;225:798–805.

62. Lambrichts DPV, Vennix S, Musters GD, Mulder IM, Swank HA, Hoofwijk AGM, Belgers EHJ, Stockmann HBAC, Eijsbouts QAJ, Gerhards MF, van Wagensveld BA, van Geloven AAW, Crolla RMPH, Nienhuijs SW, Govaert MJPM, di Saverio S, D'Hoore AJL, Consten ECJ, van Grevenstein WMU, Pierik REGJM, Kruyt PM, van der Hoeven JAB, Steup WH, Catena F, Konsten JLM, Vermeulen J, van Dieren S, Bemelman WA, Lange JF, LADIES Trial Collaborators. Hartmann's procedure versus sigmoidectomy with primary anastomosis for perforated diverticulitis with purulent or faecal peritonitis (LADIES): a multicentre, parallel-group, randomised, open-label, superiority trial. Lancet Gastroenterol Hepatol. 2019;4(8):599–610. https://doi.org/10.1016/S2468-1253(19)30174-8.

63. Dreifuss NH, Schlottmann F, Piatti JM, Bun ME, Rotholtz NA. Safety and feasibility of laparoscopic sigmoid resection without diversion in perforated diverticulitis. Surg Endosc. 2020;34(3):1336–42.

64. Lipman JM, Reynolds HL. Laparoscopic management of diverticular disease. Clin Colon Rectal Surg. 2009;22:173–80.

65. Agaba EA, Zaidi RM, Ramzy P, Aftab M, Rubach E, Gecelter G, Ravikumar TS, DeNoto G. Laparoscopic Hartmann's procedure: a viable option for treatment of acutely perforated diverticultis. Surg Endosc. 2009;23:1483–6.

66. Mazeh H, Greenstein AJ, Swedish K, Nguyen SQ, Lipskar A, Weber KJ, Chin EH, Divino CM. Laparoscopic and open reversal of Hartmann's procedure–a comparative retrospective analysis. Surg Endosc. 2009;23:496–502.

67. Harji D, Marshall H, Gordon K, Crow H, Hiley V, Burke D, Griffiths B, Moriarty C, Twiddy M, O'Dwyer JL, Verjee A, Brown J, Sagar P. Feasibility of a multicentre, randomised controlled trial of laparoscopic versus open colorectal surgery in the acute setting: the LaCeS feasibility trial protocol. BMJ Open. 2018;8(2):e018618.

68. Xia J, Paul Olson TJ, Rosen SA. Robotic-assisted surgery for complicated and non-complicated diverticulitis: a single-surgeon case series. J Robot Surg. 2019;13(6):765–72. https://doi.org/10.1007/s11701-018-00914-x.

69. Ragupathi M, Ramos-Valadez DI, Patel CB, Haas EM. Robotic-assisted laparoscopic surgery for recurrent diverticulitis: experience in consecutive cases and a review of the literature. Surg Endosc. 2011;25(1):199–206. https://doi.org/10.1007/s00464-010-1159-y.

70. Al-Temimi MH, Chandrasekaran B, Agapian J, Peters WR Jr, Wells KO. Robotic versus laparoscopic elective colectomy for left side diverticulitis: a propensity score-matched analysis of the NSQIP database. Int J Color Dis. 2019;34(8):1385–92. https://doi.org/10.1007/s00384-019-03334-x.

71. Ogilvie JW Jr, Saunders RN, Parker J, Luchtefeld MA. Sigmoidectomy for diverticulitis—a propensity-matched comparison of minimally invasive approaches. J Surg Res. 2019;243:434–9. https://doi.org/10.1016/j.jss.2019.06.018.

72. Raskin ER, Keller DS, Gorrepati ML, Akiel-Fu S, Mehendale S, Cleary RK. Propensity-matched analysis of sigmoidectomies for diverticular disease. JSLS. 2019;23(1):e2018.00073. https://doi.org/10.4293/JSLS.2018.00073.

73. Maciel V, Lujan HJ, Plasencia G, et al. Diverticular disease complicated with colovesical fistula: laparoscopic versus robotic management. Int Surg. 2014;99(3):203–10. https://doi.org/10.9738/INTSURG-D-13-00201.1.

74. Madiedo A, Hall J. Minimally invasive management of diverticular disease. Clin Colon Rectal Surg. 2021;34(2):113–20. https://doi.org/10.1055/s-0040-1716703.

75. Bilgin IA, Bas M, Benlice C, et al. Totally laparoscopic and totally robotic surgery in patients with left-sided colonic diverticulitis. Int J Med Robot. 2020;16(1):e2068. https://doi.org/10.1002/rcs.2068.

76. Beltzer C, Knoerzer L, Bachmann R, Axt S, Dippel H, Schmidt R. Robotic versus laparoscopic sigmoid resection for diverticular disease: a single-center experience of 106 cases. J Laparoendosc Adv Surg Tech A. 2019;29(11):1451–5. https://doi.org/10.1089/lap.2019.0451.

77. Bianchini M, Palmeri M, Stefanini G, Furbetta N, Di Franco G. The role of robotic-assisted surgery for the treatment of diverticular disease. J Robot Surg. 2020;14(1):239–40. https://doi.org/10.1007/s11701-019-01008-y.

78. Elliott PA, McLemore EC, Abbass MA, Abbas MA. Robotic versus laparoscopic resection for sigmoid diverticulitis with fistula. J Robot Surg. 2015;9(2):137–42. https://doi.org/10.1007/s11701-015-0503-6.

79. Cassini D, Depalma N, Grieco M, Cirocchi R, Manoochehri F, Baldazzi G. Robotic pelvic dissection as surgical treatment of complicated diverticulitis in elective settings: a comparative study with fully laparoscopic procedure. Surg Endosc. 2019;33(8):2583–90. https://doi.org/10.1007/s00464-018-6553-x.

80. Bastawrous AL, Landmann RG, Liu Y, Liu E, Cleary RK. Incidence, associated risk factors, and impact of conversion to laparotomy in elective minimally invasive sigmoidectomy for diverticular disease. Surg Endosc. 2020;34(2):598–609. https://doi.org/10.1007/s00464-019-06804-z.

81. Wunker C, Montenegro G. Use of robotic technology in the management of complex colorectal pathology. Mo Med. 2020;117(2):149–53.

82. Vasudevan V, Reusche R, Wallace H, Kaza S. Clinical outcomes and cost-benefit analysis comparing laparoscopic and robotic colorectal surgeries. Surg Endosc. 2016;30(12):5490–3. https://doi.org/10.1007/s00464-016-4910-1.

Complicated Inflammatory Bowel Disease and Colonic Non-diverticular Emergencies

Francesco Maria Carrano, Antonino Spinelli, and Hayato Kurihara

1   Introduction

Inflammatory bowel disease (IBD) are non-infectious chronic inflammatory disorders of the gastrointestinal tract with a relapsing-remitting course that primarily include Crohn's disease (CD), ulcerative colitis (UC), and indeterminate colitis. Currently, approximately nearly seven million individuals are living with IBD worldwide and the number of prevalent cases is on the rise, especially in newly industrialized countries [1]. The highest incidence of IBD is among adolescents and young adults (ages 18–35 years) with an almost 1:1 female to male ratio [2]. Although their pathogenesis is still to be uncovered, it is thought to be driven by genetics and environment, such that dysregulated mucosal immune function is associated with a dysbiotic commensal microbiome that coordinately drives a pathological inflammatory cycle [3]. CD is characterized by transmural inflammation that can occur in the entire gastrointestinal tract, and complications of poorly controlled disease include strictures, fistulae, obstruction, and perforation. The most common localizations include the terminal ileum and caecum. On the contrary, the inflammation in UC is confined to the mucosa and submucosa, usually beginning in the distal rectum and progressing to the more proximal colon. In about 25% of patients with UC, terminal ileum is also involved (backwash ileitis) [4]. Due to the nature of the disease, IBD can often manifest as acute surgical emergencies in the form of acute

F. M. Carrano · A. Spinelli
Department of Colon and Rectal Surgery, IRCCS Humanitas Research Hospital, Milan, Italy
e-mail: antonino.spinelli@hunimed.eu

H. Kurihara (✉)
Emergency Surgery and Trauma Section, Department of Surgery, IRCCS Humanitas Research Hospital, Milan, Italy
e-mail: hayato.kurihara@humanitas.it

© The Author(s), under exclusive license to Springer Nature Switzerland AG 2023
F. Coccolini et al. (eds.), *Mini-invasive Approach in Acute Care Surgery*,
Hot Topics in Acute Care Surgery and Trauma,
https://doi.org/10.1007/978-3-031-39001-2_8

severe colitis, toxic megacolon and fulminant colitis, uncontrolled bleeding, free perforation, intra-abdominal masses or abscesses with sepsis, and intestinal obstruction. In 47% of patients with CD and 16% of patients with UC, those emergent presentations lead to surgery within 10 years of diagnosis [5] with a significant morbidity and impact on the quality of life.

This chapter will discuss the main presentations of IBD in the acute setting and the relative treatment approaches.

2 Initial Assessment and Diagnosis

When a patient is admitted to the Emergency Department (ED) with abdominal pain, fever, diarrhea, bloody stools, and weight loss, the possibility of an IBD should be suspected. In case of a positive history of IBD, it is important to investigate whether patient's symptoms are related to a flare of IBD or the insurgence of a complication (i.e., C. difficile infection, cytomegalovirus infection, enteric fistulae formation) or if it's an unrelated event (i.e., acute diverticulitis, appendicitis, etc.). To achieve a proper differential diagnosis, it is important to obtain a thorough patient's medical and surgical history, physical examination, laboratory test results (including a complete blood count, electrolytes, serum albumin, C-reactive protein, and fecal calprotectin), and imaging studies. In case of Crohn's disease patients, it is important to evaluate the disease phenotype, which is usually classified following the Montreal classification [6] according to age at diagnosis (early or late onset), predominant disease location (small bowel, large bowel, or perianal), and behavior (penetrating, fibrostenotic, or inflammatory) [7, 8]. Disease severity in CD can be measured with The Crohn's disease activity index (CDAI), the International Organization for the study of IBD (IOIBD) index, and the Harvey–Bradshaw index, although their use may not be very practical in the ED setting. In case of UC, it can be divided in the active stage, with active mucosal lesions and symptoms, and in the remission stage, with resolution of symptoms and lack of active mucosal lesions at endoscopy. According to disease extent, UC can be divided into proctitis, distal colitis (up to the sigmoid colon), left-sided colitis (up to the splenic flexure), and pancolitis. The severity of UC can be graded according to Truelove-Witts criteria into mild, moderate, and severe [8, 9]. More recently, the American College of Gastroenterology proposed an updated UC activity index [10] (Table 1).

In the emergent setting, however, a complete investigation of the disease may not always be possible. Thus, of primary importance is to correctly stratify patients, in order to decide if the patient can be discharged home safely or if further studies are needed, if patients require hospitalization or emergency surgery. A series of criteria that can be used as practical guidance for this task is listed in Table 2.

Table 1 UC activity index grading proposed by the American College of Gastroenterology

	Remission	Mild	Moderate to severe	Fulminant
Stools/day (n)	Formed stools	<4	>6	>10
Blood in stools	None	Intermittent	Frequent	Continuous
Urgency	None	Mild, occasional	Often	Continuous
Hemoglobin	Normal	Normal	<75% of normal	Transfusion required
ESR	<30	<30	>30	>30
CRP (mg/L)	Normal	Increased	Increased	Increased
FC (µg/g)	<150–200	>150–200	>150–200	>150–200
Endoscopy (Mayo subscore)	0–1	1	2–3	3
UCEIS	0–1	2–4	5–8	7–8

ESR erythrocyte sedimentation rate, *CRP* C-reactive protein, *FC* fecal calprotectin, *UCEIS* Ulcerative Colitis Endoscopic Index of Severity
Adapted from Rubin DT et al. [10]

Table 2 Practical criteria for the management of IBD patients in the ED

	When to request a CT-scan	When to hospitalize
Clinical criteria	Abdominal signs or symptoms suggestive of IBD complications	Abdominal signs or symptoms suggestive of IBD complications
	Bowel obstruction	Bowel obstruction
		Fever
	Surgical bowel resection in the past 30 days	Surgical bowel resection in the past 30 days
		Vomiting
		Ano-perineal abscess
		Hemodynamic instability
Laboratory criteria		Laboratory-confirmed signs of dehydration
		Acute kidney failure
		Hemoglobin <9 g/dL or decrease of ≥2 g/dL
	Very high CRP	

Modified from Hebuterne et al. [11]

3   Acute Severe Colitis

Acute severe colitis (ASC) is a life-threating condition that can occur in both CD and UC patients. In this paragraph, we will focus mainly on acute severe ulcerative colitis (ASUC) for clarity of exposition; however, the management of ASC in CD patients is similar. ASUC requires hospital admission in up to 25% of UC patients, it is burdened by high morbidity, requires colectomy in 40% of cases [12, 13], and carries a 1% mortality [14]. In the ED, patients with a clinical suspect of ASUC should receive extensive laboratory testing, including complete blood cell counts, basic metabolic panels, liver function tests, serum albumin, and prealbumin. An abdominal radiograph should be obtained to assess the degree of bowel dilation and rule out the presence of toxic megacolon or free air. In case of recent history of bowel resection, or if abdominal signs or symptoms are suggestive of IBD complications (bowel obstruction, perforation, abscess, bleeding), patients should be studied with an abdominal CT scan with contrast. Those patients who meet admission criteria should be hospitalized with the aim of further investigating the disease activity and initiate the most appropriate treatment. At admission, stool cultures and Clostridium difficile test are fundamental to rule out enteric infection, though this should not delay initial treatment. Additionally, Hepatitis B serology and Quantiferon-y test, cytomegalovirus (CMV), human immune deficiency virus (HIV), Epstein–Barr virus (EBV) serology, and tuberculosis exposure should be considered once the emergent need for surgery is excluded to rule out latent infections, in preparation for possible rescue therapy with biologic agents. Patients should receive early endoscopy, within 24 h from the admission, without bowel preparation and using minimal air insufflation, to confirm or exclude CMV colitis, which is essential for optimal treatment [13]. After a proper diagnosis is achieved and an initial risk stratification performed, it is of upmost importance to determine which patients are at higher risk of requiring rescue therapy or emergent colectomy; several disease scores are used for this purpose. The most used criteria to predict outcomes in ASUC are those from Truelove and Witts, although they were not originally conceived for this task. In fact, it has been demonstrated that, if used alone, they may under classify those patients who have active UC without the markers of systemic disturbance, possibly leading to the undertreatment of an important subset of patients [14]. Another commonly used tool is the Oxford (or Travis) index, developed in 1996, that predicts the need for colectomy to be 85% in patients with a CRP level greater than 45 mg/L and 3–8 bowel movements a day after 3 days of intravenous corticosteroid treatment. Recent studies have shown a potential advantage of using the Ulcerative Colitis Endoscopic Index of Severity (UCEIS). A UCEIS score of 5 or more was associated with a 50% chance of requiring rescue therapy and 33% rate of colectomy compared with 27% and 9% for those with a score of less than or equal to 4 [12]. The first-line treatment for ASUC patients is high-dose intravenous steroids in both anti-TNFα-naïve and previously exposed patients, instead, infliximab and cyclosporine are the recommended drugs in case of steroid therapy failure in anti-TNFα-naïve patients [15]. The surgical option should be evaluated early in a multidisciplinary setting and not only considered when medical treatment fails, to reduce the risk of postoperative complications. The primary goal of this multimodal treatment is to avoid the onset of complications requiring an emergency operation, which is fundamental to reduce mortality (Table 3).

Urgent colectomy is required for medical treatment failure or in case of toxic megacolon with imminent perforation [13]. The goal of the operation is to restore patient's health status and create the conditions for future restorative procedures. There should be no room for single staged ileal pouch-anal anastomosis (IPAA) procedures in the urgent setting. Two- or three-stage procedures should be the primary choice. Only the first stage is performed in the urgent setting; a total abdominal colectomy with an end ileostomy is completed leaving behind the rectal stump. The operation should be ideally performed in a minimally invasive fashion whether

Table 3 ASUC treatment algorithm

Timing	Initial investigations	Additional tests	Initial treatment	Daily clinical assessment
Admission (day 0)	Full blood count, urea, creatinine, electrolytes, liver function tests, CRP, ESR, magnesium, lipid profile • C. difficile toxin • Abdominal X-ray • Stool frequency • Nutritional status assessment	CMV, hepatitis B and C serology, HIV, EBV serology, and TB exposure • CT • Early colonoscopy	IV hydrocortisone (100 mg 3–4× daily) • Prophylactic LMWH • IV fluids, consider potassium replacement • Early nutritional support	• Stool frequency • Temperature • Heart rate • Clinical abdominal examination • Full blood cell count, urea, electrolytes, CRP
Day 3	**Reevaluate** Full blood cell count, CRP, stool frequency Additional tests: • CT • Colonoscopy	**Identify high-risk patients** Stool frequency > 8/day • CRP > 45 mg/L • Require rescue therapy (ciclosporin or infliximab)	**Management decisions** • MTD consultation • Continue IV hydrocortisone • Start rescue therapy in high-risk patients (ciclosporin, infliximab)	
Days 3–7	**IV hydrocortisone responder** Full blood cell count, CRP • Stool frequency • Convert to oral prednisolone	**Rescue therapy responder** Ciclosporin (convert to oral after 5–7 days) • Infliximab, assess on day 7 for response (if non-responder MTD consultation)	**Rescue therapy non-responder** MTD consultation • Colorectal surgeon • Stoma nurse (education and necessary support) • Dietitian • Gastroenterologist • Multidisciplinary input (planning surgery and further treatment)	

Adapted from Carvello et al. [13]

conventional laparoscopy, hand-assisted laparoscopic surgery (HALS), or robotic-assisted HALS colectomy may be particularly useful to help surgeons overcome the laparoscopic learning curve, as well as in complex cases, that would otherwise require an open approach. In a recent case series, conventional laparoscopy compared to HALS total colectomy was associated with a reduced postoperative pain, lower complications and readmissions rate, and shorter length of stay, with only

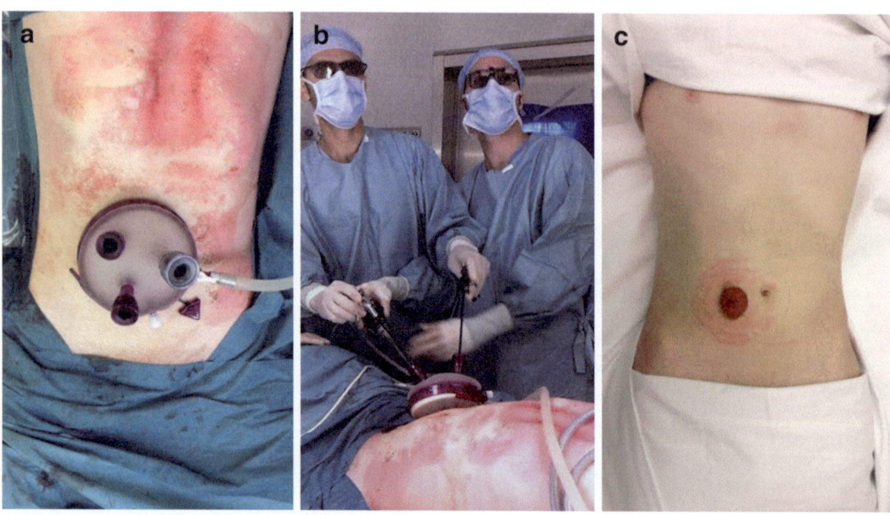

Fig. 1 Single port approach for total colectomy. (**a**) Single port platform placed at the future stoma-site; (**b**) operator positioning during surgery; (**c**) final "no-scar" result

marginal differences in operation length [16]. A possible rule of thumb of which approach to choose may be the following: if there is suspect of free perforation or the patient is hemodynamically unstable → open approach; in case of slim patients with no previous history of surgery, in good overall conditions, and with milder acute presentations → single port surgery (Fig. 1); for all the remaining → laparoscopic multi-port surgery.

Whichever the approach, this first operation provides a relatively rapid and safe resolution of the emergency while preserving intact pelvic planes for the future steps, avoiding the risk of pelvic bleeding and injury to the pelvic nerves and bladder, that may easily occur in the emergent setting. A restorative operation can then be performed at a later stage when the patient has fully recovered and is in optimal conditions. The remaining rectal stump can be managed in different ways, according to the individual patient characteristics and institutional experience, as there is no consensus in the literature on the optimal management. According to recent metanalyses, subcutaneous placement of the closed rectal stump is the least morbid [17, 18], with a pelvic sepsis rate of 2 and 0% mortality [18]. Another option is the intraperitoneal placement of the rectal stump, which is associated with the lowest wound infection rate (7.9%); however, higher rates of pelvic sepsis (5.3%), overall complications (25%), and mortality (1.5%) are reported with this technique [18].

In our opinion, mucous fistula may represent the best option in case the patient is highly compromised, with poor nutritional and performance status, and in case tissues are extremely inflamed and would not guarantee a secure management with a stapling device. Medical management after total colectomy includes topical therapy with either 5-aminosalicylic acid preparations and/or steroids or systemic therapy with thiopurines, methotrexate, infliximab, cyclosporine, and/or steroids, although there is no consensus on the best strategy [18]. The development of proctitis of the rectal stump after total colectomy occurs in most UC patients (almost 80%) and is a predictor for the development of pouchitis and therapy-refractory pouchitis [19].

4   Fulminant Colitis or Toxic Megacolon

Toxic megacolon is a more severe presentation of ASC carrying high mortality rates in case of perforation, ranging between 27 and 57%. It is identified by the same criteria as for ASC plus a radiographic evidence of total or segmental colonic distention greater than 6 cm. Unlike the typical colonic obstruction, in which cecal dilation is the area most likely to undergo perforation, in toxic megacolon the area of greatest attention is the transverse colon. Medical treatment should be started immediately and aggressively, following the same guiding principles of ASC treatment. However, toxic megacolon patients should be re-evaluated more frequently to evaluate response to therapy in the first 24–48 h, as a delay in surgery has a high risk of colonic perforation and onset of abdominal compartment syndrome that would greatly increase mortality. Colectomy should be performed when the response to the initial medical treatment is poor, and immediately in case of complicated presentations with free perforation, massive hemorrhage, toxic shock, and progression of colonic dilatation. If the patient is hemodynamically unstable, an open approach is recommended [20].

5   Bowel Perforation

Bowel perforation is another serious and potentially life-threatening complications in IBD patients and, although it occurs only in 1–3% of CD patients and 2% of UC patients, it is one of the main indications for emergency surgical intervention [21, 22]. In case of free perforation suspect, a contrast-enhanced CT-scan should be promptly obtained, and fluid resuscitation started with broad-spectrum antibiotics. In cases of a perforation blocked by omentum or neighboring structures, the first option is image-guided drainage (ultrasound or computed tomography) followed by operative or non-operative management. Positioning a drain gives the opportunity to avoid an operation in emergency conditions leading to lower morbidity and mortality rates [23]. This strategy cannot be followed in case of a diffuse peritonitis, where the only option is surgery. In CD patients, this complication occurs more frequently in the terminal ileum, often as a result of a complete small bowel obstruction due to an inflammatory stricture [22, 23].

In this case, a small bowel or ileocolic resection with primary anastomosis should be undertaken (Fig. 2). The construction of a mucous fistula should be considered in heavily contaminated fields, very inflamed tissues, poor nutritional status, and in case of multiple previous surgeries. If evidence of severe sepsis/septic shock, damage control surgery may be considered, with resection, stapled off bowel ends, and temporary abdominal closure with return to theater in 24–48 h for a second look, washout, and consideration of stoma vs anastomosis [21]. In case of perforation due to a colonic stricture causing large bowel obstruction, a subtotal colectomy

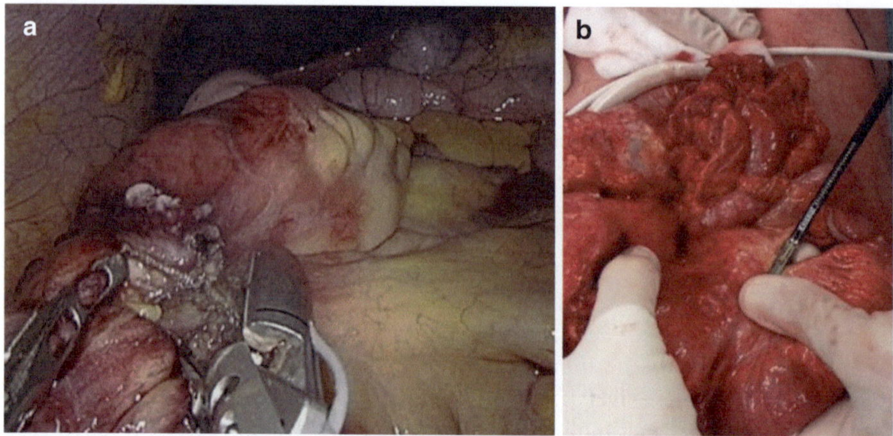

Fig. 2 Dividing the mesentery during a small bowel resection could be tricky in CD patients, and choosing the right approach is fundamental to reduce risks. In case of a mesentery that is moderately inflamed and thickened, a laparoscopic resection can be safely undertaken (**a**); when inflammation is severe and tissues are thickened and edematous, it is safer to divide the mesentery in an open fashion (**b**)

including the stricture site with the construction of an end ileostomy should be performed. A segmental colonic resection with primary anastomosis and proximal diversion or a Hartmann procedure may also be considered, however, they are associated with earlier disease recurrence [22, 23]. In UC patients, perforation typically occurs in the setting of toxic megacolon or, not rarely, due to iatrogenic injury during surveillance colonoscopy [24]. In both cases, the operation of choice would be a total abdominal colectomy with end ileostomy. Only in case of rectal perforation a proctectomy should be undertaken. Both open and laparoscopic approaches are appropriate in the emergency setting, if the patient is hemodynamically stable, otherwise an open approach is recommended [21].

6 Acute Abscess

The formation of an acute abscess is a typical manifestation of CD, with different clinical presentations, from asymptomatic to septic shock. We hereby discuss its diagnosis and management according to the site of occurrence.

6.1 Intra-abdominal

The typical presentation of intra-abdominal abscesses is characterized by fever, often associated with shivers, abdominal pain, and rebound tenderness. Alterations in blood tests show an increase in white blood cells count and increased CRP. Many times, clinical presentation may mimic that of acute appendicitis. Abscess formation is often associated with a diseased bowel tract fistulizing into another bowel segment

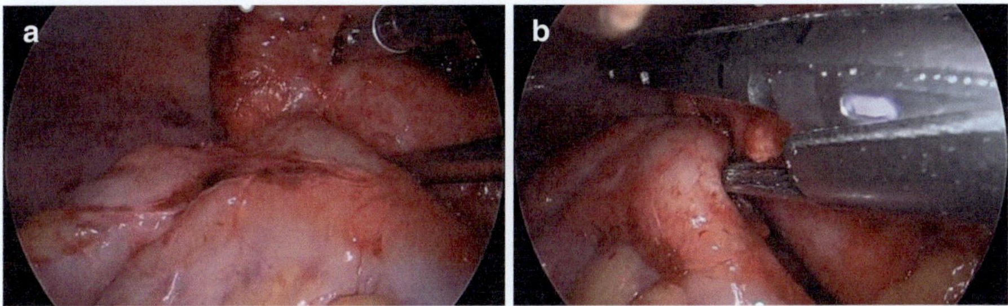

Fig. 3 An ileal fistula with sigmoid colon (**a**) can be safely managed laparoscopically with a stapled wedge resection (**b**)

(usually cecum or sigmoid colon), abdominal wall, or bladder (Fig. 3). A contrast-enhanced CT-scan or MRI should be obtained and early broad-spectrum antibiotic therapy initiated. If an abscess greater than 5 cm is demonstrated at imaging, initial management would be the placement of a percutaneous drainage with the help of interventional radiologists [23]. If patients do not respond to conservative treatment and become septic, patients should undergo a staged procedure, consisting in surgical exploration, resection of the diseased bowel segment, abscess drainage, lavage, and stoma formation. The anastomosis would be left for a secondary stage procedure when out of harm's way [25]. After bowel resection, attention should be paid to the prevention of recurrence, and a personalized therapy should be discussed in a multidisciplinary setting, see Fig. 4 for an example of possible management strategies.

Despite the increased technical demand, the presence of abscesses or inflammatory masses should not discourage from the adoption of the laparoscopic approach, which is the current treatment of choice for non-penetrating CD due to the proven reduced surgical trauma and postoperative pain, earlier bowel function, and shorter hospital stay compared to open procedures [27]. Despite the more aggressive clinical behavior of emergent cases compared to elective, often requiring more complex resections and longer hospital stays, morbidity is not higher in these patients [27]. With this approach, surgeons should clearly have in mind that chances of a conversion to open surgery are higher than usual [27].

6.2   Perianal Sepsis

Perianal disease can occur in 1 in 3 patients with CD and, sometimes, may be present at the time of diagnosis or even precede other intestinal symptoms. The most common presentation is perianal sepsis caused by an acute perianal or ischiorectal abscess, which is often associated with one or more perianal fistulae [28]. The majority of abscesses in CD develop at the level of the dentate line or may be the result of an obstructed fistula tract. In case of severe perianal pain without local clinical findings at inspection, an ischiorectal, intersphincteric, or supralevator abscess should be suspected [29]. For this reason, early diagnosis is important and an urgent MRI scan with contrast should be requested. Once precisely located,

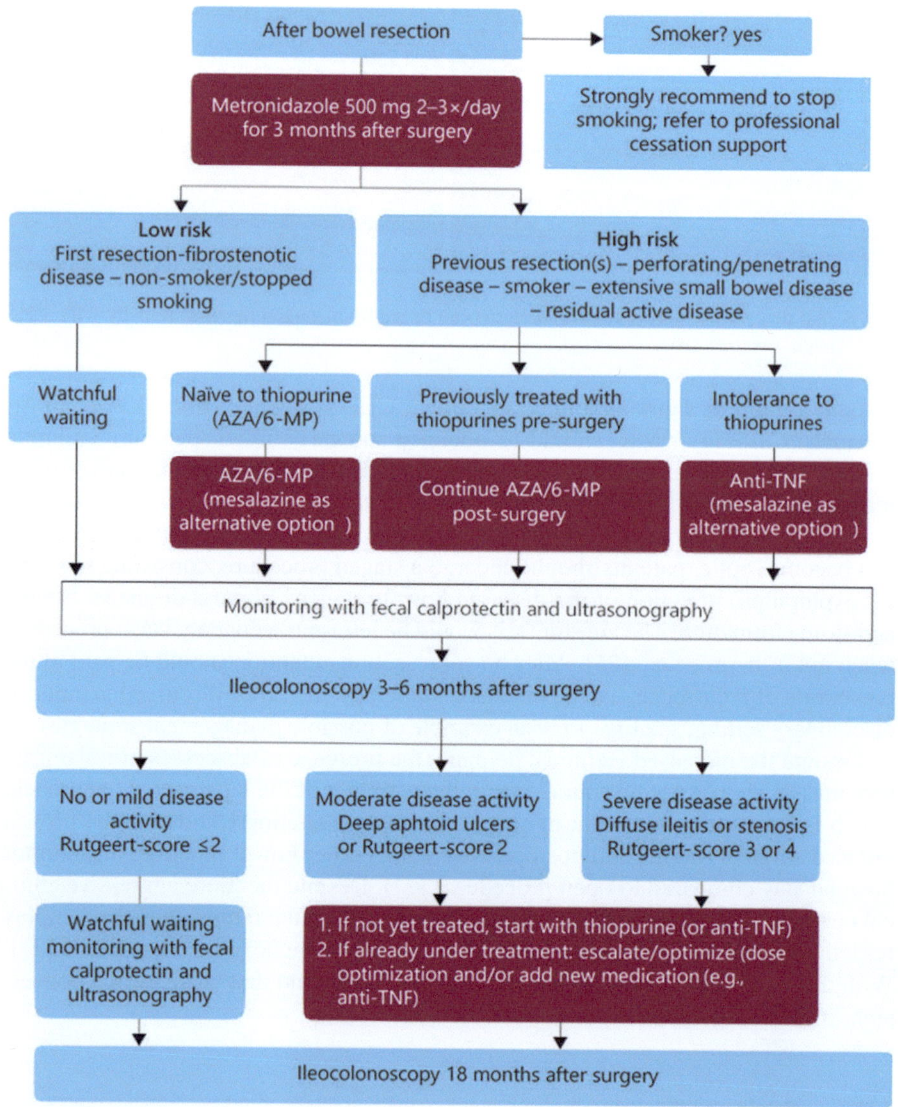

Fig. 4 Management of postoperative CD. *AZA* azathioprine, *6-MP* 6-mercaptopurine, *TNF* tumor necrosis factor. (Adapted from Sulz et al. [26])

patient should undergo examination of rectum under anesthesia (EUA) followed by adequate drainage of the abscess. In the emergent setting, the only goal should be the adequate drainage of the abscess while avoiding anal sphincter damage. Thus, the search for an underlying fistula should be discouraged, as local tissue conditions (induration and sepsis) may easily lead to probing false iatrogenic tracks which will further complicate the complexity of the disease. Only if the fistula tract can be clearly identified at the time of abscess drainage, a draining seton should be placed [20]. This approach provides the best results, allowing for a precise assessment of the perianal disease, in order to achieve an optimal outcome and avoid irreversible damage due to incomplete or inaccurate intervention. After resolution of the acute phase, both endoscopic ultrasonography-EUS and MRI are useful to accurately classify the disease (low/high fistulas, presence of undrained abscess, presence of proctitis), as well as to plan the most suitable treatment and monitor its results [30].

7   Bowel Obstruction

Bowel obstruction is characterized by nausea, vomiting, a distended abdomen, and absence of gas or stool passage per rectum. Although can occur also in UC patients, bowel obstruction is more frequent among CD patients, that typically undergo several episodes in their lives secondary to the development of fibrotic strictures combined with inflammation flares that acutely reduce the bowel lumen. A contrast CT scan should promptly be obtained. MRI may help in differentiating between a fibrotic stricture, inflammatory stricture, or mixed inflammatory and fibrotic stricture resulting precious when deciding the most appropriate treatment strategy; however, its use in the emergency setting may be limited outside referral centers. Nasogastric decompression, bowel rest, intravenous hydration, and intravenous steroids should be considered in active inflammatory disease as primary treatment. However, if there are signs of peritoneal irritation or suspected bowel ischemia, emergency surgery may be indicated, and a resection of the diseased segment should be performed [25, 31]. In cases of partial bowel obstruction nonresponsive to medical therapy, surgery can usually be scheduled after the patient is optimized [31]. If the patient is hemodynamically stable, a laparoscopic exploration may be considered as a routine starting point. If intraoperative findings allow for a safe totally laparoscopic surgery, the patient will have all the benefits of such a choice and, if a totally laparoscopic approach may not be possible, patients could benefit a lot also from hybrid procedures, in which part of the operation is performed hand-assisted or through a mini-laparotomy [32]. In case of need, there is always room for conversion. This event should not represent a failure for the surgeon in any circumstance and should not discourage from choosing the minimally invasive approach. Even in an emergency setting, proper pre-operative studies and planning are of paramount importance to choose the right intraoperative strategies and avoid unpleasant surprises while operating [32]. In case of patients at high risk of short bowel syndrome due to several previous resections or in case of extensive fibrostenosing disease, strictureplasty may be a viable solution, with effective and durable long-term results [22]. An alternative to surgery, if there are no signs of bowel ischemia and peritoneal irritation, endoscopic balloon dilation is an effective alternative solution, with short-term success rates of 89–91% [22]. In case of upper abdominal pain, nausea and vomiting, weight loss, diarrhoea, hematemesis. and anemia, a primary CD of the stomach and duodenum should be suspected. The strictures are typically located in the distal stomach and duodenal bulb in 50–60% of patients and are commonly treated by a distal gastrectomy with Roux-en-Y reconstruction. Duodenal strictures are best treated with stricturoplasty, as there is no possibility of a blind loop, dumping, or anastomotic ulcerations [31]. For the treatment of stenotic segments up to 68 cm, the technique of choice is the Heineke-Mikulicz stricturoplasty, while a Michelassi stricturoplasty should be preferred for multiple and close strictures [25, 31]. In case of large bowel obstructions, especially in UC, high suspicion for malignancy should be raised and, if an emergent colectomy is required, oncologic principles should be followed.

8   Uncontrolled Intestinal Hemorrhage

Gastrointestinal bleeding is a common complication in patients with UC or CD and is caused by inflammation/ulceration of the bowel; however, uncontrolled, life-threatening gastrointestinal bleeding occurs in less than 6% of cases [20]. Patients with suspect ongoing bleeding or already with hemodynamic instability should receive immediate fluid resuscitation and packed red blood cells transfusions to maintain hemoglobin levels above 7 g/dL, or 9 g/dL in case of massive bleeding or if cardiovascular comorbidities are present [20].

The causes of bleeding, and related treatment, differ between UC and CD. In UC patients, bleeding is usually caused by large areas of mucosal ulceration and hemorrhage. When massive bleeding occurs, endoscopic assessment and management of the bleeding source may not be possible, due to the reduced visuals and considering the ulceration extent (Fig. 5). In case of ASUC, the bleeding could involve all colonic mucosa and, after ruling out any rectal bleeding source endoscopically, an emergent subtotal colectomy with end ileostomy should be performed [20]. Causes of bleeding in CD patients are more insidious and complex to localize, due to the segmental nature

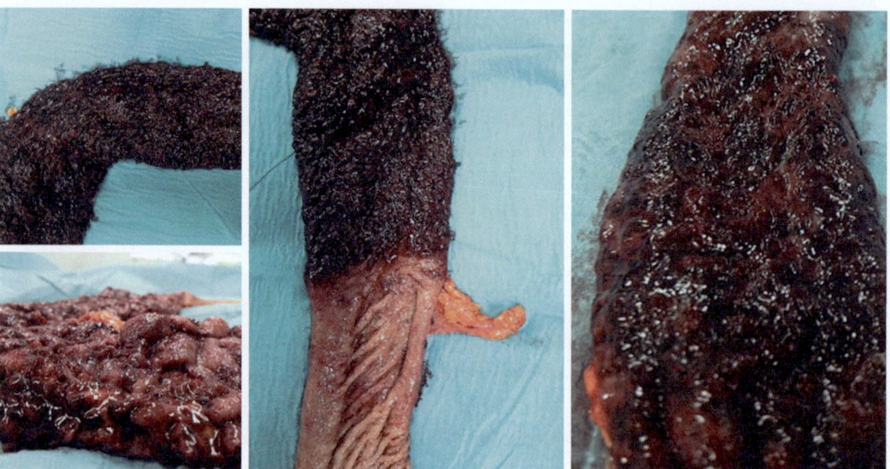

Fig. 5 Massive bleeding in UC patient requiring multiple blood transfusions without hemodynamic stabilization

of the disease. Most of the times, bleeding comes from the erosion of an intestinal vessel and, especially in case of massive bleeding, multiple segments of the gastrointestinal tract could be involved. For this reason, it is of paramount importance to localize bleeding sources preoperatively, thus great effort should be given to patient stabilization first. Subsequently, if an upper GI bleeding is suspect, an esophagogastroduodenoscopy should be promptly performed (eventually in the operating room if there's a serious risk that the patient cannot be stabilized for long), otherwise, if a lower GI bleeding is suspect, a complete colonoscopy should be carried out [20]. In case of more subtle or suspect extraluminal bleeding, CT-angiography may be useful as a noninvasive diagnostic tool to identify bleeding at rates of at least 0.3 mL/min. In case of failure to detect the active bleeding source, a possible alternative solution is the use of a nuclear medicine labeled red cell scans. Once the bleeding source has been detected, if the patient is hemodynamically stable and a conservative option is feasible (e.g., embolization, endoscopic hemostasis, etc.), it should be the preferred first treatment approach. In case of treatment failure, or in case the patient is unstable even after significant resuscitation, an open surgical exploration is mandatory [20]. In this scenario, there is insufficient evidence to support the laparoscopic approach.

9   Conclusions

Acute surgical emergencies in patients with IBD may be life threatening and carry a high degree of morbidity if not treated promptly in the appropriate way. Most emergencies in patients with CD that are hemodynamically stable, should be initially treated conservatively, and definitive treatment postponed in the elective setting after the patient has been optimized, so that the resection would be as minimal as possible. On the contrary, in case of UC complicated patients, surgical treatment should be pursued earlier and with a curative intent. With sufficient expertise, the laparoscopic approach is safe and feasible even in the emergency setting, carrying positive benefits for IBD patients. In case of hemodynamic instability and previous history of surgeries with complicated postoperative courses, an open approach would better serve the patient. Regardless of the underlying disease, the management of surgical emergencies in patients with IBD should be discussed in a multidisciplinary setting for optimal results.

References

1. Alatab S, Sepanlou SG, Ikuta K, Vahedi H, Bisignano C, Safiri S, et al. The global, regional, and national burden of inflammatory bowel disease in 195 countries and territories, 1990–2017: a systematic analysis for the global burden of disease study 2017. Lancet Gastroenterol Hepatol. 2020;5:17–30.
2. Kaplan GG, Windsor JW. The four epidemiological stages in the global evolution of inflammatory bowel disease. Nat Rev Gastroenterol Hepatol. 2021;18:56–66.
3. Graham DB, Xavier RJ. Pathway paradigms revealed from the genetics of inflammatory bowel disease. Nature. 2020;578:527–39.

4. Erden A, Kuru Oz D, Gursoy Coruh A, Erden I, Ozalp Ates FS, Toruner M. Backwash ileitis in ulcerative colitis: are there MR enterographic features that distinguish it from Crohn disease? Eur J Radiol. 2019;110:212–8.

5. Frolkis AD, Dykeman J, Negron ME, Debruyn J, Jette N, Fiest KM, et al. Risk of surgery for inflammatory bowel diseases has decreased over time: a systematic review and meta-analysis of population-based studies. Gastroenterology. 2013;145:996–1006.

6. Silverberg MS, Satsangi J, Ahmad T, Arnott ID, Bernstein CN, Brant SR, et al. Toward an integrated clinical, molecular and serological classification of inflammatory bowel disease: report of a working party of the 2005 Montreal world congress of gastroenterology. Can J Gastroenterol. 2005;19:5A–36A.

7. Mak JWY, Ng SC. Epidemiology of fibrostenosing inflammatory bowel disease. J Dig Dis. 2020;21:332–5.

8. Spekhorst LM, Visschedijk MC, Alberts R, Festen EA, van der Wouden EJ, Dijkstra G, et al. Performance of the Montreal classification for inflammatory bowel diseases. World J Gastroenterol. 2014;20:15374–81.

9. Matsuoka K, Kobayashi T, Ueno F, Matsui T, Hirai F, Inoue N, et al. Evidence-based clinical practice guidelines for inflammatory bowel disease. J Gastroenterol. 2018;53:305–53.

10. Rubin DT, Ananthakrishnan AN, Siegel CA, Sauer BG, Long MD. ACG clinical guideline: ulcerative colitis in adults. Am J Gastroenterol. 2019;114:384–413.

11. Hebuterne X, Peyrin-Biroulet L, Hausfater P. The management of emergency hospital visits for inflammatory bowel diseases: a French national expert consensus report. Dig Liver Dis. 2020;52:420–6.

12. Pabla BS, Schwartz DA. Assessing severity of disease in patients with ulcerative colitis. Gastroenterol Clin North Am. 2020;49:671–88.

13. Carvello M, Watfah J, Wlodarczyk M, Spinelli A. The management of the hospitalized ulcerative colitis patient: the medical-surgical conundrum. Curr Gastroenterol Rep. 2020;22:11.

14. Gupta V, Mohsen W, Chapman TP, Satsangi J. Predicting outcome in acute severe colitis—controversies in clinical practice in 2021. J Crohns Colitis. 2021;15:1211.

15. D'Amico F, Peyrin-Biroulet L, Danese S. Tofacitinib for acute severe colitis: when the going gets tough, the tough get going. J Crohns Colitis. 2020;14:883–5.

16. Chough I, Zaghiyan K, Ovsepyan G, Fleshner P. It is not just cosmesis: straight laparoscopy with stoma site extraction improves outcomes in ulcerative colitis patients undergoing total colectomy. Am Surg. 2019;85:1194–7.

17. Lawday S, Leaning M, Flannery O, Summers S, Antoniou GA, Goodhand J, et al. Rectal stump management in inflammatory bowel disease: a cohort study, systematic review and proportional analysis of perioperative complications. Tech Coloproctol. 2020;24:671–84.

18. Bedrikovetski S, Dudi-Venkata N, Kroon HM, Liu J, Andrews JM, Lewis M, et al. Systematic review of rectal stump management during and after emergency total colectomy for acute severe ulcerative colitis. ANZ J Surg. 2019;89:1556–60.

19. Wasmann KA, van der Does de Willebois EM, Koens L, Duijvestein M, Bemelman WA, Buskens CJ. The impact of rectal stump inflammation after subtotal colectomy on pouch outcomes in ulcerative colitis patients. J Crohns Colitis. 2020;15:299.

20. De Simone B, Davies J, Chouillard E, Di Saverio S, Hoentjen F, Tarasconi A, et al. WSES-AAST guidelines: management of inflammatory bowel disease in the emergency setting. World J Emerg Surg. 2021;16:23.

21. Coccolini F, Perrone G, Chiarugi M, Di Marzo F, Ansaloni L, Scandroglio I, et al. Surgery in COVID-19 patients: operational directives. World J Emerg Surg. 2020;15:25.

22. Goldstone RN, Steinhagen RM. Abdominal emergencies in inflammatory bowel disease. Surg Clin North Am. 2019;99:1141–50.

23. Gomes CA, Podda M, Veiga SC, do Vale Cabral T, Lima LV, Miron LC, et al. Management of inflammatory bowel diseases in urgent and emergency scenario. J Coloproctol. 2021;40: 083–8.

24. DiCaprio D, Lee-Kong S, Stoffels G, Shen B, Al-Mazrou A, Kiran RP, et al. Management of iatrogenic perforation during colonoscopy in ulcerative colitis patients: a survey of gastroenterologists and colorectal surgeons. Int J Color Dis. 2018;33:1607–16.

25. Adamina M, Bonovas S, Raine T, Spinelli A, Warusavitarne J, Armuzzi A, et al. ECCO guidelines on therapeutics in Crohn's disease: surgical treatment. J Crohn's Colitis. 2020;14:155–68.
26. Sulz MC, Burri E, Michetti P, Rogler G, Peyrin-Biroulet L, Seibold F, et al. Treatment algorithms for Crohn's disease. Digestion. 2020;101(Suppl 1):43–57.
27. Kristo I, Stift A, Argeny S, Mittlböck M, Riss S. Minimal-invasive approach for penetrating Crohn's disease is not associated with increased complications. Surg Endosc. 2016;30:5239–44.
28. Marzo M, Felice C, Pugliese D, Andrisani G, Mocci G, Armuzzi A, et al. Management of perianal fistulas in Crohn's disease: an up-to-date review. World J Gastroenterol. 2015;21:1394–403.
29. Lewis RT, Bleier JI. Surgical treatment of anorectal Crohn disease. Clin Colon Rectal Surg. 2013;26:90–9.
30. Spinelli A, Armuzzi A, Ciccocioppo R, Danese S, Gionchetti P, Luglio G, et al. Management of patients with complex perianal fistulas in Crohn's disease: optimal patient flow in the Italian clinical reality. Dig Liver Dis. 2020;52:506–15.
31. Bemelman WA, Warusavitarne J, Sampietro GM, Serclova Z, Zmora O, Luglio G, et al. ECCO-ESCP consensus on surgery for Crohn's disease. J Crohns Colitis. 2018;12:1–16.
32. Spinelli A, Fiorino G, Bazzi P, Sacchi M, Bonifacio C, De Bastiani S, et al. Preoperative magnetic resonance enterography in predicting findings and optimizing surgical approach in Crohn's disease. J Gastrointest Surg. 2014;18:83–90; discussion 90–1.

Gastroduodenal Perforation

Amit Sharma and Mansoor Ali Khan

1 Introduction

Learning Goals
- **Be able to readily identify the causes of gastroduodenal perforation**
- **Have the knowledge basis to initiate immediate treatment of gastroduodenal perforation**
- **Identify the spectrum of treatment modalities available dependent on physiology of the patient**

Acute gastroduodenal perforation can either be spontaneous or secondary to trauma. The former is primarily due to underlying peptic ulcer disease. The incidence of peptic ulcer disease has declined over the years due to medical treatment with histamine 2 receptor blockers (H2RBs) and proton pump inhibitors (PPI) and, the use of eradication treatment for a Helicobacter pylori (H. pylori) infection [1]. The lifetime risk of benign gastroduodenal perforation is 10% in patients with untreated peptic ulcer disease [2–4]. However, the need for surgical intervention for gastroduodenal perforation remains stable and may be increasing [3, 4]. This in part related to increasing use of medications such as non-steroidal anti-inflammatory drugs (NSAIDs)/aspirin and to the ageing population [1]. Therefore, management of peptic ulcer remains a significant healthcare issue. Furthermore, iatrogenic duodenal perforations are becoming more common following the widespread use of endoscopic procedures [1]. Yet there are several controversies regarding evidence-based management for acute gastroduodenal perforations including the role of non-operative management, type of surgical approach, type of repair, and the role of gastric diversion procedures, such as a pyloric exclusion [1, 4].

A. Sharma · M. A. Khan (✉)
Brighton and Sussex University Hospitals NHS Trust, Brighton, UK
e-mail: a.sharma1@nhs.net; mansoorkhan@nhs.net

2   Causes of Gastroduodenal Perforation

Peptic ulcer disease accounts for the majority of acute gastroduodenal perforations. Underlying causes of peptic ulcer disease include H. pylori infection, medications (steroids, NSAIDs, and aspirin), and acid hypersecretion. Infection with H. pylori is highly prevalent amongst the patients with peptic ulcer disease. As many as 90–100% of patients with uncomplicated peptic ulcer disease and 65–70% of patients with perforated peptic ulcers are infected with H. pylori [2]. NSAIDs related ulcer perforations occur in 30–50% of patients [2–4]. Duodenal ulcers are four times more common than gastric ulcers below the age of 40 years and are more common in men [2]. The anterior surface of the duodenal bulb is the most common site of disease (60%) followed by the gastric antrum (20%) and the lesser curvature of the stomach (20%) [4]. Benign gastric ulcers occur predominantly on the lesser curve in elderly patients. Ulcers on the greater curve, fundus, and in the antrum are more commonly malignant [2].

Other causes of acute gastroduodenal perforation include malignancy, trauma (blunt or penetrating), foreign body ingestion (by direct trauma or distal luminal obstruction), iatrogenia from endoscopic procedures, marginal ulcer formation following bariatric surgery, prolonged fasting, illicit drug consumption, Zollinger-Ellison syndrome, stress ulcers in critically ill patients (Curling's ulcer), and chemotherapy with angiogenesis inhibitors such as bevacizumab [5, 6]. Blunt trauma accounts for only 5% of hollow viscus perforations. Malignancy causes perforation by necrosis, or involution response to chemotherapy or due to distal luminal obstruction [3]. Gastric cancers account for 10–16% of perforations [4]. Iatrogenic duodenal perforations with ERCP occur in around 1% patients [1]. Gastric volvulus in setting of large hiatus hernia can cause strangulation and perforation secondary to ischaemia [2].

Duodenal perforations can also occur in people with conditions such as duodenal diverticula, duodenal ischemia, infectious disease, and autoimmune conditions, including Crohn's disease, scleroderma, and vasculitis (e.g., abdominal polyarteritis nodosa) [1]. Impacted gallstones in the duodenum have also been associated with perforations [1]. Gastroduodenal perforation has also been reported as a complication of a variety of abdominal operations including the commonly performed laparoscopic cholecystectomy (0.015%) [1].

3   Presentation and Diagnosis

A diagnosis of gastroduodenal perforation is frequently made based on good clinical history and examination. Patients classically present with sudden onset acute upper abdominal pain that commonly radiates to the shoulder due to diaphragmatic irritation from free air or gastric contents. Nausea and vomiting are present in around 50% of patients [7]. Shock is detected in 5–10% of patients [7]. A previous history of peptic ulcer disease is present in 60–70% of patients who present with perforation [8]. Other important risk factors in the medical history include gastroesophageal reflux disease, use of NSAIDs, smoking, and a recent history of upper GI endoscopy. A recent history of trauma should also be sought from the medical history.

On clinical examination, patients generally show classical signs of peritonitis due to irritation from gastric contents leakage with rigid board-like abdomen secondary to recti muscle spasm. However, only two-thirds of patients present with frank peritonitis which might explain the diagnostic delay in some patients [6]. This can occur when the perforation has managed to conceal or be contained to locally surrounding tissues or into the retroperitoneal space. Examination findings in the obese, elderly, or immunocompromised patients can also be challengingly non-specific and mild [1, 2]. In addition, if perforation is in the thorax as in the case of strangulated hiatus hernia, then the patient is likely to have chest symptoms and general signs of severe sepsis, with little or no evidence of peritonitis [2].

An upright chest X-ray is the first choice of investigation to detect pneumoperitoneum with evidence of air under the diaphragm (Fig. 1). However, pneumoperitoneum on the erect chest X-ray is absent in 20–30% of cases [2, 6]. Therefore, a negative erect chest X-ray should prompt further investigations in the form of contrast enhanced CT scan, which has sensitivity of 98% (Fig. 2). Adding water soluble oral contrast enables further assessment of perforation [6]. In addition, CT scan enables assessment of other synchronous intra-abdominal pathologies. Suspicious findings on CT scan include unexplained intraperitoneal fluid, pneumoperitoneum, bowel wall thickening, mesenteric fat stranding, and extravasation of oral contrast.

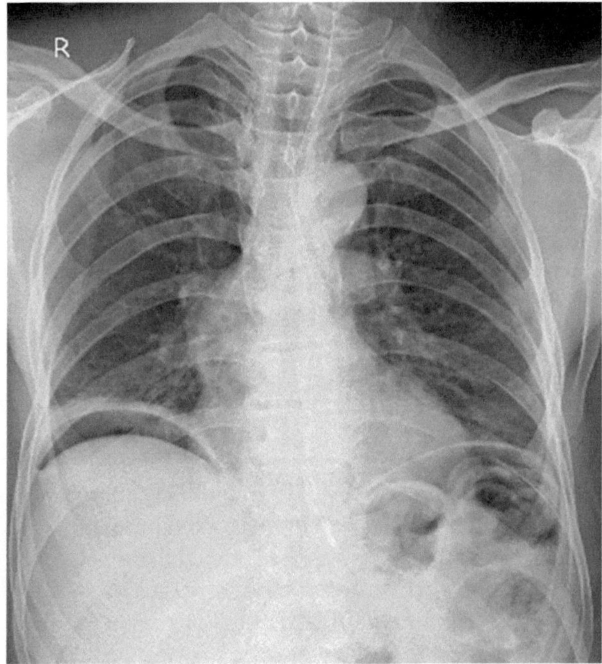

Fig. 1 Erect chest X-ray showing bilateral air under the diaphragm diagnostic of pneumoperitoneum. (Courtesy of Dr. Kewal Arunkumar Mistry [9])

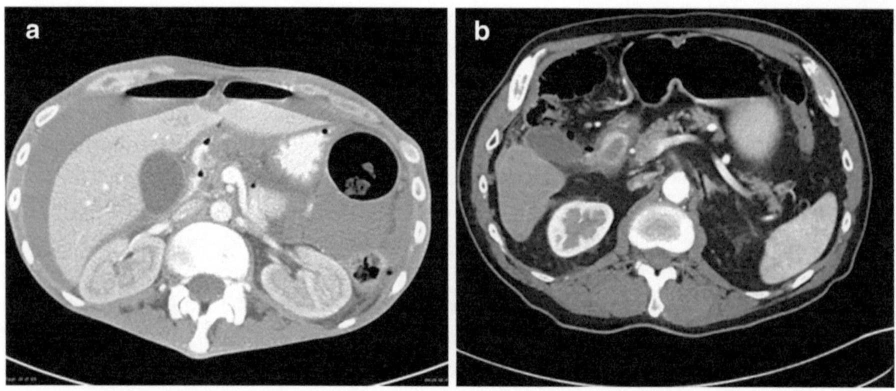

Fig. 2 Contrast-enhanced axial images of gastroduodenal perorations. (**a**) Double contrast-enhanced (intravenous and oral) axial image of upper abdomen. There is evidence of free perihepatic fluid and air. In addition, multiple locules of free gas are seen medial to the gallbladder. (**b**) Contrast-enhanced axial image of upper abdomen with locules of free air around a thickened gastroduodenal junction. Image erect chest X-ray showing bilateral air under diaphragm diagnostic of pneumoperitoneum. (Courtesy of Associate Professor Fran Gaillard [10])

Up to 12% of patients with traumatic perforations may have a normal initial CT scan [6]. Although in a patient with penetrating trauma with signs of peritonitis, surgical intervention is the key; and in both blunt and penetrating trauma patients that are clinically stable, trauma CT scanning is the standard of care for diagnosis [3].

Other markers that help physicians in assessing a patient's clinical state include leukocytosis, metabolic acidosis, high lactate levels, a negative base excess, and reduced levels of consciousness. There is usually an associated hyperamylasaemia. Patients with reduced GCS may be difficult to assess on examination [3].

4   Management

Delays of greater than 12 h result in a three-fold increase in mortality, while delays of 24 h are associated with a nine-fold increase.

4.1   Conservative Management

Also known as the Taylor method named after author who proposed this form of management first in 1946. Approximately half of the perforations spontaneously seal [5]. This occurs with fibrin, omentum, or by fusion of the duodenum to the underside of the liver between the gallbladder and the falciform ligament [1]. Various retrospective observational studies show variable rate of success in non-operative management of perforated peptic ulcer disease (Table 1). However, there is a high degree of heterogeneity in methodology and selection bias in these reports.

Table 1 Retrospective data on conservative management of perforated peptic ulcer disease

Study	Number of patients	Failed conservative treatment
Cao et al. (2014) [11]	132	25 (19%)
Songne et al. (2004) [12]	82	38 (46%)
Marshall et al. (1999) [13]	49	8 (16%)
Croft et al. (1989) [14]	40	11 (28%)
Berne et al. (1989) [15]	35	2 (6%)
Asanasak (2019) [16]	38	2 (5%)
Shashi et al. (2018) [17]	30	4 (13%)
Gul et al. (1999) [18]	28	6 (18%)
Zedan et al. (2020) [19]	24	6 (25%)
Karabulut et al. (2019) [20]	6	0

The difficulty is identifying those patients who have sealed without compromising the outcomes for those who have not sealed while one observes them for signs of clinical deterioration. Early oral contrast CT scan or gastroduodenogram can help in detecting self-sealed perforations. In patients under 70 years of age with very few or localised symptoms who are haemodynamically stable and with an onset of symptoms of less than 24 h, the choice to operate might be delayed deliberately in favour of an observation period [3, 6]. However, it has been clearly demonstrated that observation periods of longer than 12 h without improvement worsen the outcomes from perforated peptic ulcers and should be avoided [3, 5]. In surgically unfit patients, conservative treatment is an option but has a mortality of 30% [4]. Initial conservative management consists of nil by mouth, intravenous fluid therapy, broad-spectrum antibiotics, intravenous PPIs, nasogastric tube insertion, and H. pylori eradication [1]. However, conservative management has now been largely abandoned even in high-risk cases because the conversion to operative treatment is required in up to a third [2]. The use of such an observation period can obviate the need for emergency surgery in more than 70% of patients [14].

Another issue with non-operative treatment is the risk of missing a perforated gastric cancer [4]. Conservative management does not allow for the assessment of a possible differential diagnosis or histologic assessment of gastric ulcers. Therefore, non-operative management should be followed by upper endoscopy within 6 weeks to identify the site of perforation, confirm healing of the ulcer, and allow for gastric biopsy to rule out malignancy (Table 1).

4.2 Surgical Management

Surgical management still remains the mainstay of treatment for gastroduodenal perforations. Various surgical techniques have been described to deal with the perforated site including: primary closure by interrupted sutures, primary closure by interrupted sutures covered with pedicled omentopexy, Cellan-Jones repair with pedicled omentoplasty without closure of the primary defect (described in 1929), or Graham omental patch repair without closure of the primary defect (described in 1937) (Fig. 3).

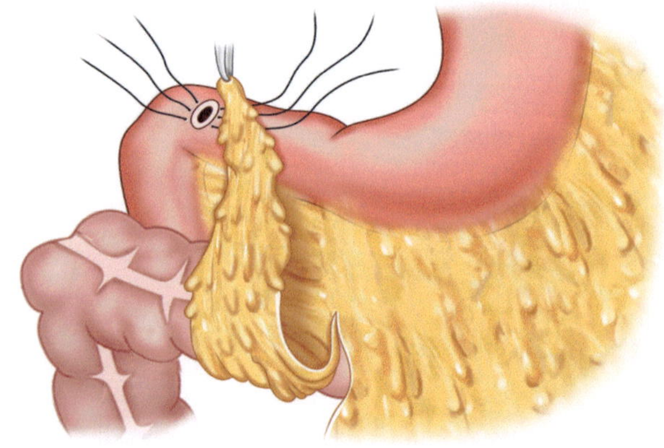

Fig. 3 Diagrammatic representation of pedicled omental patch repair of anterior duodenal bulb perforation [2]

Infrequent radical surgical approach includes distal gastrectomy and vagotomy (truncal, selective, or highly selective) combined with antrectomy or pyloroplasty [4]. Currently, principal emergency indication for this approach is massive haemorrhage with perforation, for perforated gastric ulcer with significant loss of substance, >10–20 mm diameter. In patients with a history of chronic ulcer disease and prior failed medical therapy, a definitive ulcer operation may be indicated [4]. A 2003 questionnaire of nearly 700 British surgeons reported that the use of selective vagotomy during urgent surgery for perforation had been abandoned in favour of medical therapy with PPIs and eradication of H. pylori infection [4]. One could consider performing urgent gastrectomy in well-selected stable patients but a two-stage procedure should be performed in most cases, consisting of emergency suture closure of the perforation followed by a second-stage oncologic gastrectomy. This two-stage approach was proposed by Lehnert et al. in 2000 in a prospective study of 23 patients with perforated gastric cancer [21].

4.2.1 Open Vs Laparoscopic Approach

Open surgical procedure with midline laparotomy wound remains the most commonly practiced surgical technique for the last several decades [6]. The first laparoscopic repair for a perforated duodenal ulcer was reported in 1990 [1]. Since then, numerous studies have compared open versus laparoscopic surgery for perforated duodenal ulcer and have demonstrated both the feasibility and efficacy of the laparoscopic approach. Quah et al. recently conducted large meta-analysis based on RCTs have shown a significant benefit in performing laparoscopic repair with a significant reduction in the overall postoperative morbidity, wound infection, and a shorter LOS with no difference in mortality rate, re-operation rate, intra-abdominal abscess formation, and respiratory complications [22]. In addition, Zhang et al. showed reductions in the intraoperative blood loss, ileus, postoperative pain with laparoscopic approach [23]. Finally, the recommendations of the European Association of Endoscopic Surgery have concluded that the diagnostic laparoscopy is useful when the clinical presentation suggests the diagnosis of perforated peptic ulcer, and they recommend laparoscopic repair (Grade B recommendation) [4]. In a large United Kingdom based propensity-matched study of the National Emergency Laparotomy Audit (NELA), there was no difference in 90-day mortality, re-operation rate, and re-admission rate to critical care unit between a laparoscopic and open repair of peptic ulcer perforations [24]. However, the author reported a 35% conversion to open rate.

As no difference in mortality has been shown for open surgery versus the laparoscopic technique, the local surgeons' experience and patient assessment must be considered in deciding optimal surgical approach for a particular patient. In terms of the actual surgical technique of the repair, Ellatif et al. showed difference in laparoscopic simple repair vs patch repair with mean perforation size of 7 mm in each group [25].

5   Prognosis

Mortality is reported up to 30%, and morbidity rates are around 60% [1, 6]. Again, mortality increases with every hour by which surgery is delayed [6]. Therefore, early resuscitation and timely diagnosis and appropriate management are crucial. Prognosis is worse in elder and co-morbid patients. Gastric perforations are associated with worse two- to three-fold increased risk of mortality [7]. Boey score is based on shock, patient comorbidities, and duration of symptoms prior to surgery (>24 h) predicts postoperative outcome with score of 0:1.5%, 1:14%, 2:32%, 3:100% [7].

Postoperative morbidity is generally infectious, with pneumonia as the most common complication (up to 30%), followed by superficial and deep surgical site infections [3].

Routine postoperative endoscopy is advised to rule out malignancy in gastric ulcers or when precise location of perforation was not known.

Dos and Don'ts
- Early diagnosis and timely management are key.
- Mainstay treatment remains surgical and if in doubt, operate.
- Type of surgical approach and repair remain debated and should follow surgeons' experience.
- Gastric perforations or conservatively manged patients need follow-up endoscopy to exclude sinister aetiology.

Conflict of Interest None declared.

References

1. Ansari D, Torén W, Lindberg S, Pyrhönen H-S, Andersson R. Diagnosis and management of duodenal perforations: a narrative review. Scand J Gastroenterol. 2019;54(8):939–44.
2. Weledji E. The surgical management of benign gastroduodenal perforation. J Gastric Surg. 2020;2(3):84–91.

3. Lui F, Davis K. Gastroduodenal perforation: maximal or minimal intervention? Scand J Surg. 2010;99(2):73–7.

4. Mouly C, Chati R, Scotté M, Regimbeau J-M. Therapeutic management of perforated gastroduodenal ulcer: literature review. J Visc Surg. 2013;150(5):333–40.

5. Nirula R. Gastroduodenal perforation. Surg Clin North Am. 2014;94(1):31–4.

6. Søreide K, Thorsen K, Harrison EM, Bingener J, Møller MH, Ohene-Yeboah M, et al. Perforated peptic ulcer. Lancet. 2015;386(10000):1288–98.

7. Bertleff MJ, Lange JF. Perforated peptic ulcer disease: a review of history and treatment. Dig Surg. 2010;27(3):161–9.

8. Morris A, Midwinter MJ. Chapter 8. Perforated peptic ulcer. In: Emergency surgery. Hoboken: Wiley-Blackwell; 2010. p. 43.

9. Radiopaedia. Subdiaphragmatic free gas. https://radiopaedia.org/articles/subdiaphragmatic-free-gas?lang=gb.

10. Radiopaedia. Pneumoperitoneum. https://radiopaedia.org/articles/pneumoperitoneum?lang=us.

11. Cao F, Li J, Li A, Fang Y, Wang Y-J, Li F. Nonoperative management for perforated peptic ulcer: who can benefit? Asian J Surg. 2014;37(3):148–53.

12. Songne B, Jean F, Foulatier O, Khalil H, Scotté M, editors. Non operative treatment for perforated peptic ulcer: results of a prospective study. Annales de chirurgie; 2004.

13. Marshall C, Ramaswamy P, Bergin F, Rosenberg I, Leaper D. Evaluation of a protocol for the non-operative management of perforated peptic ulcer. Br J Surg. 1999;86(1):131–4.

14. Crofts TJ, Park KG, Steele RJ, Chung SS, Li AK. A randomized trial of nonoperative treatment for perforated peptic ulcer. N Engl J Med. 1989;320(15):970–3.

15. Berne TV, Donovan AJ. Nonoperative treatment of perforated duodenal ulcer. Arch Surg. 1989;124(7):830–2.

16. Asanasak P. The case series of peritonitis due to perforated peptic ulcer: how does conservative management play role? Int J Surg Case Rep. 2019;58:74–6.

17. Shashi SS, Hossain AS, Bar D, Rahman A, Reza AM, Rashid MHA. Outcome of non-operative management of perforated peptic ulcer disease. J Surg Sci. 2018;22(2):95–8.

18. Gul Y, Shine M, Lennon F. Non-operative management of perforated duodenal ulcer. Ir J Med Sci. 1999;168(4):254–6.

19. Zedan AM, Head MH, Hussein BG. Conservative versus surgical treatment of perforated peptic ulcer. Ann Trop Med Health. 2020;23:231–22.

20. Karabulut K, Dinçer M, Liman RK, Usta S. Non-operative management of perforated peptic ulcer: a single-center experience. Turkish J Trauma Emerg Surg. 2019;25(6):585–8.

21. Lehnert T, Buhl K, Dueck M, Hinz U, Herfarth C. Two-stage radical gastrectomy for perforated gastric cancer. Eur J Surg Oncol. 2000;26(8):780–4.

22. Quah GS, Eslick GD, Cox MR. Laparoscopic repair for perforated peptic ulcer disease has better outcomes than open repair. J Gastrointest Surg. 2019;23(3):618–25.

23. Zhang H, Chen J, Li Y-J. Systematic review of curative effect between laparoscopic and open repair for perforated gastroduodenal ulcer. 2018;29.

24. Coe PO, Lee MJ, Boyd-Carson H, Lockwood S, Saha A. Open versus laparoscopic repair of perforated peptic ulcer disease: a propensity-matched study of the national emergency laparotomy audit. Ann Surg. 2021;275:928.

25. Abd Ellatif M, Salama A, Elezaby A, El-Kaffas H, Hassan A, Magdy A, et al. Laparoscopic repair of perforated peptic ulcer: patch versus simple closure. Int J Surg. 2013;11(9):948–51.

Adhesive Small Bowel Obstruction (ASBO)

Gabriele Luciano Petracca, Vittoria Pattonieri, Concetta Prioriello, Gennaro Perrone, Antonio Tarasconi, and Fausto Catena

1 Introduction

Adhesive small bowel obstruction (ASBO) is one of the most frequent diagnoses of patients with abdominal pain that are admitted in the emergency department (ED). The diagnosis of small bowel obstruction (SBO) is a combination of clinical presentation, laboratory studies, and radiological findings. Signs and symptoms with different grades of intensity include abdominal pain and distension, diffuse tenderness, nausea, vomiting, and progressive failure to pass stool and flatus. The plain film radiological signs of a SBO are air/fluid levels in the small intestine, gastrectasia, and the presence of conniventes valvulae.

The most frequent cause of SBO is abdominal adhesions occurring approximately 50–60% of the time. Other causes include abdominal hernias, which is the most frequent cause in patients who have not had previous abdominal surgery, cancer, inflammatory bowel disease, intussusception, radiation, endometriosis, infections, and foreign bodies (to include gallstones and bezoars). The diagnosis is primarily related to the past medical history of a patient, his physical examination, the findings on the radiological studies (abdominal radiography, CT scan), and the consideration of the likely causes. Definitive treatment is related to the cause and degree of obstruction, duration of symptoms, and if medical therapy fails.

G. L. Petracca · V. Pattonieri · C. Prioriello · G. Perrone
Azienda Ospedaliera-Universitaria di Parma, Dipartimento Interaziendale Urgenza-Emergenza. U.O. Chirurgia d'Urgenza, Parma, Italy

A. Tarasconi
Azienda Ospedaliera-Universitaria di Parma, Dipartimento Interaziendale Urgenza-Emergenza. U.O. Chirurgia d'Urgenza, Parma, Italy

ASST Cremona, Ospedale di Cremona, UO Chirurgia Generale, Cremona, Italy

F. Catena (✉)
Azienda Unità Sanitaria Locale della Romagna, Ospedale "Bufalini" di Cesena, U.O. Chirurgia Generale d'Urgenza, Cesena, Italy

© The Author(s), under exclusive license to Springer Nature Switzerland AG 2023
F. Coccolini et al. (eds.), *Mini-invasive Approach in Acute Care Surgery*,
Hot Topics in Acute Care Surgery and Trauma,
https://doi.org/10.1007/978-3-031-39001-2_10

2   Physiopathology of SMO

Intestinal obstruction determines a series of consequences that alter the homeostasis of the intestinal contents (gas, liquids, electrolytes, microbial flora). The nature and location of the occlusion characterize different pathophysiological changes of the intestine. The digestive tract produces approximately 6–8 L of secretions in 24 h (saliva, gastric juices, pancreatic-duodenal juices, bile, ileal juices). To these is added the dietary intake through food and drink (1.5–2 L/day). Therefore, the reabsorption of liquids represents an important mechanism of homeostasis of the organism that influences the general state of the individual (cardiovascular, respiratory, nervous, and urinary systems). About 9 of the 10 liters that pass through the intestine are reabsorbed by the ileum, about 900 cc are absorbed by the colon, so only 100 cc are expelled with the feces.

In addition to the fluids in the intestine, there is also a large amount of gas that comes mainly from oral ingestion during meals and from bacterial metabolism. The bacterial flora is present in preponderant quantities in the colon; therefore, the amount of gas present is greater in this part of the intestine than in the ileum. The microbial flora is made up of more than 500 different species and varies according to the location. In the mouth, anaerobes predominate on teeth and gums. From the stomach to the terminal ileum, the microbial load, consisting of Gram positive, is very low due to gastric acidity which destroys many bacteria.

The intestinal mucous membranes have efficient means to counteract the absorption of bacteria and toxins. The main defense mechanism is characterized by the presence of type A immunoglobulins (IgA), lymphocytes, and macrophages that do not allow bacterial intestinal translocation. When there is a mechanical or physical obstacle to the progression of intestinal contents, this causes an accumulation of liquids and gases upstream of the occlusion with a subsequent increase in the bacterial load, interrupting the normal balance between growth and elimination of germs.

The jejunoileal and small bowel occlusions reduce the hydro-electrolytic absorption both for the exclusion of the distal tract to the occlusion and for the ileal distension which determines alterations of the microcirculation and venous return to the parietal level with inversion of the flow of liquids through the mucosa moving from the intravascular to the intraluminal compartment. Consequently, there is an intraluminal sequestration of liquids, electrolytes, and proteins to which the parietal edema and the exudation of the serous side toward the peritoneal cavity (third space) are added. Additionally and often in complete occlusions, the patient vomits and loses fluids to the outside. Thus, dehydration is established with hyponatremia, hypokalemia, hypochloremia, and metabolic alkalosis. If the site of the intestinal obstruction is proximal, dehydration will occur faster (early vomiting). In distal ileal occlusions, on the other hand, vomiting is later, but abdominal distension may be more conspicuous.

The hydro-electrolytic alterations, when severe, can lead in the most cases to hypovolemic shock with a septic component due to intestinal bacterial translocation (septic-toxemic shock). This occurs above all in blind loop occlusions (volvulus, strangulated hernias) where a rapid alteration of the microcirculation is caused by acute and sudden parietal tension. Other alterations that occur in the patient with SBO are the changes in blood coagulation system linked to the reduced absorption of vitamin K and due to the interruption of the enteropoietic circulation of bile salts (in the biliary ileum or due to distal ileal occlusions).

Finally, the occlusive state can lead to cardiovascular and respiratory disorders. Hypokalemia led to heart rhythm alterations: ST segment elevation, T wave depression, and U wave elevation. These electrocardiographic changes are the instrumental manifestation of ventricular and supraventricular tachyarrhythmias, second and third degree up to ventricular fibrillation.

Bowel obstruction can lead to death whether it is treated surgically or not. Mortality appears to be related more to the speed of treatment, medical and/or surgical, than to its etiological cause. The main causes of death are cardiac failure, respiratory failure, and septic complications.

3   Clinical Presentation

ASBO results like the combination of different clinical signs and symptoms. The degree of intensity in clinical presentation gives an indication about the severity and the level of obstruction, sometimes the cause, even related to the history of the patient. Therefore, the degree of abdominal pain, tenderness and distension, amount and feature of vomiting, or nasogastric tube outputs (bilious vs feculent) could address to the level of the obstruction. A proximal bowel obstruction (duodenal-jejunal) is characterized by sudden, acute pain, and early vomiting with bile characteristics and absence of abdominal distention. On the other hand, a lower intestinal obstruction (ileum) is characterized by colic-like pain, abdominal distension, tenderness, and late vomiting with initially biliary and later feculent characteristics. In both cases, there can be a normal passage of stools especially at the beginning of the occlusion due to the emptying of the intestines distal to the occlusion.

ASBO can also occur with recurrent or chronic sub-occlusive syndromes. Patients who complain about digestive difficulties may have adhesive disease making the passage of food difficult. Patients may also present with a partial obstruction, which is often just a less severe clinical presentation of complete SBO.

The increase in the number of abdominal surgeries has led to an increased incidence of SBOs, although with the advent of laparoscopy, it seems that the incidence of obstructions due to postoperative adhesions has decreased. However, the laparoscopic techniques that use >10 mm trocars can cause SBOs due to hernia at the trocar site. The patient's surgical history should therefore always be carefully investigated, focusing on previous abdominal surgeries and the surgical technique used. Because hernias represent the most frequent cause of obstruction in non-operated patients, a meticulous inspection of all possible hernia sites is mandatory in every patient with clinical features of intestinal obstruction.

4 Laboratory Findings

Leukocytosis, usually greater than 10,000/mm^3, is almost always present with an SBO. White blood cell (WBC) counts greater than 20,000/mm^3 should prompt concern for bowel compromise or perforation in cases of ASBO.

The deficit of electrolytes can help us identify the level of obstruction (if intestinal obstruction is proximal, there is a greater loss of H+ ions). In pyloric occlusions, for instance, there is a metabolic alkalosis due to the great losses of gastric acids, while in proximal jejunal or duodenal occlusions, there is a metabolic acidosis due to the loss of the alkaline contents of the pancreatic and biliary secretions. It is useful to investigate renal function. The increase in blood urea nitrogen (BUN) and creatinine levels indicates a state of dehydration which can also lead to acute renal failure and even require dialysis treatment. Furthermore, the dilation of the intestinal loops and therefore the abdominal distension leads to the elevation of the diaphragm with a consequent reduction of the total lung volume and an increase in CO_2 levels with subsequent respiratory acidosis. Elevated levels of CRP (C-reactive protein) are a non-specific indicator of systemic inflammation of the organism and non-specific of intestinal obstruction, while high blood levels of procalcitonin may indicate peritoneal sepsis, for example, due to perforation of the intestine. Resulting from global hypoperfusion, a lactate level may be elevated.

5 Radiologic Diagnosis

Radiological examinations are essential for the diagnosis of mechanical intestinal obstruction and help us, more than anything else, to identify its localization. The first diagnostic step consists in performing an abdominal radiograph in the upright position and in the supine position. This simple and inexpensive test can quickly give us information about the presence of an occlusive picture. In a patient with a proximal intestinal obstruction, abdominal radiographs may show stomach distention only. When the site of the occlusion becomes distal, the presence of dilated intestinal loops with multiple air-fluid levels can be seen. The more numerous they are, more distal the occlusion site likely is. Furthermore, in the first hours immediately following the onset of the occlusive picture, direct examination of the abdomen can highlight the presence of mucous folds occupying the entire transverse diameter of the loops (conniving valves) which indicate an important peristaltic activity. Usually in cases of complete ASBO, gas in the large colon and rectum is absent. In the case of perforations, the radiograph can highlight the presence of extraluminal fluid or free abdominal air in the subdiaphragmatic area on upright films.

The second most performed diagnostic test in emergency rooms around the world in patients with acute abdominal pain is abdominal ultrasound. This examination, operator dependent, plays a secondary role in the diagnosis of intestinal obstruction because in the patient with an obstructive picture, the loops are so stretched by liquid and gas that the examination does not have a good diagnostic sensitivity and specificity. The importance of ultrasound, however, remains in the simplicity and speed of execution. An urgent/emergency ultrasound scan in a patient with a distended abdomen can demonstrate the presence of free air and endoperitoneal liquid. In addition, ultrasound can give us useful information to exclude pathologies of parenchymatous organs (kidneys, liver and biliary tract, adrenal gland, pancreas if visible) and is therefore an important test for the differential diagnosis in the acute abdomen.

Computed tomography (CT) with oral and intravenous contrast is an important examination in the patient with an occlusive picture. The CT gives us information about the site of the obstruction, the degree of severity, the presence of endoperitoneal fluid, and free abdominal air. Through CT, the location (jejunum, ileus, colorectal) and the cause of the occlusion (bridle, adhesion syndrome, ileal or colic stenosis, volvulus, invagination) can be determined. Furthermore, the CT allows us to study all the abdominal parenchymatous organs at the same time to search for any concomitant pathologies to the occlusive picture (primary, secondary, or benign tumors). Through CT, it is also possible to define whether there is ischemic distress in the affected intestine as it may show pneumatosis. CT can accurately predict the etiology of obstruction in 70–90% of patients. CT is most valuable when there are systemic signs suggesting infection, bowel infarction, or an associated palpable mass. CT signs of SBO (small bowel obstruction) include:

1. Dilated/distended air-filled or fluid-filled small bowel greater than 2.5–3 cm seen proximal to collapsed loops
2. Air-fluid levels greater than 2.5 cm or at disparate levels within the same loop that transverse the entire lumen of the obstructed bowel loops or trapped air bubbles between folds at the top of a fluid-filled bowel loop known as the string of pearls sign.
3. Gastric distention
4. Small bowel dilated out of proportion to colon
5. Absence of paucity of colorectal gas

Other radiological tests that can help us in the diagnosis of intestinal obstruction are transit X-ray with iodinated contrast medium (Gastrografin→) or barium taken orally. The presence of an ileal obstruction is demonstrated with stagnation of the contrast medium upstream of the occlusion. If the contrast arrives at the cecum in about 24 h, the obstruction is partial and presumably, it will resolve without operation.

Nuclear magnetic resonance is not used often in the emergency department and does not give us any further information than CT. However, it can be used in cases of sub-occlusions or recurrent mechanical obstruction, especially in Crohn's disease, to determine the localization of the stenosis and the degree of activity of the disease.

It is established by a multivariate analysis that the following factors predict the need for surgical resection: free peritoneal fluid at CT scan (more than 500 mL), reduction of CT bowel enhancement, abdominal pain persisting for 4 or more days, abdominal tenderness with guarding, WBC count >10,000/mm^3, and C-reactive protein >75 mg/L. In the analysis, all the patients with four or more variables required resection. In another multivariate analysis conducted to determine predictors of the need of operation in ASBO, it was found that vomiting, mesenteric edema on CT scan, and the lack of the small bowel feces sign are independent factors.

6   Treatment

ASBO is not necessarily a surgical indication, and it is not an urgency in any case. The most important factor to consider is the possible or suspected ischemic suffering of the intestine. If this possibility can be excluded thanks to the clinical signs and symptoms, laboratory and radiological tests, medical conservative therapy is the first therapeutic option. All patients with intestinal obstruction must be monitored from a clinical and vital functions by treating the hydro-electrolytic and volume alteration. The possibility of being able to delay the surgery, or in the best cases not to perform it, allows to stabilize the patient, his vital functions and to improve his general clinical condition.

If, on the other hand, intestinal ischemic suffering cannot be excluded, the intervention must not be postponed, but all those therapeutic strategies must still be started as soon as possible to rebuild body homeostasis.

6.1   Conservative Management

6.1.1   Patients' Selection

For patients presenting with acute adhesive small bowel obstruction (ASBO) without signs of strangulation, peritonitis, or severe intestinal impairment, there is good evidence to support nonoperative management (NOM).

Free intraperitoneal fluid, mesenteric edema, lack of the "small bowel feces sign" at CT scan, history of vomiting, severe abdominal pain, abdominal guarding, raised white cell count (WCC), and devascularized bowel at CT scan predict the need for emergent surgery.

Moreover, patients with repeated ASBO episodes, many prior laparotomies for adhesions, and prolonged conservative treatment should be cautiously selected to find out only those who may benefit of early surgical interventions.

At present, there is no consensus about when conservative treatment should be considered unsuccessful and the patient should undergo surgery: in fact the use of surgery to solve ASBO is controversial, as surgery induces the formation of new adhesions.

Data have shown that NOM can be successful in up to 90% of patients without peritonitis.

As a counterpart, a delay in operation for ASBO places patients at higher risk for bowel resection. A retrospective analysis showed that in patients with a $\leq$24-h wait time until surgery, only 12% experienced bowel resection, and in patients with a $\geq$24-h wait time until surgery, 29% required bowel resection.

Schraufnagel et al. showed that in their huge patient cohort complications, resection, prolonged length of stay, and death rates were higher in patients admitted for ASBO and operated on after a time period of ≥ 4 days.

The World Society of Emergency Surgery (WSES) 2018 guidelines stated that NOM in the absence of signs of ischemia or peritonitis can be prolonged up to 72 h. After 72 h of NOM without resolution, surgery is recommended.

There are no objective criteria that identify those patients who are likely to respond to conservative treatment. Less clear, in fact, is the way to predict between progression to strangulation and resolution of ASBO. Some authors suggested strong predictors of NOM failure: the presence of ascites, complete ASBO, increased serum creatine phosphokinase, and ≥ 500 mL from nasogastric tube on the third NOM day.

However, at any time, if there is an onset of signs of strangulation, peritonitis, or severe intestinal impairment, NOM should be discontinued, and surgery is recommended.

So, it's difficult to predict the risk of operation among those patients with ASBO initially undergone to NOM.

6.1.2 Medical Treatment

Medical conservative therapy consists of

1. Patient monitoring
2. Support of his vital functions
3. Bowel decompression upstream of the occlusion

Monitoring must be initiated immediately, especially in polypathological patients in critical general conditions. The measurement of blood pressure, body temperature, and 1-h diuresis are indispensable parameters. In the occluded patient, the positioning of the bladder catheter helps us not only to define the patient's diuresis but also to reduce the abdominal pressure. Adequate peripheral venous access is essential to start supportive therapy which consists of intravenous hydration with isotonic crystalloid liquids (for example, Ringer's lactate) whose infusion rate must be defined based on the characteristics of the patient and the central venous pressure which in any case must be maintained below 10 cm H_2O. The electrolyte deficit should be corrected with suitable intravenous solutions. The lack of Na^+ with isotonic physiological solution at 0.9% while a deficiency of K^+ with physiological solution added to KCl in an adequate quantity to correct the deficit.

The administration of antibiotics is not always necessary, especially in the absence of leukocytosis or increased inflammation indices. If there is fever and leukocytosis or in view of surgery, the infusion of first-line large-spectrum antibiotic therapy is indicated.

Supportive therapy alone helps to improve the patient's general clinical condition by re-establishing a valid diuresis and restoring acid-base balance by improving blood concentration.

Together with clinical monitoring and supportive therapy, a series of maneuvers must be implemented to decompress the intestine upstream of the obstruction. The placement of a nasogastric tube is useful for emptying the stomach and avoiding repeated episodes of vomiting, also reducing the risk of aspiration pneumonia. For challenging cases of ASBO, the long tube should be placed as soon as possible.

The administration of water-soluble contrast agent (WSCA) showed to be effective in several randomized studies and meta-analysis. Three meta-analyses showed no advantages in waiting longer than 8 h after the administration of WSCA and demonstrated that the presence of contrast in the colon within 4–24 h is predictive of AASBO resolution. Moreover, for patients undergoing nonoperative management, water-soluble contrast decreased the need for surgery and reduced the length of hospital stay.

The duration of conservative therapy varies from 12 to 72 h, after this time the patient enters in the emergency room. In this period, we can witness either the resolution of the occlusive picture or its persistence. In the first case, the patient will have passed stool and gas and will be able to resume an adequate oral diet. In the second case, the patient may be a candidate for surgery.

6.2 Surgical Treatment

According to the WSES evidence-based guidelines on diagnosis and management of ASBO, nonoperative management should always be tried in patients with adhesive small bowel obstruction, unless there are signs of peritonitis, strangulation, or bowel ischemia.

Historically, abdominal exploration through laparotomy has been the standard treatment for adhesive small bowel obstruction. In recent years, however, laparoscopic surgery for ASBO has been introduced. Surgical therapy varies according to the location of the obstruction and the underlying cause. If the surgery is performed in an emergency regime with the patient in critical general conditions, an important obstruction and the suspicion of vascular ischemic suffering, usually the most used surgical approach is the open surgery with median incision, though laparoscopy is not contraindicated, especially by surgeons with good expertise in emergency laparoscopic surgery (di saverio).

The potential benefits of laparoscopy include less extensive adhesion (re)formation, earlier return of bowel movements, reduced postoperative pain, and shorter length of stay.

The use of the laparoscopic technique in ASBO still seems to have a minority use in interventions made in the USA in emergency regime. In the analysis performed by Patel in 2018 on the data of the American College of Surgeons (ACS) through the National Surgical Quality Improvement Program, the data of 24,028 patients undergoing emergency surgery for ASBO from 2005 to 2011 were analyzed. Only 3391 interventions were performed laparoscopically, showing that the use of this technique in emergency for ASBO is still relatively low.

Laparoscopic adhesiolysis for small bowel obstruction has a number of potential advantages: less postoperative pain, faster return of intestinal function, shorter hospital stay, reduced recovery time, allowing an earlier return to full activity, fewer wound complications, and decreased postoperative adhesion formation.

In a recent international, multicentric, and randomized study on laparoscopic versus open adhesiolysis for adhesive small bowel obstruction (LASSO), 100 patients were included (49 in the open surgery group; 51 in the laparoscopy group). This study shows that the postoperative length of hospital stay for open surgery group was longer than that in the laparoscopy group and had most postoperative complications within 30 days. Laparoscopic adhesiolysis provides quicker recovery in selected patients with adhesive small bowel obstruction than open adhesiolysis.

Further recent reports confirmed that laparoscopic surgical management of acute ASBO is associated with quicker GI recovery, shorter LOS, and reduced overall complications compared to open surgery, without significant differences in operative times.

All recent meta-analyses published in the last 3 years (2018–2021) agree that laparoscopy is the treatment of choice in the treatment of ASBO in selected patients. The metanalysis of Quah in 2018 were studied a sample of 38,927 patients undergoing surgery for ASBO (5729 in the laparoscopic group and 33,389 in the open group). This study demonstrated that patients undergoing open surgery have more overall postoperative morbidity, respiratory complications, cardiac complications, wound complications, postoperative sepsis, intra-abdominal abscess venous thromboembolism (VTE), incisional hernia, urinary tract infections (UTI), renal complications, and mortality.

Similarly, Kriellen's 2020 meta-analysis demonstrated similar results on a total population of 37,007 patients. All the most recent studies agree in recommending laparoscopy as the technique of first choice in selected patients. It therefore becomes essential to understand which patients to offer this surgical technique compared to the traditional open technique. The study that most of all identified the characteristics of the patient suitable for undergoing laparoscopic surgery for ASBO is that of Valverde in 2019. Analyzing retrospectively the characteristics of the population undergoing laparoscopic surgery compared to the open one, it was seen that the patients who benefited from the laparoscopic approach were younger, with lower ASA, with fewer previous abdominal surgery operations and finding less adhesions at the time of intervention.

Although laparoscopic adhesiolysis requires a specific skill set and may not be appropriate in all patients, the laparoscopic approach demonstrates a clear benefit in 30-day morbidity and mortality even after controlling for preoperative patient characteristics.

Patient selection is still a controversial issue. From a recent consensus conference, a panel of experts recommended that the only absolute exclusion criteria for laparoscopic adhesiolysis in ASBO are those related to pneumoperitoneum [e.g., hemodynamic instability or cardiopulmonary impairment]; all other contraindications are relative and should be judged on a case-to-case basis, depending on the laparoscopic skills of the surgeon.

Nonetheless, it is now well known that the immune response correlates with inflammatory markers associated with injury severity and, as a consequence, the magnitude of surgical interventions may influence the clinical outcomes through the production of molecular factors, ultimately inducing systemic inflammatory response, and the beneficial effect of minimally invasive surgeries and of avoiding laparotomy is even more relevant in the frail patients.

Laparoscopic adhesiolysis is technically challenging, given the bowel distension and the risk of iatrogenic injuries if the small bowel is not appropriately handled. The technical steps consist in how to establish peritoneal access, how to do a safe bowel handling, and when to consider converting to open procedure.

It is very important to evaluate preoperative imaging, inspect the abdomen, and avoid previous surgical incisions. The open access in the abdominal cavity is the gold standard, usually away from previous surgical scars. The use of Veress technique is almost never recommended, but if the surgeon is familiar with this approach, the Veress needle is used in right upper quadrant or left upper quadrant. When the access is done, inspect the anterior abdominal wall with the laparoscopic camera for additional safe entry points. After the positioning of the trocar is important to use sharp dissection of adhesion and where it is possible avoid energy use. It is also mandatory to fully explore the small bowel starting from the cecum and running the small bowel distal to proximal until the transition point is found and the band/transition point identified. After the release of the band, the passage into distal bowel is restored, and the strangulation mark on the bowel wall is visible and should be carefully inspected. The intestine must never be manipulated directly if it is very distended due to the risk of iatrogenic perforation. If distended bowel must be grasped, ensure large bites that use the entire jaw of the grasper and always prefer the use of laparoscopic forceps with long bite to distribute the tension of the grip over a larger surface and always grasp the intestinal loops in two different places. Approximately 30% of cases that are initiated laparoscopically for SBO are converted to an open procedure. There are several critical moments in which the decision to convert to an open procedure should be considered, to avoid or repair injured bowel. If it is not possible to place trocars in correct positions, the conversion is mandatory. In addition, other causes of conversion are as follows: distal collapse bowel is not identified and grasped, the procedure is not advance for significant dilatation of the bowel, the intestine is ischemic, and a bowel resection is necessary when a bowel injury has occurred.

As a precaution and in the absence of advanced laparoscopic skills, a low threshold for open conversion should be maintained when extensive and matted adhesions are found.

6.3   Prevention of Adhesion After Adhesiolysis and Classification

Strategies for reduction of adhesions are based on their pathophysiological mechanisms of origin. Factors that may limit adhesion formation include preference for tissue-sparing and microinvasive surgical techniques, minimization of operating time and of heat, covering anastomosis and raw peritoneal surfaces and light and avoidance of peritoneal trauma by superfluous contact and coagulation. Before closure of the abdominal wall, therefore, it is advisable to perform careful—though not excessive, to avoid necrosis—hemostasis and irrigate repeatedly with saline and Ringer solution. In high-risk patients, the use of adjuvants that reduce adhesions can be applied. The 4% glucose polymer icodextrin is an adhesion-inhibiting peritoneal instillate. By virtue of its osmotic activity, it is thought to retain fluid in the peritoneal cavity for 3–4 days and keep organs and injured peritoneal surfaces separated from each other until it is eliminated via the kidneys. Comparison of icodextrin and Ringer's lactate revealed an advantage for the former with regard to the reduction of incidence (52% vs. 32%), extent (52% vs. 47%), and severity (65% vs. 37%) of adhesions. Clinical improvement was observed in 49% of patients following treatment with icodextrin, against 38% after Ringer's lactate. Carboxymethylcellulose (CMC) and polyethylene oxide (PEO) form a gel-like resorbable barrier to adhesions.

There is no universal classification of the severity of peritoneal adhesions. Adhesion's quantification and scoring may be useful for achieving standardized assessment of adhesions severity and for further research in prevention and treatment of ASBO. Among the numerous scores proposed for quantifying the severity of peritoneal adhesions, the one proposed by Coccolini and colleagues is one of the most comprehensive and simple to use. The Peritoneal Adhesion Index (PAI) in based on the macroscopic appearance of adhesion and their diffusion to different regions of the abdomen (See Fig. 1). Using these criteria, the PAI ranges from 0 to 30 describing in a detailed manner the abdominal adhesions pattern. By using a detailed and universal score, like the one proposed by Coccolino et al., surgeons from different centers will be able to compare the different patterns of peritoneal adhesion and employ the most appropriate treatment approach for each patient, distinguishing those at high risk and implementing adhesion-reducing adjuvants.

PERITONEAL ADHESION INDEX:

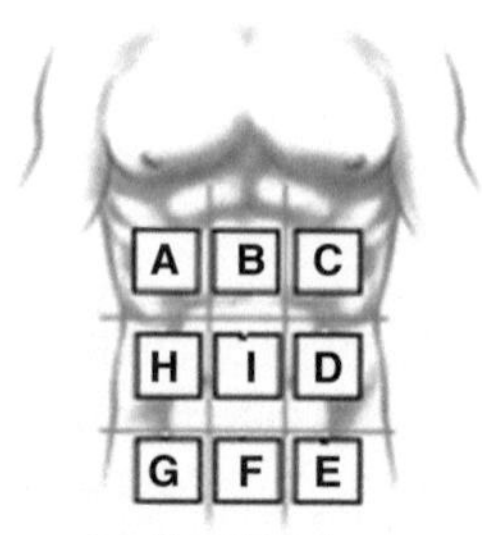

Regions:	Adhesion grade:	Adhesion grade score:
A Right upper	____	**0** No adhesions
B Epigastrium	____	**1** Filmy adhesions, blunt dissection
C Left upper	____	**2** Strong adhesions, sharp dissection
D Left flank	____	**3** Very strong vascularized adhesions, sharp dissection, damage hardly preventable
E Left lower	____	
F Pelvis	____	
G Right lower	____	
H Right flank	____	
I Central	____	
L Bowel to bowel	____	

PAI

Fig. 1 Peritoneal adhesion index: by ascribing to each abdomen area an adhesion related score as indicated, the sum of the scores will result in the PAI. (From Coccolini et al.: Peritoneal adhesion index (PAI): proposal of a score for the "ignored iceberg" of medicine and surgery. World Journal of Emergency Surgery 2013 8:6. Published under CC BY 4.0 https://creativecommons.org/licenses/by/4.0/legalcode)

Recommended Readings

1. ten Broek RPG, Issa Y, van Santbrink EJP, Bouvy ND, Kruitwagen RFPM, Jeekel J, Bakkum EA, Rovers MM, van Goor H. Burden of adhesions in abdominal and pelvic surgery: systematic review and met-analysis. BMJ. 2013;347:–f5588.
2. Loftus T, Moore F, VanZant E, et al. A protocol for the management of adhesive small bowel obstruction. J Trauma Acute Care Surg. 2015;78:13–21.

3. Millet I, Ruyer A, Alili C, Curros Doyon F, Molinari N, Pages E, Zins M, Taourel P. Adhesive small-bowel obstruction: value of CT in identifying findings associated with the effectiveness of nonsurgical treatment. Radiology. 2014;273:425–32.

4. Parker MC, Ellis H, Moran BJ, et al. Postoperative adhesions. Dis Colon Rectum. 2001;44:822–9.

5. Shi H, Wu B, Wan J, Liu W, Su B. The role of serum intestinal fatty acid binding protein levels and D-lactate levels in the diagnosis of acute intestinal ischemia. Clin Res Hepatol Gastroenterol. 2015;39:373–8.

6. Gerhardt RT, Nelson BK, Keenan S, Kernan L, MacKersie A, Lane MS. Derivation of a clinical guideline for the assessment of nonspecific abdominal pain: the guideline for abdominal pain in the ED setting (GAPEDS) phase 1 study. Am J Emerg Med. 2005;23:709–17.

7. Cook K. Evaluating acute abdominal pain in adults. J Am Acad Phys Assist. 2005;18:1–8.

8. Di Saverio S, Tugnoli G, Orlandi PE, Casali M, Catena F, Biscardi A, Pillay O, Baldoni F. A 73-year-old man with long-term immobility presenting with abdominal pain. PLoS Med. 2009;6:e1000092.

9. Mullan CP, Siewert B, Eisenberg RL. Small bowel obstruction. Am J Roentgenol. 2012;198:W105–17.

10. Jaffe TA, Martin LC, Thomas J, Adamson AR, DeLong DM, Paulson EK. Small-bowel obstruction: coronal reformations from isotropic voxels at 16-section multi–detector row CT. Radiology. 2006;238:135–42.

11. Branco BC, Barmparas G, Schnüriger B, Inaba K, Chan LS, Demetriades D. Systematic review and meta-analysis of the diagnostic and therapeutic role of water-soluble contrast agent in adhesive small bowel obstruction. Br J Surg. 2010;97:470–8.

12. Trésallet C, Lebreton N, Royer B, Leyre P, Godiris-Petit G, Menegaux F. Improving the management of acute adhesive small bowel obstruction with CT-scan and water-soluble contrast medium: a prospective study. Dis Colon Rectum. 2009;52:1869–76.

13. Grassi R, Romano S, D'Amario F, Giorgio Rossi A, Romano L, Pinto F, Di Mizio R. The relevance of free fluid between intestinal loops detected by sonography in the clinical assessment of small bowel obstruction in adults. Eur J Radiol. 2004;50:5–14.

14. Di Saverio S, Catena F, Ansaloni L, Gavioli M, Valentino M, Pinna AD. Water-soluble contrast medium (Gastrografin) value in adhesive small intestine obstruction (Asio): a prospective, randomized, controlled, clinical trial. World J Surg. 2008;32:2293–304.

15. ten Broek RPG, Krielen P, Di Saverio S, et al. Bologna guidelines for diagnosis and management of adhesive small bowel obstruction (ASBO): 2017 update of the evidence-based guidelines from the world society of emergency surgery ASBO working group. World J Emerg Surg. 2018;13:24. https://doi.org/10.1186/s13017-018-0185-2.

16. Farid M, Fikry A, El Nakeeb A, Fouda E, Elmetwally T, Yousef M, Omar W. Clinical impacts of oral Gastrografin follow-through in adhesive small bowel obstruction (SBO). J Surg Res. 2010;162:170–6.

17. Leung AM, Vu H. Factors predicting need for and delay in surgery in small bowel obstruction. Am Surg. 2012;78:403–7.

18. Schraufnagel D, Rajaee S, Millham FH. How many sunsets? Timing of surgery in adhesive small bowel obstruction. J Trauma Acute Care Surg. 2013;74:181–9.

19. Diaz JJ, Bokhari F, Mowery NT, et al. Guidelines for management of small bowel obstruction. J Trauma. 2008;64:1651–64.

20. Abbas S, Bissett I, Parry B. Oral water soluble contrast for the management of adhesive small bowel obstruction. Cochrane Database Syst Rev. 2004.

21. Chen S-C, Chang K-J, Lee P-H, Wang S-M, Chen K-M, Lin F-Y. Oral urografin in postoperative small bowel obstruction. World J Surg. 1999;23:1051–4.

22. Vettoretto N, Carrara A, Corradi A, et al. Laparoscopic adhesiolysis: consensus conference guidelines. Color Dis. 2012;14:e208–15.

23. Di Saverio S. Emergency laparoscopy. J Trauma Acute Care Surg. 2014;77:338–50.

24. Catena F, Di Saverio S, Ansaloni L, Pinna A, Lupo M, Mirabella A, Mandalà V. Adhesive small bowel obstruction. In: The role of laparoscopy in emergency abdominal surgery. Milan: Springer Milan; 2012. p. 89–104.
25. Catena F, Saverio SD, Ansaloni L, Coccolini F, Sartelli M. CT scan in abdominal emergency surgery. Springer; 2018.
26. Saverio SD, Catena F, Ansaloni L, Coccolini F, Velmahos G. Acute care surgery handbook, vol. 2. Common gastrointestinal and abdominal emergencies. Springer; 2017.
27. Di Saverio S, Birindelli A, Broek RT, Davies JR, Mandrioli M, Sallinen V. Laparoscopic adhesiolysis: not for all patients, not for all surgeons, not in all centres. Updates Surg. 2018;70:557–61.
28. Sallinen V, Di Saverio S, Haukijärvi E, et al. Laparoscopic versus open adhesiolysis for adhesive small bowel obstruction (LASSO): an international, multicentre, randomised, open-label trial. Lancet Gastroenterol Hepatol. 2019;4:278–86.
29. Sebastian-Valverde E, Poves I, Membrilla-Fernández E, Pons-Fragero MJ, Grande L. The role of the laparoscopic approach in the surgical management of acute adhesive small bowel obstruction. BMC Surg. 2019;19:40. https://doi.org/10.1186/s12893-019-0504-x.
30. Behman R, Nathens AB, Byrne JP, Mason S, Look Hong N, Karanicolas PJ. Laparoscopic surgery for adhesive small bowel obstruction is associated with a higher risk of bowel injury. Ann Surg. 2017;266:489–98.
31. Behman R, Nathens AB, Karanicolas PJ. Laparoscopic surgery for small bowel obstruction. Adv Surg. 2018;52:15–27.
32. Quah GS, Eslick GD, Cox MR. Laparoscopic versus open surgery for adhesional small bowel obstruction: a systematic review and meta-analysis of case–control studies. Surg Endosc. 2018;33:3209–17.
33. Hackenberg T, Mentula P, Leppäniemi A, Sallinen V. Laparoscopic versus open surgery for acute adhesive small-bowel obstruction: a propensity score–matched analysis. Scand J Surg. 2016;106:28–33.
34. Kelly KN, Iannuzzi JC, Rickles AS, Garimella V, Monson JRT, Fleming FJ. Laparotomy for small-bowel obstruction: first choice or last resort for adhesiolysis? A laparoscopic approach for small-bowel obstruction reduces 30-day complications. Surg Endosc. 2013;28:65–73.
35. Krielen P, Di Saverio S, ten Broek R, Renzi C, Zago M, Popivanov G, Ruscelli P, Marzaioli R, Chiarugi M, Cirocchi R. Laparoscopic versus open approach for adhesive small bowel obstruction, a systematic review and meta-analysis of short term outcomes. J Trauma Acute Care Surg. 2020;88:866–74.
36. Mazzetti CH, Serinaldi F, Lebrun E, Lemaitre J. Early laparoscopic adhesiolysis for small bowel obstruction: retrospective study of main advantages. Surg Endosc. 2017;32:2781–92.
37. Miyake H, Seo S, Pierro A. Laparoscopy or laparotomy for adhesive bowel obstruction in children: a systematic review and meta-analysis. Pediatr Surg Int. 2017;34:177–82.
38. Patel R, Borad NP, Merchant AM. Comparison of outcomes following laparoscopic and open treatment of emergent small bowel obstruction: an 11-year analysis of ACS NSQIP. Surg Endosc. 2018;32:4900–11.
39. Pei KY, Asuzu D, Davis KA. Will laparoscopic lysis of adhesions become the standard of care? Evaluating trends and outcomes in laparoscopic management of small-bowel obstruction using the American College of Surgeons National Surgical Quality Improvement Project Database. Surg Endosc. 2016;31:2180–6.
40. Sajid MS, Khawaja AH, Sains P, Singh KK, Baig MK. A systematic review comparing laparoscopic vs open adhesiolysis in patients with adhesional small bowel obstruction. Am J Surg. 2016;212:138–50.
41. Catena F, De Simone B, Coccolini F, Di Saverio S, Sartelli M, Ansaloni L. Bowel obstruction: a narrative review for all physicians. World J Emerg Surg. 2019;14:20. https://doi.org/10.1186/s13017-019-0240-7.
42. Frago R, Ramirez E, Millan M, Kreisler E, del Valle E, Biondo S. Current management of acute malignant large bowel obstruction: a systematic review. Am J Surg. 2014;207:127–38.

43. Downes TJ, Cheruvu MS, Karunaratne TB, De Giorgio R, Farmer AD. Pathophysiology, diagnosis, and management of chronic intestinal pseudo-obstruction. J Clin Gastroenterol. 2018;52:477–89.

44. UpToDate. https://www.uptodate.com/contents/management-of-small-bowel-obstruction-in-adults?search=adhesive%20small%20bowel%20obstruction&source=search_result&selectedTitle=2~13&usage_type=default&display_rank=2. Accessed 13 June 2021.

45. UpToDate. https://www.uptodate.com/contents/etiologies-clinical-manifestations-and-diagnosis-of-mechanical-small-bowel-obstruction-in-adults?search=adhesive%20small%20bowel%20obstruction&source=search_result&selectedTitle=3~13&usage_type=default&display_rank=3. Accessed 13 June 2021.

46. diZerega GS, Verco SJS, Young P, et al. A randomized, controlled pilot study of the safety and efficacy of 4% icodextrin solution in the reduction of adhesions following laparoscopic gynaecological surgery. Hum Reprod. 2002;17:1031–8.

47. Kossi J, Gronlund S, Uotila-Nieminen M, Crowe A, Knight A, Keranen U. The effect of 4% icodextrin solution on adhesiolysis surgery time at the Hartmann's reversal: a pilot, multicentre, randomized control trial vs lactated Ringer's solution. Color Dis. 2009;11:168–72.

48. Brüggmann D, Tchartchian G, Wallwiener M, Münstedt K, Tinneberg HR, Hackethal A. Intra-abdominal adhesions: definition, origin, significance in surgical practice, and treatment options. Dtsch Arztebl Int. 2010;107(44):769–75. https://doi.org/10.3238/arztebl.2010.0769.

49. Coccolini F, et al. Peritoneal adhesion index (PAI): proposal of a score for the "ignored iceberg" of medicine and surgery. World J Emerg Surg. 2013;8:6.

Large Bowel Obstructions

Elisa Reitano, Aleix Martínez-Pérez, and Nicola de'Angelis

1 Introduction

Large bowel obstructions (LBOs) are defined as a partial or complete interruption of the normal flow of the luminal continent of the colon. LBO can be secondary to both mechanical and functional diseases [1]. They are less frequent than small bowel obstructions (SBO), but they still represent the 25% of all intestinal obstructions [2]. Patients with LBO frequently exhibit abdominal pain and abdominal distension, nausea, vomiting, and constipation. Depending on the clinical scenario, different management strategies could be required to achieve a successful resolution [3]. The present chapter provides an overview of LBOs, describing the most common causes, the diagnosis, and the different therapeutic alternatives. A multidisciplinary teamwork is pivotal to mitigate the risk of severe complications and the long-term morbidity after LBO.

1.1 Epidemiology

Bowel obstructions are a relevant cause of morbidity and mortality, resulting in 30,000 deaths every year, and more than $3 billion/year of direct medical costs [3]. LBOs account for approximately 2–4% of the overall emergency surgical

E. Reitano
Division of General Surgery, Department of Translational Medicine, Maggiore della Carità Hospital, University of Eastern Piedmont, Novara, Italy
e-mail: 20042156@studenti.uniupo.it

A. Martínez-Pérez · N. de'Angelis (✉)
Service de Chirurgie Colorectale et Digestive, DMU DIGEST, Hôpital Universitaire Beaujon, AP-HP, Clichy, and Faculty of Medecine, Université Paris Cité, Paris, France
e-mail: aleix.martinez@campusviu.es

F. Coccolini et al. (eds.), *Mini-invasive Approach in Acute Care Surgery*,
Hot Topics in Acute Care Surgery and Trauma,
https://doi.org/10.1007/978-3-031-39001-2_11

admissions. Different predictors for LBOs have been described, and they include prior abdominal surgery, colorectal cancer, inflammatory bowel disease (IBD), abdominal wall and inguinal hernias, irradiation, and foreign body ingestion [4]. There is no difference between the sex, and they can occur at any age. However, LBO are more frequent in the elderly, as cancer constitutes its commonest cause [5].

1.2 Etiology

The etiopathology of LBOs is substantially different from SBOs. LBO can occur secondary to a functional disorder or due to mechanical obstruction. The main causes of LBOs are listed in Table 1 [6–8]. Colorectal cancer (CRC) is the responsible of 60% of LBO cases [9]. In 3/4 of them, the obstruction is placed distally to the splenic flexure, with the commonest location being the sigmoid colon. According to the National Institute for Clinical Excellence (NICE), up to 30% of cases of CRC are diagnosed in the emergency setting, and approximately 15% of these patients present with LBO [6, 7]. Mechanical LBOs are mainly produced by cancer, diverticulitis, volvulus, hernias, and adhesions. Endometriosis, bezoars, chronic ischemia, inflammatory bowel disease (IBD), intussusception, irradiation, post-anastomotic stenosis, gallstones, foreign bodies, and tuberculosis have been also described [3].

Functional LBOs are characterized by the development of signs and symptoms of mechanical obstruction, without appreciable anatomical condition altering the normal flow of the intestinal content [6, 10]. Functional LBOs are often related to

Table 1 Common and uncommon causes of LBOs

Causes of mechanical LBO	
Common (>95%)	**Uncommon (<5%)**
• Primary colon carcinoma (60–80%) • Volvulus (11–15%) of the sigmoid, cecum, or transverse colon • Complicated diverticulitis (4–10%)	• Intussusception • Hernia • Inflammatory bowel disease • Extrinsic compression (e.g., abscess) • Fecal impaction • Bezoars • Lymphoma • Peritoneal carcinomatosis • Foreign body ingestion • Endometriosis • Stenosis (ischemia, radiation, anastomosis) • Post-operative adhesions • Gallstones • Tuberculosis • Trauma • Neurofibromatosis
Causes of functional LBO	
Common	**Uncommon**
• Narcotic/medication use (opiates, anticholinergics, amphetamines, steroids) • Ogilvie's syndrome	• Autoimmune diseases • Infection diseases

narcotic use, medication intake (e.g., opiates, anticholinergics, amphetamines, steroids), systemic illnesses such as sepsis or toxic megacolon (e.g., *Clostridium Difficile* infection), and severe acute colitis [1]. A particular form of functional LBOs is the Ogilvie's syndrome, which is an acute colonic pseudo-obstruction characterized by a massive colonic dilatation. This syndrome is related to abnormalities involving the autonomic control system of the colonic motility [6, 7].

1.3   Classification

Mechanical LBOs can be classified as a partial, complete, or closed loop occlusions. In this latter type, there is a complete obstruction proximal and distal to a given colonic segment [10]. LBO can be similarly classified in simple or complicated forms. In complicated obstructions, the vascular supply of the colon is compromised, then implying a subsequent risk of ischemia, necrosis, and ultimately, colonic perforation [7].

1.4   Pathophysiology

The presentation of LBO depends on the competency of the ileocecal valve [8]. When this valve is not competent, the large bowel is decompressed toward the small bowel. A competent ileocecal valve is present in the 75% of cases, hampering the colonic decompression and leading to a closed loop obstruction. This result in a marked increase of the intraluminal pressure leading to wall distension and finally to perforation [6, 8]. Following Laplace's law, the intraluminal pressure required to stretch the wall of a tube is inversely proportional to its radius. Given its larger diameter, the cecum is the segment with the highest risk of perforation [3, 9, 10].

2   Diagnosis

2.1   Clinical Presentation

LBO may develop acutely or over a protracted period [2]. However, the clinical presentation is most often sudden and associated with acute signs and symptoms, such as abdominal pain and distension. Vomiting is relatively a late symptom of LBO and is more common in SBO [1]. Patients with LBO may present with signs of hypovolemia due to fluid loss into the dilated bowel. They can be accompanied by electrolyte imbalances and metabolic alkalosis as a consequence of vomiting and dehydration [11]. Laboratory tests including blood cell count, renal function, and electrolytes are of paramount importance to help the diagnosis. Marked leukocytosis and acidosis with low bicarbonate and high lactic levels could be reflecting an ongoing intestinal ischemia [1, 3]. A prompt diagnosis and establishing the cause of LBO is of paramount important given the high associated morbidity and mortality.

Indeed, the nature of the obstruction will influence the treatment choice, which ranges from medical and endoscopic therapies to surgical resections or bowel decompressions via an ostomy formation [9].

2.2   Tests

2.2.1   Abdominal Plain Radiography and Ultrasound

Abdominal plain X-ray represents the first imaging evaluation when LBBO is suspected. The examination should include supine and upright or left-lateral decubitus projections to diagnose LBO and its possible complications such as pneumatosis and pneumoperitoneum [6]. Abdominal radiography has shown a sensitivity of 84% and a specificity of 72% in the diagnosis of LBO [3, 6]. Normal colonic caliber ranges from 3 to 8 cm, with the largest diameter in the cecum. Colonic dilatation is diagnosed when the caliber is >9 cm in the cecum or >6 cm in any other segment. In the setting of an LBO, abdominal radiography usually shows the dilation of the colon proximally to the site of the obstruction and the absence of distal gas [6, 7]. The presence of air-fluid levels in the dilated colon suggests an acute obstruction since the colonic fluid has not been present enough time to be absorbed [6] (Figs. 1 and 2).

The main disadvantage of plain radiology is that it usually does not provide an etiological diagnosis [3]. Administration of water-soluble contrasts increases the sensitivity to 96% and the specificity to 98% but obtaining the etiological diagnosis is usually unfeasible [12]. This exploration has been widely used in the diagnosis

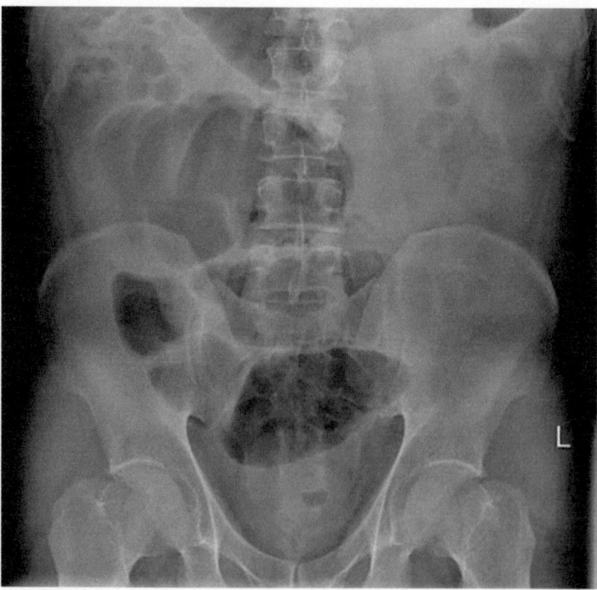

Fig. 1 Anteroposterior supine abdominal radiograph in a 72-year-old man with LBO showing dilated transverse and descending colon due to an ascending colon carcinoma

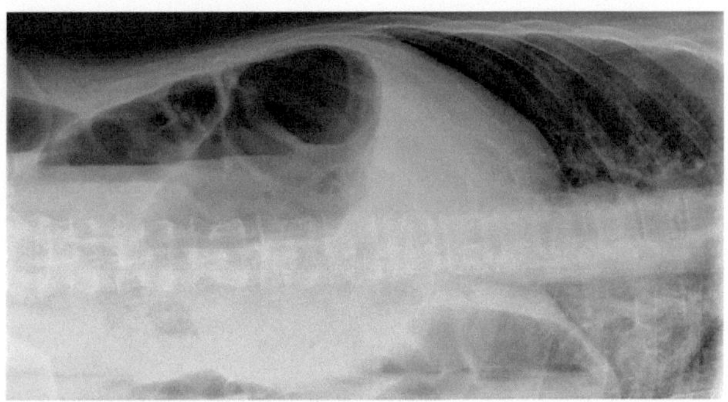

Fig. 2 Right lateral decubitus radiograph in LBO due to an ascending colon carcinoma

and management of adhesive SBO. The inability of the contrast agent to reach the colon during 24 h at a plain X-ray is highly indicative of the failure of a non-operative management for SBO [12, 13]. Abdominal ultrasound, conversely, allows to establish an etiological diagnosis of LBO. However, the success of the exploration highly depends on the experience of the radiologist and on the physical characteristics of the patient [14].

2.2.2 Computed Tomography and Magnetic Resonance Imaging

Computed tomography (CT) with intravenous contrast administration is superior to both plain X-ray and ultrasound to provide an etiological diagnosis of LBO, allowing for a more accurate preoperative management [6, 15]. The administration of water-soluble rectal contrast may be useful if diagnostic doubts persist after the CT [15]. Moreover, CT allows to perform an accurate staging of the neoplastic bowel obstructions and identify possible complications, such as a perforation [16]. Despite the disadvantage of an increased irradiation compared to the previously described techniques, CT is the gold standard imaging exploration for LBO having a high sensitivity (96%) and specificity (93%) [17]. Intravenous contrast agent is recommended to identify the presence of masses, signs of inflammation, and bowel wall ischemia. Iodinated intravenous contrast agent can be administrated following a weight-based protocol, or in a routine volume (e.g., 150 mL) and 3 mL/s rate with a delay of 70 s, to allow portal venous phase imaging [6, 16, 17].

Beyond the risk linked to radiation exposure, allergic reactions to intravascular iodinated contrasts and renal failure in patients with underlying kidney diseases must be considered. According to the current guidelines, prophylaxis with corticosteroid and antihistamine should be administered in patients with a history of moderate/severe allergic reactions to iodinated contrast or when the reaction severity is unknown [18]. Hydration therapy should be administered in patients with kidney diseases due to the risk of contrast induced nephropathy [19]. In children and during pregnancy, magnetic resonance imaging (MRI) should be preferred over CT to avoid the exposure to ionizing radiations [20]. MRI had a sensitivity of 95% and specificity of 100% for LBO diagnosis [20] (Fig. 3).

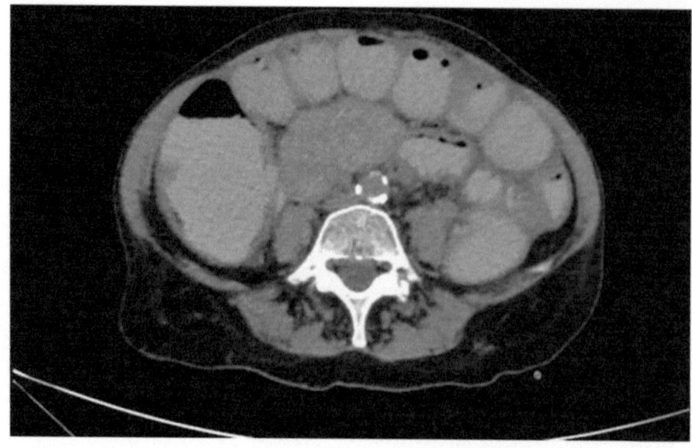

Fig. 3 CT scan showing a LBO with dilated transverse, descending, and ascending colon due to a rectal carcinoma

2.2.3 Colonoscopy

CRC may present with LBO in 15–20% of cases [17]. According to the American Society for Gastrointestinal Endoscopy (ASGE), the colonoscopy is contraindicated in patients with severe unremitting pain or peritoneal signs with a complete colonic obstruction or presenting with bowel ischemia [21]. Patients with partial colonic obstruction may undergo endoscopy after IV hydration, electrolytes correction, and nasogastric tube placement. Endoscopic evaluation of a left-side colonic obstruction by flexible sigmoidoscopy or a limited colonoscopy allows to confirm the site of obstruction, to apply anal tubes, stents, or endoscope decompression with no bowel preparation [21]. Endoscopic evaluation of the right side of the colon is challenging and requires an adequate bowel preparation with a higher risk of perforation [21]. If contrast enemas are used, water-soluble are of choice, to avoid barium peritonitis in patients with an unrecognized perforation. Colonoscopy facilitates a histological diagnosis of the bowel occlusion providing tissue biopsy for analysis [3]. Moreover, tattooing of the pathologic segment could guide the surgeon during further surgical procedure.

3 Therapy

3.1 Medical Treatment

In hemodynamically stable patients without signs of sepsis or peritonitis, the initial treatment consists of fluid resuscitation with correction of electrolyte imbalances, gastrointestinal decompression through a nasogastric tube, and close monitoring of the diuresis [3]. The conservative treatment is not indicated in patients with mechanical LBO with severe pain or in those with signs of peritonitis: in these cases, surgery should be considered as the first therapeutic option [3]. Patients with malignant LBO could undergo surgery or endoscopic/interventional radiology treatment, after restoring the electrolyte unbalance (Fig. 4). Non-operative management could be the definitive treatment in cases of inflammatory LBO (e.g., IBD or acute diverticulitis without peritonitis) [22]. Complicated abdominal hernias without signs of

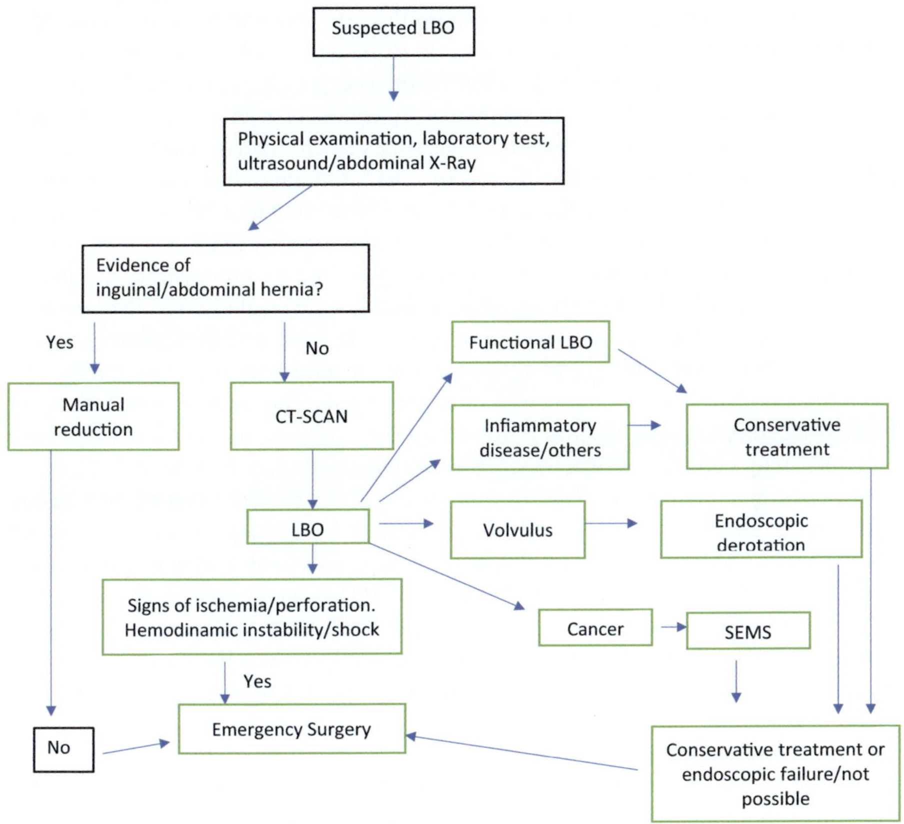

Fig. 4 Flowchart of diagnosis and treatment of LBO

ischemia/perforation can be reduced manually, reserving surgery for unsuccessful cases [23].

In Ogilvie's syndrome, the treatment aims to relieve the patient's discomfort and to prevent colonic complications, consisting in supportive care for 24–48 h. If failure occurs, different options may be considered such as neostigmine and erythromycin use, endoscopic decompression, or surgery, which is mandatory in patients who develop signs of peritonitis [6].

3.1.1 Endoscopy

The endoscopic management has a role in selected patients presenting with LBO secondary to malignant or benign conditions. Endoscopic placement of a transanal tube for decompression in malignant colonic obstructions represents an alternative to diverting decompressive stoma, allowing for 78–100% of patients to undergo one-stage surgery [21]. However, it is noteworthy to recognize that these tubes are not routinely used because of different limitations such as tube malfunction, expulsion, or severe patient discomfort.

Sigmoid volvulus can be treated with endoscopic derotation, while surgery is indicated in cases of endoscopic failure, or in patients with cecal volvulus [24]. Patients with IBD, diverticulitis, previous colonic surgery, or radiation therapy may develop colon stenosis. They can be treated by endoscopic dilation or stent placement [21, 24]. The endoscopic stenting constitutes an alternative strategy to manage colonic obstructions, especially in case of CRC. Colonic stent for malignancies were first used in the early 1990s, and they have been used as a bridge to surgery or with palliative intention [25]. Self-expandable metal stents (SEMS) allow for the decompression of the proximal colon, making possible to administrate a standard bowel preparation and to further perform an endoscopic evaluation of the proximal colon. This can be useful to detect synchronous lesions and to perform a quasi-elective surgery [25]. Elective resections are associated with lower morbidity and mortality compared with emergency procedures [3]. The main complications of SEMS placement are perforation followed by stent migration, and cancer regrowth into the stent causing obstruction [26]. According to the European Society of Gastrointestinal Endoscopy (ESGE) guidelines, given the high risk of perforation with cancer cell dissemination, SEMS placement as a bridge to surgery should always be discussed within a multidisciplinary team as a treatment option in patients with potentially curable left-sided obstructing CRC as an alternative to emergency surgery [26]. SEMS, however, are the preferred palliative treatment in malignant left-colon obstructions [25]. SEMS cannot be considered as a long-term solution in benign obstructions, but they could be helpful as a bridge to surgery [25, 26].

3.1.2 Interventional Radiology

In the last years, several studies suggested the placement of colonic self-expanded stent under fluoroscopic guide as a palliative treatment in oncologic patients not fit for surgery [26]. This minimal-invasive technique allows the stent placement without the need of colonic preparation [27]. Moreover, angiographic catheters with variable head shapes and easily shapeable guidewires can overcome the angulated obstructions, allowing the placement of stents otherwise not possible to place endoscopically [27, 28]. A hybrid approach with combined endoscopy and fluoroscopy could be used in technically challenging cases. Indeed, most of the malignant strictures are located distal to the splenic flexure. In this segment, endoscopy allows an easier negotiation of tortuous bowel loops and SEMS delivery to other locations such as the ascending or transverse colon [28].

Finally, some authors suggested the possibility to perform cecostomy or colostomy under image-guidance, with high technical success [29]. Despite the data is still limited, interventional radiology could represent a relevant tool for decompressive or palliative purposes in selected patients.

3.2 Surgery

Surgery is the treatment of choice of mechanical LBO. The type of surgery depends on the underlying disease. Non-reducible abdominal and inguinal hernias must undergo prosthetic repair. In some cases with associated perforation and highly contaminated surgical field, a direct suture can be considered to avoid mesh infection [30]. Explorative laparoscopy can be performed to assess the vitality of the bowel after the reduction of complicated hernias [30].

CRC determining bowel occlusion and benign obstruction irresponsive to medical therapy may require surgery and bowel resection as well. The type of surgery to performed depend on the patient's and disease characteristics, which are detailed below.

3.2.1 Right-Sided Obstruction

Right-sided obstruction can be treated with right-hemicolectomy with ileocolic anastomosis. It is considered the treatment of choice with low rates of anastomotic leak (AL) [1]. When a primary anastomosis is judged unsafe, a terminal ileostomy or an ileo-colostomy can be performed [31]. In the event of unresectable cancers causing obstruction, a loop ileostomy, or an ileocolic bypass (i.e., between the terminal ileum and the transverse colon), is the treatment of choice [32, 33]. Cecostomy with decompressive purpose is no longer performed due to the high complications rate [31]. Endoscopic stent placement is not recommended in right colic occlusions due to its technical difficulty, and the high migration and complications rates [26–28].

3.2.2 Left-Sided Obstruction

Left-sided obstruction can be treated with resection and primary anastomosis [33]. The current literature shows no evidence that a diverting stoma decreases the risk of AL [33–35]. However, in patients with high surgical risk, the Hartmann procedure (HP) should be preferentially considered. It consists in the resection of the primary lesion and the creation of a left colostomy [36]. A HP avoids the risk of AL while insuring an oncologic resection during the first operation [36]. However, HP reversal surgery is associated with high morbidity and mortality rates, and the effective stoma reversion rate after HP for CRC is limited (approximately 20%) [37, 38]. Patients unfit to major surgery or with unresectable lesions can be treated with loop colostomy as a bridge to surgery or with palliative purposes (when endoscopic stent placement is unfeasible) [35, 36]. Subtotal colectomy (SC) with ileo-sigmoid or ileo-rectal anastomosis is an alternative to stoma creation in patients with left-sided obstructions with the advantage to remove any possible compromised and dilated segment of the colon and any possible synchronous colonic neoplasms [39]. However, SC is burdened by a strong impact on the quality of life, a risk of dehydration, the need for dietary restrictions, and a reduction in the daily activity [40]. Therefore, it should be reserved to selected patients. Figure 4 reported the flowchart of LBO diagnosis and treatment.

3.3 Prognosis

LBO are usually an abdominal emergency, with relevant morbidity and mortality rates, if left untreated, due to the high risk of perforation and subsequent peritonitis

[6]. Recent studies reported a morbidity rate of 42–46% and a mortality rate of 13–19% following surgery for LBO [6].

The prognosis the LBO patients depends on the cause of the obstruction, with a life expectancy of 1–9 months for patients with malignant LBO [2, 3]. However, different factors (e.g., previous surgery, age $\geq$ 75 years old, male sex, comorbidities) may impact on the prognosis [6]. Recognizing the cause of LBO and providing a timely and appropriate treatment are pivotal for the patient's prognosis.

Take Home Messages
- LBO remain as one of the most frequent abdominal emergency conditions, with several different underlying causes.
- CT scan is the gold standard radiologic exploration to diagnose an LBO, providing etiological and anatomical information to choose the best treatment strategy.
- Endoscopic or interventional radiology are treatments which can be applied in selected patients. Surgery is required in the majority of the cases.
- The best strategy to adopt should be discussed in a multidisciplinary staff.

References

1. Sawai R. Management of colonic obstruction: a review. Clin Colon Rectal Surg. 2012;25(4):200–3. https://doi.org/10.1055/s-0032-1329533.
2. Markogiannakis H, Messaris E, Dardamanis D, et al. Acute mechanical bowel obstruction: clinical presentation, etiology, management and outcome. World J Gastroenterol. 2007;13:432–7. https://doi.org/10.3748/wjg.v13.i3.432.
3. Catena F, De Simone B, Coccolini F, et al. Bowel obstruction: a narrative review for all physicians. World J Emerg Surg. 2019;14:20. https://doi.org/10.1186/s13017-019-0240-7.
4. Andersen P, Jensen KK, Erichsen R, Frøslev T, Krarup PM, Madsen MR, Laurberg S, Iversen LH. Nationwide population-based cohort study to assess risk of surgery for adhesive small bowel obstruction following open or laparoscopic rectal cancer resection. BJS Open. 2017;1(2):30–8.
5. Doshi R, Desai J, Shah Y, Decter D, Doshi S. Incidence, features, in-hospital outcomes and predictors of in-hospital mortality associated with toxic megacolon hospitalizations in the United States. Intern Emerg Med. 2018;13(6):881–7.
6. Jaffe T, Thompson WM. Large-bowel obstruction in the adult: classic radiographic and CT findings, etiology, and mimics. Radiology. 2015;275(3):651–63. https://doi.org/10.1148/radiol.2015140916.
7. Farkas NG, Welman TJP, Ross T, Brown S, Smith JJ, Pawa N. Unusual causes of large bowel obstruction. Curr Probl Surg. 2019;56(2):49–90.
8. Ramanathan S, Ojili V, Vassa R, Nagar A. Large bowel obstruction in the emergency department: imaging spectrum of common and uncommon causes. J Clin Imaging Sci. 2017;7:15.
9. Kim YJ. Surgical treatment of obstructed left-sided colorectal cancer patients. Ann Coloproctol. 2014;30:245–6. https://doi.org/10.3393/ac.2014.30.6.245.
10. Smothers L, Hynan L, Fleming J, et al. Emergency surgery for colon carcinoma. Dis Colon Rectum. 2003;46:24–30. https://doi.org/10.1007/s10350-004-6492-6.
11. Van Oudheusden TR, Aerts BAC, de Hingh IHJT, et al. Challenges in diagnosing adhesive small bowel obstruction. World J Gastroenterol. 2013;19(43):7489–93. https://doi.org/10.3748/wjg.v19.i43.7489.

12. Ceresoli M, Coccolini F, Catena F, et al. Water-soluble contrast agent in adhesive small bowel obstruction: a systematic review and meta-analysis of diagnostic and therapeutic value. Am J Surg. 2016;211(6):1114–25. https://doi.org/10.1016/j.amjsurg.2015.06.012.

13. Branco BC, Barmparas G, Schnüriger B, et al. Systematic review and meta-analysis of the diagnostic and therapeutic role of water-soluble contrast agent in adhesive small bowel obstruction. Br J Surg. 2010;97(4):470–8. https://doi.org/10.1002/bjs.7019.

14. Hollerweger A, Wüstner M, Dirks K. Bowel obstruction: sonographic evaluation. Ultraschall Med. 2015;36:216–38. https://doi.org/10.1055/s-0034-1399292.

15. Frager D. Intestinal obstruction role of CT. Gastroenterol Clin North Am. 2002;31(3):777–99. https://doi.org/10.1016/s0889-8553(02)00026-2.

16. Hayakawa K, Tanikake M, Yoshida S, et al. Radiological diagnosis of large-bowel obstruction: neoplastic etiology. Emerg Radiol. 2013;20(1):69–76. https://doi.org/10.1007/s10140-012-1088-2.

17. Frago R, Ramirez E, Millan M, et al. Current management of acute malignant large bowel obstruction: a systematic review. Am J Surg. 2014;207(1):127–38. https://doi.org/10.1016/j.amjsurg.2013.07.027.

18. American College of Radiology (ACR) Committee on Drugs and Contrast Media. ACR manual on contrast media, version 10.2. 2016. http://www.acr.org/quality-safety/resources/contrast-manual. Accessed 2 Aug 2016.

19. Isaka Y, Hayashi H, Aonuma K, Horio M, Terada Y, Doi K, et al. Guideline on the use of iodinated contrast media in patients with kidney disease. Circ J. 2019;83(12):2572–607. https://doi.org/10.1253/circj.CJ-19-0783.j.

20. Beall DP, Fortman BJ, Lawler BC, et al. Imaging bowel obstruction: a comparison between fast magnetic resonance imaging and helical computed tomography. Clin Radiol. 2002;57:719–24. https://doi.org/10.1053/crad.2001.0735.

21. American Society for Gastrointestinal Endoscopy (ASGE). The role of endoscopy in the management of patients with known and suspected colonic obstruction and pseudo-obstruction. https://www.asge.org/docs/default-source/education/practice_guidelines/doc-the-role-of-endoscopy-in-the-management-of-patients-with-known-and-suspected-colonic-obstruction-and-pseudo-obstruction.pdf.

22. Lamb CA, Kennedy NA, Raine T, et al. British Society of Gastroenterology consensus guidelines on the management of inflammatory bowel disease in adults. Gut. 2019;8(Suppl 3):s1–s106. https://doi.org/10.1136/gutjnl-2019-318484.

23. Birindelli A, Sartelli M, Di Saverio S, et al. 2017 update of the WSES guidelines for emergency repair of complicated abdominal wall hernias. World J Emerg Surg. 2017;12:1–16.

24. Gingold D, Murrell Z. Management of colonic volvulus. Clin Colon Rectal Surg. 2012;25:236–43. https://doi.org/10.1055/s-0032-1329535.

25. Saida Y. Current status of colonic stent for obstructive colorectal cancer in Japan; a review of the literature. J Anus Rectum Colon. 2019;3:99–105.

26. Van Hooft JE, Van Halsema EE, Vanbiervliet G, et al. Self-expandable metal stents for obstructing colonic and extracolonic cancer: European Society of Gastrointestinal Endoscopy (ESGE) clinical guideline. Endoscopy. 2014;46:990–1002. https://doi.org/10.1055/s-0034-1390700.

27. Sato KT, Takehana C. Palliative nonvascular interventions. Semin Intervent Radiol. 2007;24(4):391–7. https://doi.org/10.1055/s-2007-992327.

28. Katsanos K, Sabharwal T, Adam A. Stenting of the lower gastrointestinal tract: current status. Cardiovasc Intervent Radiol. 2011;34:462–73. https://doi.org/10.1007/s00270-010-0005-x.

29. Tewari SO, Getrajdman GI, Petre EN, et al. Safety and efficacy of percutaneous cecostomy/colostomy for treatment of large bowel obstruction in adults with cancer. J Vasc Interv Radiol. 2015;26:182–8. https://doi.org/10.1016/j.jvir.2014.09.022.

30. Álvarez JA, Baldonedo RF, Bear IG, et al. Incarcerated groin hernias in adults: presentation and outcome. Hernia. 2004;8:121–6. https://doi.org/10.1007/s10029-003-0186-1.

31. Farinha HT, Melloul E, Hahnloser D, et al. Emergency right colectomy: which strategy when primary anastomosis is not feasible? World J Emerg Surg. 2016;11:19. https://doi.org/10.1186/S13017-016-0073.

32. Chang GJ, Kaiser AM, Mills S, et al. Practice parameters for the management of colon cancer. Dis Colon Rectum. 2012;55:831–43. https://doi.org/10.1097/DCR.0b013e3182567e13.
33. Lee YM, Law WL, Chu KW, et al. Emergency surgery for obstructing colorectal cancers: a comparison between right-sided and left-sided lesions. J Am Coll Surg. 2001;192:719–25. https://doi.org/10.1016/s1072-7515(01)00833-x.
34. Kube R, Granowski D, Stübs P, et al. Surgical practices for malignant left colonic obstruction in Germany. Eur J Surg Oncol. 2010;36(1):65–71. https://doi.org/10.1016/j.ejso.2009.08.005.
35. Hsu TC. Comparison of one-stage resection and anastomosis of acute complete obstruction of left and right colon. Am J Surg. 2005;189:384–7. https://doi.org/10.1016/j.amjsurg.2004.06.046.
36. Zorcolo L, Covotta L, Carlomango N, et al. Safety of primary anastomosis in emergency colorectal surgery. Color Dis. 2003;5:262–9. https://doi.org/10.1046/j.1463-1318.2003.00432.x.
37. Meyer F, Marusch F, Koch A, et al. Emergency operation in carcinomas of the left colon: value of Hartmann's procedure. Tech Coloproctol. 2004;8:s226–9. https://doi.org/10.1007/s10151-004-0164-3.
38. Melkonian E, Heine C, Contreras D, et al. Reversal of the Hartmann's procedure: a comparative study of laparoscopic versus open surgery. J Minim Access Surg. 2017;13:47–50. https://doi.org/10.4103/0972-9941.181329.
39. You YN, Chua HK, Nelson H, et al. Segmental vs. extended colectomy: measurable differences in morbidity, function, and quality of life. Dis Colon Rectum. 2008;51:1036–43. https://doi.org/10.1007/s10350-008-9325-1.
40. Duclos J, Lefevre JH, Lefrançois M, et al. Immediate outcome, long-term function and quality of life after extended colectomy with ileorectal or ileosigmoid anastomosis. Color Dis. 2014;6(8):O288–96. https://doi.org/10.1111/codi.12558.

Minimally Invasive Approach to Treatment of Acute Pancreatitis

Christopher Goljan, Jesse Bandle, and Matthew J. Martin

1 Introduction

The surgical management of complicated acute pancreatitis (AP) has significantly evolved over the last 20 years. The introduction of several novel minimally invasive techniques has given the modern general surgeon an increasing number of options to counter a highly morbid disease. Early and aggressive surgical intervention with open necrosectomy had been the standard of care for many years, which unfortunately resulted in extremely high rates of morbidity and mortality. This chapter will bring the general surgeon up to date on several key concepts targeted specifically to improve outcomes for patients with AP. We will start with background epidemiological information about AP and further discuss severity scoring, disease-specific definitions, as well as recommendations for radiographic investigation. We will review the initial goals of supportive care for patients with AP, their nutrition optimization, and examine several minimally invasive surgical techniques. The surgical review will examine the relative strengths and weakness of each procedure with clinical pearls based on our personal experience. The integration of a multidisciplinary team approach for the treatment of AP has made great progress over the past 20 years helping patients overcome a challenging disease process.

All authors declare that they have no conflicts of interest or other disclosures.

C. Goljan · J. Bandle
Department of Surgery, Naval Medical Center San Diego, San Diego, CA, USA
e-mail: christopher.goljan.mil@mail.mil; jesse.bandle.mil@mail.mil

M. J. Martin (✉)
Division of Trauma and Acute Care Surgery, Department of Surgery, Los Angeles County + USC Medical Center, Los Angeles, CA, USA
e-mail: matthew.martin@med.usc.edu

© The Author(s), under exclusive license to Springer Nature Switzerland AG 2023
F. Coccolini et al. (eds.), *Mini-invasive Approach in Acute Care Surgery*,
Hot Topics in Acute Care Surgery and Trauma,
https://doi.org/10.1007/978-3-031-39001-2_12

2 Prevalence and Etiology

AP in the United States accounts for roughly 300,000 hospital admissions a year with an estimated incidence of 4.9–73.4 cases per 100,000 in the worldwide population [1]. The most common causative agents of pancreatitis in the United States are gallstones, followed by alcohol, medications, infection, and metabolic derangements. The initial assessment for patients with suspected AP should include a detailed history, abdominal ultrasound, and basic labs including lipase, alcohol, and triglyceride level in order to elucidate the inciting agent [2]. Regardless of the etiology, AP has up to a 20% incidence of progression to necrotizing pancreatitis (NP) which is generally regarded as the most severe form of AP [3, 4]. Approximately 30% of NP patients will develop an infection of the necrotic material which will typically require a percutaneous, surgical, or endoscopic intervention [5]. Although the number of benign cases of AP far outweigh the severe, the management of NP and its sequelae can be some of the most challenging cases faced by modern practitioners. For the surgeon, it is critical to understand the natural history of this disease as well as the optimal type and timing of surgical interventions in order to optimize the chances for a successful outcome.

3 Predicting Severity

Determining the eventual severity of acute pancreatitis from information available at the time of admission is challenging because of wide variation in the intensity of each patient's inflammatory reaction. Patients may clinically decompensate over the first 48 h of their hospital admission as localized inflammation becomes systemic. There are several models available to assist in objectively evaluating AP severity and standardize initial care. Ranson's criteria utilize objective data at admission and after 48 h of treatment which gives practitioners an objective measurement of disease severity as well as response to initial treatment. Other important scoring systems to note are Acute Physiology and Chronic Health Evaluation (APACHE), Bedside Index of Severity in Acute Pancreatitis (BISAP), and the CT-severity score. These scores focus on admission parameters to provide a quick estimate of the patient's status, disease severity, and physiologic response to initial treatments. In our experience, the most clinically useful of these scoring systems is the BISAP (Table 1), which provides a rapid clinical snapshot of the patient and their physiology. This couples well with the CT-severity score (Table 2) that can add more objective detail. There can be large disparities between the patient's clinical appearance and the findings on radiologic imaging. Utilizing several modalities provides a diverse assessment of a patient's status and gives the care team the best chance for a timely analysis and effective management.

Focused pancreatic perfusion CT scan is a newer diagnostic method for predicting the development of necrosis [6]. This CT modality predicts necrosis by timing its contrast administration for post-processing into color-coded maps showing

Table 1 Bedside Index of Severity in acute pancreatitis [23]

	Yes	No
BUN > 25 mg/dL	1	0
Impaired mental status	1	0
SIRS	1	0
Age > 60	1	0
Pleural effusion	1	0
Score Total	0–5	
	Mortality %	
Score < 2	0–0.5	
Score = 2.2%	2	
Score = 3	4	
Score = 4	12.7	
Score = 5	22	

Table 2 CT-severity index [24]

CT findings		Points	Necrosis %	Points	Severity index
A	Normal pancreas	0	0	0	0
B	Pancreatic enlargement	1	0	0	1
C	Pancreatic inflammation and/or peri-pancreatic fat	2	<30	2	4
D	Single peri-pancreatic fluid collection	3	30–50	4	7
E	Two or more fluid collections and/or retroperitoneal air	4	>50	6	10

parameters such as blood flow, blood volume, and peak enhancement. The method has yet to be incorporated into any major studies, however, and will require further prospective validation.

4 Pancreatitis Classifications and Definitions

The history of categorization and descriptions of pancreatitis and related local complications has been characterized by confusing and poorly defined terms. The recently revised Atlanta classification is the gold standard for codifying AP as it provides a three-tier severity scale based on uniform clinical and radiographic nomenclature over two set phases of time. It is important for the modern surgeon to understand each phase and severity definition as recommended interventions and goals of care will change depending on the patient's progression. Starting with the phases of AP, the classification divides its pathophysiology into an early and late phase. The early phase is the first 7 days of an episode, and the late phase is any time beyond the initial 7 days for a single attack [7]. The three-tier severity scale is based on the presence of organ failure during the early phase of an AP episode; separating AP into three main classifications: mild, moderate, and severe. For example, an AP episode changes from mild to moderate if there is any evidence of organ failure. Similarly, moderate severity transitions to severe if the organ failure persists over

48 h. Disease severity can be further described by inclusion of local complications such as pancreatic or peri-pancreatic fluid collections. Patients can have moderately severe disease if they do not have organ failure but have findings consistent with necrotizing pancreatitis requiring ongoing supportive care [7].

Most importantly for the surgeon managing AP, the working group broke AP into two broad groups, interstitial edematous pancreatitis (IEP) and NP, along with clinical sub-groups based on imaging characteristics and the time elapsed from the initial presentation:

- **Interstitial Edematous Pancreatitis (IEP)**—Pancreatitis with parenchymal and surrounding inflammation and edema, but no evidence of necrosis.
  - **Acute Peri-pancreatic Fluid Collection** (APFC)—Peri-pancreatic fluid collection that occurs within the first 4 weeks of pancreatitis in the setting of IEP, without a well-defined wall.
  - **Pancreatic Pseudocyst** (PP)—APFC that has persisted more than 4 weeks and now has evidence of well-defined wall.
- **Necrotizing Pancreatitis** (NP)—Pancreatitis with parenchymal, peri-pancreatic, or combined necrosis, identified by contrast-enhanced imaging.
  - **Acute Necrotic Collection** (ANC)—Collection of both fluid and necrotic solid material, in NP, within the first 4 weeks, without a well-defined wall.
  - **Walled-Off Necrosis** (WON)-ANC that has persisted more than 4 weeks and has developed a well-defined wall [7, 8].

5 The Role of Contrast-Enhancing Imaging in Classification and Treatment

There is limited general utility for CT scanning in the early phase of routine AP but an essential role in the late phase when delineating the possible complications of IEP or NP. Mild AP is usually clinically diagnosed and treated based on abdominal pain and elevated lipase without the assistance of advanced imaging. Enhanced CT scan during the early phase is appropriate in cases of severe pancreatitis that are not responding to standard supportive care or when there is concern for other complicating abdominal pain etiologies. However, a CT scan will not change AP treatment goals during the early phase because both IEP and NP share such similar radiological findings during the initial presentation. Distinguishing radiographic characteristics of the different categories of AP requires time from the initial inflammation, allowing the findings to mature and differentiate on advanced imaging. Therefore, other than ruling out other etiologies of abdominal pain, it is prudent to delay the first CT imaging for at least 2–7 days from diagnosis to increase the diagnostic and clinical yield [7]. However, advanced imaging is the only way to differentiate IEP from NP and to accurately characterize local complications, making its appropriate application an essential component for effective, targeted treatment (see Fig. 1).

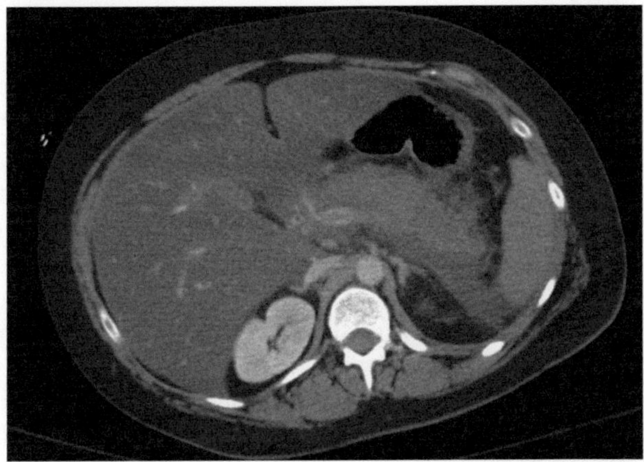

Fig. 1 CT scan with intravenous contrast showing areas of non-perfusion of the pancreas consistent with early acute necrotizing pancreatitis

6   Advanced Imaging Severity Grading

It is important to assess NP severity based on the percent burden of necrotic tissue and for evidence of infected necrosis. NP commonly effects the surrounding fat and retroperitoneal tissues in addition to the actual pancreatic tissue. There are three potential presentations of NP based on the location of effected tissue: primarily parenchymal, peri-pancreatic, or combined. The most common presentation of NP is combined necrosis, followed by peri-pancreatic and lastly isolated parenchymal disease. Patients who have more viable remaining pancreatic tissue generally have improved outcomes [8]. An infection can develop in the late phase of disease within necrotic tissue and dramatically increase the severity. Symptoms of infected necrosis include fever, tachycardia, and leukocytosis related to bacteria seeding the necrotic material or surrounding fluid collections [8]. Distinguishing infected NP can be challenging in severe cases as many patients will have similar symptoms at outset. A CT scan demonstrating air in the retroperitoneum/necrotic material or an image-guided Fine Needle Aspiration (FNA) of the necrosis confirming the presence of bacteria is the diagnostic marker for infected NP. FNA has fallen out of favor in recent years due to the benefits of diagnostic and therapeutic percutaneous drainage (PD) procedures [9].

7   Initial Management Strategies: Optimizing Medical Management

The early phase of AP represents a significant inflammatory reaction which can rapidly progress to severe multisystem end organ failure. The universal initial management of AP focuses on supportive care to blunt the systemic inflammatory response. Patients may warrant ICU level monitoring based on the disease severity and need for closer monitoring or interventions.

8   Intravenous Fluid Resuscitation

There is strong support in the literature for aggressive IV fluid resuscitation within the first 24 h of admission [10]. Resuscitation with 250–500 mL per hour of LR using the normalization of BUN as an objective target is a generally accepted guideline. An elevated BUN in AP is a useful marker for hypo-perfused kidneys and estimate of overall intravascular volume depletion. Aggressive resuscitation can produce improvement in clinical markers as early as 6–12 h from initiation. Care teams should be wary of patients who do not respond to early intervention and monitor them closely for signs of volume overload, pulmonary edema, and abdominal compartment syndrome [2]. There are two ways to administer high volume resuscitation: continuous high rate and bolus dosing. The drawback to running high-rate continuous IV fluid is it can lead to inadvertent administration of higher fluid volumes than originally intended if not monitored closely. We prefer a strategy of continuous IV fluids at a standard maintenance rate and boluses of crystalloid or colloid as needed for volume expansion. Regardless of the IV fluid strategy, the care team should closely follow a uniform metric to track volume responsiveness and overall intravascular volume in patients requiring significant resuscitation.

9   Nutrition

The role of nutrition in acute pancreatitis has evolved significantly over time. Traditionally, it was thought placing a patient on a NPO diet and "resting" the pancreas was appropriate. More recent evidence suggests that resuming enteral nutrition as early as possible helps decrease the risk of infection. Early enteral nutrition reduces the breakdown and sloughing of the gut mucosa, decreasing the incidence of transmural infection by protecting the possible bacterial seeding of necrotic material [4]. Total parenteral nutrition should not be initiated before enteral feeds as it carries a higher risk of infection and does not provide any of the benefit to the gut mucosa. Enteral nutrition, either PO or via an NG/NJ tube, in more severe forms of pancreatitis should be initiated within 72 h of treatment to preserve the gut and maximize the protective effects [2].

10   Role of Antibiotics

The use of prophylactic antibiotics for AP has been a matter of debate for years. The only evidence supported indication for the administration of antibiotics that has shown any benefit is a confirmed infection of NP on CT scan or tissue analysis. There is significant disagreement in the literature on the role of routine antibiotic administration for sterile NP. A recent large meta-analysis of early prophylactic antibiotics, within 72 h of onset of NP specifically, found that prophylactic antibiotics were associated with decreased mortality and reduced incidence of infected necrosis [11]. As there is high associated morbidity and mortality with NP, and the lack of any strong evidence of harm with this approach, it is reasonable to initiate antibiotics in patients who demonstrate significant NP with a worsening clinical picture. Although FNA is often advocated to confirm or rule-out infected NP, most clinicians now base that determination on a combination of clinical (fever, WBC count) and imaging characteristics.

Once the care team establishes the diagnosis of infected NP and starts antibiotics, some surgeons advocate for an early source control intervention rather than observing the patient on antibiotics alone. This concept has been challenged with some accumulating evidence that patients with proven or suspected infected necrosis may resolve with antibiotics alone [12]. In the right situation, an otherwise stable patient can safely undergo a period of observation on antibiotics alone. Infection of NP significantly complicates the disease course, and close observation for any clinical decline is warranted if antibiotics are selected as the primary treatment method. This is particularly important in early NP, when surgical interventions such as necrosectomy should be delayed whenever possible to at least 4–6 weeks from presentation.

11   Types and Timing of Surgical Interventions

During the early phase of AP, less than 7 days, surgical interventions are increasingly rare thanks to improvements in early diagnosis and supportive care. When AP becomes complicated by NP and advances beyond the scope of medical support, ongoing treatment requires a procedural intervention for improved source control. Table 3 lists and compares the common interventional procedures for necrotizing pancreatitis including their strengths, weaknesses, and technical details. Despite advances in minimally invasive techniques, patients with peritonitis and rapid decompensation will warrant an emergent open exploration and necrosectomy. The historically high morbidity and mortality from this operation have remained unchanged over the years but should not dissuade the surgeon from intervening on an acutely decompensating patient. Classically a complication of the late phase, development of infected NP in the early phase should be treated with antibiotics and if indicated, percutaneous or surgical drainage. Of the possible source control procedures, PD is a well-tolerated and minimally invasive procedure that can provide source control, culture data, and can ultimately be curative for some patients without need for further surgery [13].

In the late phase, ANC and APFC may progress to WON and PP, respectively. Procedural treatment should be considered for those who demonstrate infection, severe pain, mechanical obstruction, or other complications. The care team should select a surgical debridement procedure that will best target the findings demarcated on advanced imaging (Fig. 2). Although advanced imaging may show an actionable disease process, patients will have improved outcomes if intervention is delayed until at least 4–6 weeks after the initial episode. Inflammatory changes may complicate the surgical approach and make identification of healthy vs necrotic tissue challenging. The optimal treatment is a procedure that de-bulks and obtains source

Table 3 Interventional procedures/techniques for necrotizing pancreatitis

Technique	Pros	Cons	Technical details
Percutaneous drainage (PD)	– Least invasive, minimal risk – Upsize/add more catheters for improve drainage – No anesthesia	– Inadequate drainage of debris/necrotic tissue – DRAINS clog, dislodge	– Usually placed via a retroperitoneal approach – Image-guided (IR suite)
Endoscopic drainage	– Minimally invasive – No surgery – Can drain large simple fluid collections	– Sedation/intubation – Collection must abut stomach – Often requires frequent scopes – High failure rate in NP	– Upper endoscopy – Locate fluid collection through posterior gastric wall – Place drain and/or stent
Endoscopic necrosectomy	– Minimally invasive – Remove necrotic debris as well as fluid – Avoids enterocutaneous access, reduced fistula complication	– Sedation/intubation – Requires a gastrotomy and removal of large fragments using limited instruments – Commonly requires frequent procedures	– Create gastrotomy into cavity – Endoscopic instruments to remove solid material and fluid – Option to leave nasojejunal drain for ongoing lavage/drainage
Laparoscopic approach	– Less invasive than open – Excellent visualization and debridement – Variety of instruments available	– No tactile feedback – Difficult with dense adhesions – Iatrogenic injuries	– Standard laparoscopy – Exposure via the lesser sac or trans-gastric – Remove all necrosis and – Leave large drains
Video-assisted retroperitoneal debridement (VARD)	– Less invasive than open – Does not violate peritoneal cavity – Direct visualization/excellent drainage and debridement – Small incision	– Narrow operative field – No tactile feedback – Risk of iatrogenic injuries/bleeding – Wound complications/fistulas	– Requires well placed percutaneous drain that will be followed safely down to the cavity – Use deep retractors and laparoscopic instruments – Debride and leave large drains
Sinus tract endoscopy (STE)	– Minimally invasive – Does not violate peritoneal cavity – Debridement/drainage procedure can access most any fluid pocket with a percutaneous drain	– Limited scope of view – Limited instruments – Can require multiple repeat procedures	– Requires previously placed percutaneous drain – Upsize the PD catheter with a working sheath to fit a nephroscope/small manual grasper

(continued)

Table 3 (continued)

Technique	Pros	Cons	Technical details
Open necrosectomy	– Complete visualization – Tactile feedback – Easiest to remove large amounts of necrotic tissue – No specialized equipment	– Large incision – Difficult to identify safe planes – Postop ileus – Incisional hernia risk – High morbidity	– Midline or chevron incision – Expose lesser sac and manually debride all necrotic tissue – Use "suction dissection" – Leave large irrigating drains

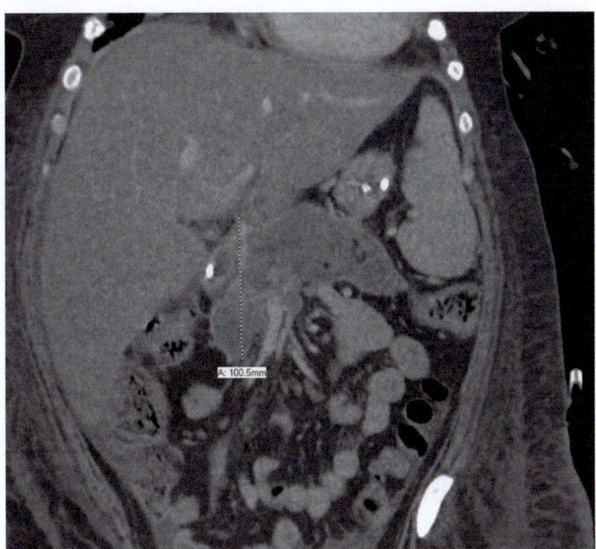

Fig. 2 CT scan at 5 weeks shows well demarcated fluid collection consistent with walled-off necrosis

control, without sacrificing the remaining healthy pancreas function [13, 14]. Ideally fluid collections are, or become, asymptomatic and can be observed without an intervention. When an intervention is needed, there are several methods for operative drainage available to the modern multidisciplinary team.

12 Minimally Invasive Step-up Approach Vs Open Necrosectomy

In 2010, a randomized trial utilizing the step-up approach was published in the New England Journal of Medicine from the Dutch Pancreatitis Study Group and has changed the standard of care for NP. They conducted a 3-year multicenter study randomly assigning 88 patients with NP to undergo primary open necrosectomy vs a step-up approach starting with PD or endoscopic drainage and progressing to minimally invasive retroperitoneal necrosectomy if the patient failed to improve after at least two procedures performed in a 6-day period [15]. While the overall mortality of each arm was unchanged, their study showed a significant reduction in secondary organ failure, hernias, and new onset diabetes in the step-up approach arm [15]. Multiple other studies have confirmed their findings and demonstrated possible decreased mortality as well [13]. These studies show that NP patients tolerate a minimal invasive approach better, while still receiving an equal if not improved overall outcome.

13 Which Minimally Invasive Technique Is Best?

There are several minimally invasive alternatives to an open exploration with necrotic debridement which embraces the NP step-up method (see Table 3). These can be divided into three main categories based on the equipment required or their manner of approach: radiographic, endoscopic, or laparoscopic. Modern treatment for NP requires a multidisciplinary approach to evaluate and match the full spectrum of interventional specialty techniques to a particular patient's disease process. Availability of specialty equipment and trained providers will also influence the choice of procedures at individual facilities. It is important to note that an open necrosectomy does not require more specialized equipment or expertise than a well-trained general surgeon and ICU admitting privileges. While an unquestionably morbid procedure, the relative lack of need for specialized equipment for an open necrosectomy is also its greatest strength for the surgeon when new techniques or endoscopic/interventional options are not available or fail.

14 Minimally Invasive Interventions

14.1 Percutaneous Catheter Drainage

PD is now a well-established first-line intervention for many AP complications due to its inherent low risk and a growing body of literature showing that patients can recover with this least invasive option [13]. PD placement should be considered when patients either have non-infected, but symptomatic, collections despite weeks of supportive therapy or for infection source control. PD is a well-tolerated and frequently successful procedure when performed by qualified and experienced interventional radiologists. Most fluid collections from AP can be accessed with acceptable risk even in significantly ill patients. Should the patient fail to improve, care teams can utilize the prior PD placement for more invasive procedures which rely on a catheter for initial access [9]. PD's greatest disadvantage is that there is minimal actual debridement of infected material. This may lead to insufficient source control in severe cases of NP, with a large burden of disease necessitating a secondary drainage procedure or surgical debridement [15].

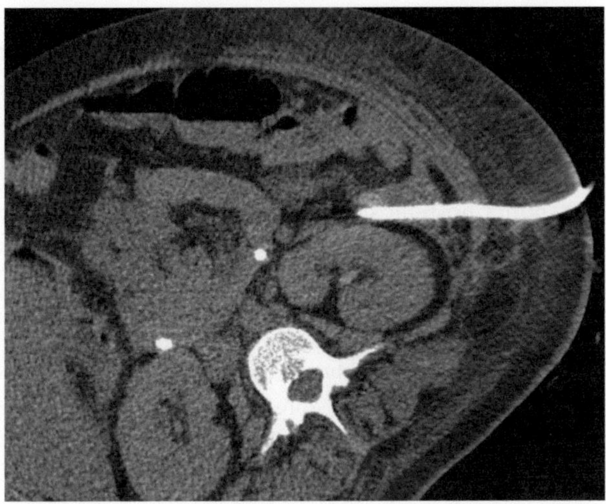

Fig. 3 Percutaneous drain placement from the left flank for walled-off necrosis

PD can be performed via a transperitoneal or retroperitoneal approach. The retroperitoneal approach can bypass vital intra-abdominal structures, avoiding potential enteric leaks, and facilitate any possible future retroperitoneal surgical procedures. If a step-up approach is being pursued, then percutaneous drain placement should always be done using a retroperitoneal approach typically from the left flank, as the drain will serve as a guide for the surgical approach into the infected collection (Fig. 3). Typical catheter sizes range from a 12 to 30 Fr and can be upsized at repeat procedures for improved drainage. Catheters require daily care with flushes to maintain patency and provide some debridement [9]. If the patient fails to improve after single catheter, a second catheter may be placed and/or the original catheter may be upsized before moving to a more invasive debridement procedure [15]. Whether as a primary treatment or as an adjunct to more aggressive therapy, PD is proven therapy for NP that should be incorporated into a modern treatment algorithm and can avoid the need for surgery in up to 50% of cases (Fig. 3).

14.2   Transoral Endoscopy

Endoscopic drainage (ED) is an excellent minimally invasive option in centers with access to advanced endoscopy and interventional capabilities. The endoscopist will access the fluid collection through the wall of an enteral structure, most commonly the stomach, and drain the fluid/necrotic material via a tract created with deployment of one or more stents. If the fluid collection is a pseudocyst, the placement of a pigtail catheter or stent is usually sufficient for decompression. The advantage of endoscopic drainage vs PD is the potential for debridement via the endoscope for collections typically seen in WON. Frequently a trans-gastric large bore stent is placed for access. The endoscope is then passed directly into the cavity through the stent so that the proceduralist can perform debridement [9]. ED debridement may be limited, and studies have found that a mean of four (range 1–23) endoscopies were required per case for a successful treatment in 81% of patients, with a low mortality (6%) and acceptable complication rate (36%) [16]. Comparing this to surgical debridement, a recent meta-analysis published in 2020 concluded that endoscopic treatment carries a lower risk of perforation, enterocutaneous fistula, organ failure, and shorter hospital stay without a significant difference in overall mortality [17]. Limitations of this technique are the availability of a specialized endoscopic provider, the higher likelihood for repeat procedures, and the anatomical restrictions based on the location of the fluid collection. This technique is completely dependent on the WON sharing a wall with the stomach or another enteral structure. While some centers perform advanced endoscopic drainage procedures such as cystoduodenostomy or cystojejunostomy, this is an even more advanced technique and therefore typically restricted to specific large volume academic centers.

14.3 Video-Assisted Retroperitoneal Debridement (VARD)

Video-Assisted Retroperitoneal Debridement (VARD) utilizes the familiar laparoscopic tools of the general surgeon to perform a minimally invasive large volume debridement without entering the peritoneal cavity. When employed in a step-up approach, VARD is an effective treatment in treating WON with significantly less morbidity than open necrosectomy [15]. This procedure couples with prior PD placement well, as this technique uses the catheter to guide a cut down to the necrotic collection before placement of the laparoscope and instruments. Preoperative review of a recent CT scan showing the course of the percutaneous drain and its relationship to key anatomic structures (most notably the stomach, left kidney, spleen, and transverse colon) is critical to ensuring a successful procedure and avoiding iatrogenic injuries (Fig. 4a and b). VARD is typically performed with the patient in partial right lateral decubitus position with a 5–8 cm incision (Fig. 5). The incision can either be centered on the existing PD or slightly offset from the

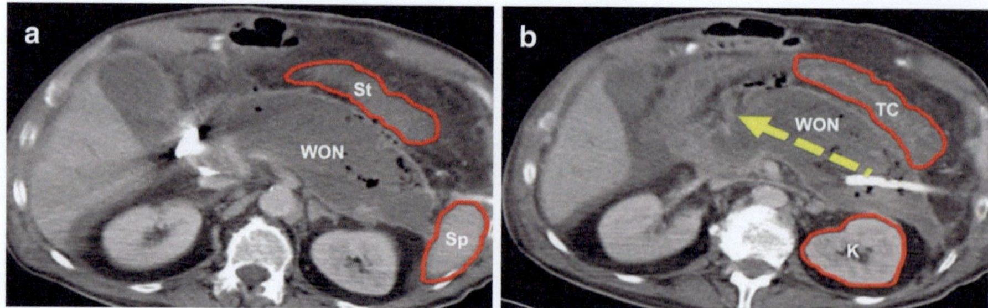

Fig. 4 Preoperative CT scan review prior to VARD for walled-off necrosis (WON) is critical to identify the course of the percutaneous drain (yellow arrow) and critical associated organs including (**a**) the stomach (St) and spleen (Sp), and (**b**) the transverse colon (TC) and left kidney (K)

Fig. 5 Patient in partial right lateral decubitus position for VARD, with suggested incision shown with the dotted white line

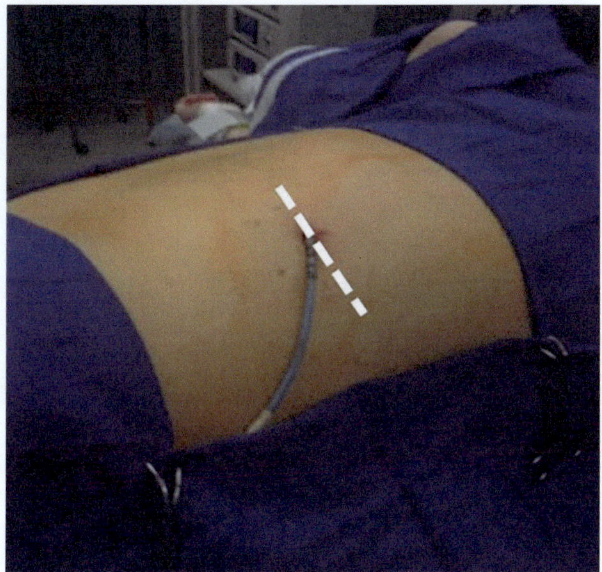

Fig. 6 View through the laparoscope during the deeper phase of dissection during VARD. Note that dissection follows the percutaneous drain, and exposure is facilitated by the use of long and narrow manual retractors

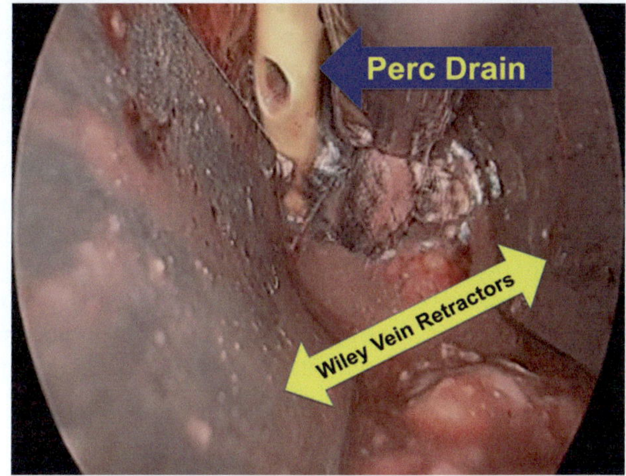

drain, but in either case the drain is exposed in the subcutaneous position and then followed as the dissection is progressively deepened. The necrotic cavity is initially debrided with suction aspiration of all fluid and then free pieces of necrotic tissue and pancreas. Subsequent debridement is then performed with rings forceps or laparoscopic graspers under initial direct visualization and then switching to the use of a laparoscope and deep narrow retractors for the deeper parts of the dissection (Fig. 6). After complete debridement, a separate incision is made to leave one or more drains for continued postoperative lavage and drainage [18]. A postoperative CT scan at 1–2 weeks is recommended to assess the adequacy of the debridement and evaluate for any persistent undrained or recurrent fluid collection (Fig. 7).

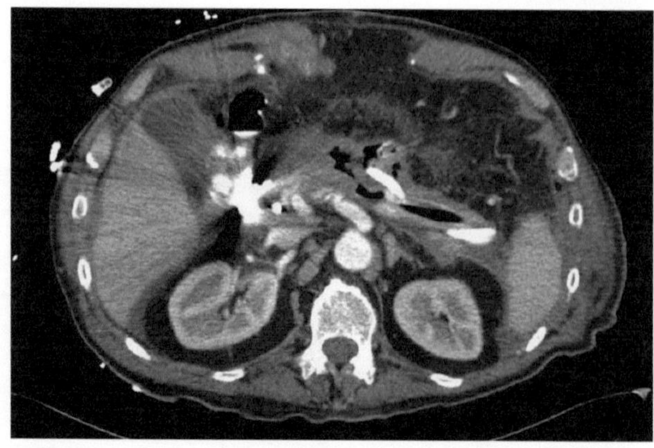

Fig. 7 Postoperative CT scan at 5 days after VARD showing resolution of walled-off necrosis and surgical drain in position in the pancreatic bed

From a surgeon's perspective, the advantage of VARD over other MIS techniques is its familiarity to other laparoscopic surgical procedures and the ability to perform a single operation with wide debridement done under direct visualization. VARD is an ideal technique in the patient with a large necrotic collection who cannot tolerate multiple endoscopic washouts or a large open procedure. The main limitation to the VARD approach is the anatomical location of the WON and its proximity to vital structures. The visualization in a VARD is limited, and any inadvertent damage to surrounding structures is difficult to correct. The VARD approach is not recommended for centromedial collections extending into the root of the small-bowel mesentery due to the inherent difficulty in operating that close to critical structures in a significantly reduced space [19]. Common complications from the VARD procedure are injury to critical surrounding structures, treatment failure, chronic wound complications, and fistula formation. Minor bleeding can be dealt with laparoscopically with pressure and clips. Larger volume hemorrhage can be initially controlled with packing the cavity and then proceeding with either interventional radiologic or surgical control of the bleeding source. Although uncommon, intraoperative injury to bowel or other adjacent intraperitoneal structures will necessitate conversion to an open exploration and repair [19].

14.4 Sinus Tract Endoscopy (STE)

Sinus tract endoscopy is a newer and more flexible innovative retroperitoneal approach to access difficult collections that utilizes a similar approach to VARD but performed with an endoscope and endoscopic instruments. While VARD is performed via a cut down procedure to gain access, STE upsizes that same percutaneous catheter with a working sheath to fit an endoscope and its associated accessories. Visualization is maintained with continuous irrigation via a nephroscope which also serves to help with debridement as the operator removes debris with a small manual grasper. The advantage of this technique comes from the operator's ability to use it anywhere there is percutaneous access, such as between ribs or within a narrow window beside vital structures. STE provides the opportunity to treat previously inaccessible collections of necrotic debris using a minimal invasive technique. Additionally, STE may reduce wound complications compared to VARD or open necrosectomy as the entire operation is in effect a drain site. It is important to note that STE is impractical as a primary modality for large volume debridement as the operator would likely need several returns to the OR for completion compared to a single VARD procedure. STE is an excellent alternative to open necrosectomy for pockets of necrotic debris previously unapproachable via a trans-gastric or a cut-down approach [18]. However, this technique requires a significantly advanced endoscopic and minimally invasive skillset that is currently not available at most centers.

14.5 Laparoscopic Transperitoneal

The laparoscopic transperitoneal technique gives the surgeon an excellent view and access to the upper abdomen to perform direct debridement. Although laparoscopic necrosectomy may be a technically more difficult operation than open necrosectomy, it can offer improved exposure and detailed visualization than the open approach. In addition, for the experienced surgeon, laparoscopy reduces length of stay and post-infectious complication rates when compared to the open approach [20]. There are essentially three ways to approach the retroperitoneum and pancreatic necrosis/fluid collections: through the lesser sac, infra-mesocolic, or trans-gastric. Accessing via the lesser sac or trans-mesocolic approach directly opens the retroperitoneum and exposes the pancreas where debridement can be performed similar to an open necrosectomy. Initial gentle suction dissection is preferred and can remove all free fluid and tissue components without injury to viable pancreatic tissue or surrounding structures. Subsequent blunt necrosectomy with laparoscopic graspers is then performed and should focus on only removing tissue that readily separates from the cavity with gentle traction. Once debridement is complete, the cavity should be irrigated and then large bore closed-suction drains are placed. These approaches do expose the intrabdominal contents to necrotic or infected material which likely correlates with the increased rates of wounds complications and fistula formation described in some series [17]. In contrast, the trans-gastric approach involves initial access via an anterior gastrotomy followed by a target gastrotomy through the posterior wall and directly into the pancreatic cavity. This ideally spares the peritoneum of any further contamination or spillage after closure of the gastrotomy. Like endoscopy, this technique relies on the offending necrosis being directly posterior to the stomach which limits its utility to those presentations. If the exposure is difficult laparoscopically, a small hand-assist port can provide the benefits of minimal invasive surgery while improving exposure and dissection capabilities.

There are several benefits of laparoscopic drainage which should prompt its consideration. Patients with gallstone pancreatitis can have a concurrent cholecystectomy during their drainage procedure provided there are no contraindications. This may significantly increase operative time and should only be considered in the stable patients without prohibitive inflammation of the gallbladder that would compromise a safe cholecystectomy. Similar to the endoscopic approach, laparoscopic techniques allow for internal drainage between the WON and the stomach or small-bowel facilitating continued drainage. The advantage of laparoscopic drainage is that the surgeon has two or more instruments in the abdomen and can directly manipulate the stomach into position for the anastomosis, allowing the surgeon to perform a single operation with wide debridement and continued postoperative drainage [21]. Overall, the transperitoneal laparoscopic approach is a better tolerated surgery than open necrosectomy. It is, however, technically challenging and is a more invasive than a percutaneous/endoscopic drain, which may make it a less attractive primary operation at a fully equipped multidisciplinary center.

14.6 Laparoscopic Pseudocyst Treatment

While studies suggest that up to 70% of pseudocysts spontaneously resolve, a significant portion of this population will develop symptoms requiring surgical intervention. Typical indications for an intervention are symptoms of pain, obstruction, or a concern for cystic neoplasm. The laparoscopic approach changes based on the location of the pseudocyst and its adjacent structures available for drainage. The basic principle is to create an anastomosis between an epithelial lined enteral structure and the granulation tissue of the pseudocyst. The location of the cyst guides the surgical approach; a posterior stomach cyst may be accessed via a trans-gastric cystogastrostomy, a pancreatic head cyst via a cystoduodenostomy, and a distal cyst via a cystojejunostomy. The surgeon has the option of a stapled or sewn anastomosis with either technique having good success rates and frequently complete resolution of the pseudocyst. The enterotomy into the epithelial lined structure will close as the pseudocyst drains, typically without long-term complications [22].

14.7 Open Necrosectomy

Open surgical debridement was the standard of care for years despite the high morbidity and mortality of the approach. Multiple studies have demonstrated high postoperative risk of multi-organ failure, perforation of hollow viscus, wound infections, and fistula formation requiring re-operation. However, this technique does retain significant value in select patients. Surgeons must consider the open approach for any rapidly decompensated patient with peritonitis, for the patient who has failed MIS techniques, or when MIS techniques result in unintentional damage to critical intra-abdominal structures [9]. The benefit of open necrosectomy is that the surgeon has the best access and visualization of the diseased tissue. It is imperative that all diseased tissue is removed to minimize any further abdominal explorations. Intraoperative technique during open debridement should focus on gentle, blunt dissection of necrosis rather than formal resection as the general inflammatory state of the abdomen creates a high-risk environment for inadvertent damage to surrounding structures. After an open procedure, the abdomen may be left open with packing in preparation for future explorations before formal closure or there are several variations to fascial closure at the index operation with large bore drain access. One technique utilizes large bore drains to continuously flush and drain sterile irrigation through the retroperitoneum. While there are no studies directly compare these techniques, minimizing operative interventions can be achieved through large volume irrigation and debridement and therefore should be considered [9]. Open necrosectomy carries significant risk but can be a lifesaving measure for the right patient.

References

1. Fagenholz PJ, et al. Increasing United States hospital admissions for acute pancreatitis, 1988-2003. Ann Epidemiol. 2007;17(7):491–7.
2. Tenner S, et al. American College of Gastroenterology guideline: management of acute pancreatitis. Am J Gastroenterol. 2013;108(9):1400–15; 1416.
3. Baron TH, Morgan DE. Acute necrotizing pancreatitis. N Engl J Med. 1999;340(18):1412–7.
4. Al Mofleh IA. Severe acute pancreatitis: pathogenetic aspects and prognostic factors. World J Gastroenterol. 2008;14(5):675–84.
5. Banks PA, Freeman ML. Practice guidelines in acute pancreatitis. Am J Gastroenterol. 2006;101(10):2379–400.
6. Yadav AK, et al. Perfusion CT: can it predict the development of pancreatic necrosis in early stage of severe acute pancreatitis? Abdom Imaging. 2015;40(3):488–99.
7. Banks PA, et al. Classification of acute pancreatitis—2012: revision of the Atlanta classification and definitions by international consensus. Gut. 2013;62(1):102–11.
8. Shyu JY, et al. Necrotizing pancreatitis: diagnosis, imaging, and intervention. Radiographics. 2014;34(5):1218–39.
9. Freeman ML, et al. Interventions for necrotizing pancreatitis: summary of a multidisciplinary consensus conference. Pancreas. 2012;41(8):1176–94.
10. Warndorf MG, et al. Early fluid resuscitation reduces morbidity among patients with acute pancreatitis. Clin Gastroenterol Hepatol. 2011;9(8):705–9.
11. Ukai T, et al. Early prophylactic antibiotics administration for acute necrotizing pancreatitis: a meta-analysis of randomized controlled trials. J Hepatobiliary Pancreat Sci. 2015;22(4):316–21.
12. Mouli VP, Sreenivas V, Garg PK. Efficacy of conservative treatment, without necrosectomy, for infected pancreatic necrosis: a systematic review and meta-analysis. Gastroenterology. 2013;144(2):333–340.e2.
13. van Santvoort HC, et al. A conservative and minimally invasive approach to necrotizing pancreatitis improves outcome. Gastroenterology. 2011;141(4):1254–63.
14. Besselink MG, et al. Timing of surgical intervention in necrotizing pancreatitis. Arch Surg. 2007;142(12):1194–201.
15. van Santvoort HC, et al. A step-up approach or open necrosectomy for necrotizing pancreatitis. N Engl J Med. 2010;362(16):1491–502.
16. van Brunschot S, et al. Endoscopic transluminal necrosectomy in necrotising pancreatitis: a systematic review. Surg Endosc. 2014;28(5):1425–38.
17. Haney CM, et al. Endoscopic versus surgical treatment for infected necrotizing pancreatitis: a systematic review and meta-analysis of randomized controlled trials. Surg Endosc. 2020;34(6):2429–44.
18. Fong ZV, Fagenholz PJ. Minimally invasive debridement for infected pancreatic necrosis. J Gastrointest Surg. 2019;23(1):185–91.

19. Horvath K, et al. Safety and efficacy of video-assisted retroperitoneal debridement for infected pancreatic collections: a multicenter, prospective, single-arm phase 2 study. Arch Surg. 2010;145(9):817–25.
20. Tan J, et al. Short-term outcomes from a multicenter retrospective study in China comparing laparoscopic and open surgery for the treatment of infected pancreatic necrosis. J Laparoendosc Adv Surg Tech A. 2012;22(1):27–33.
21. Melman L, et al. Primary and overall success rates for clinical outcomes after laparoscopic, endoscopic, and open pancreatic cystgastrostomy for pancreatic pseudocysts. Surg Endosc. 2009;23(2):267–71.
22. Townsend CM Jr. Sabiston textbook of surgery: the biological basis of modern surgical practice. 20th ed. Philadelphia: Elsevier Saunders; 2017.
23. Wu BU, et al. The early prediction of mortality in acute pancreatitis: a large population-based study. Gut. 2008;57(12):1698–703.
24. Balthazar EJ. Acute pancreatitis: assessment of severity with clinical and CT evaluation. Radiology. 2002;223(3):603–13.

Complicated Hiatal Hernia

Siobhan Rooney, Victoria Hudson, and Stavros Gourgiotis

1　Definition

A *hernia* is an abnormal protrusion of a cavity's contents through a weakness in the wall of the cavity containing it. Hernias often take the linings of its cavity with it and these contents and linings are often markedly attenuated. A *Hiatus hernia (HH)* is an anatomical abnormality in which part of the peritoneum and the stomach protrudes upwards into the mediastinum through an aperture in the diaphragmatic known as the oesophageal hiatus, which has pathologically widened. A *complex HH* describes the herniation of any abdominal structure in addition to the stomach (e.g., omentum, colon, small bowel, spleen) into the thorax through a lax diaphragmatic oesophageal hiatus.

2　Anatomy

The oesophageal hiatal orifice is an elliptical opening in the diaphragm through which the oesophagus, vagus nerves, the left inferior phrenic vessels, and some small oesophageal arteries pass from the left gastric artery. The oesophageal hiatus is created by arching fibres of right diaphragmatic crus. The diaphragmatic crura arise from tendinous fibres extending from the anterior longitudinal ligament overlying the upper lumbar vertebrae. Both left and right crural fibres move superiorly closely adherent to the vertebral bodies, then move anteriorly to and separate to allow the lower oesophagus to pass through. These crural muscle fibres then loop to form a sling around the lower oesophagus. While the medial fibres form the

S. Rooney · V. Hudson · S. Gourgiotis (✉)
Cambridge Oesophago-gastric Centre, Addenbrooke's Hospital, Cambridge University Hospitals NHS Foundation Trust, Cambridge, UK
e-mail: victoria.hudson@addenbrookes.nhs.uk; stavros.gourgiotis@nhs.net

© The Author(s), under exclusive license to Springer Nature Switzerland AG 2023　　　157
F. Coccolini et al. (eds.), *Mini-invasive Approach in Acute Care Surgery*,
Hot Topics in Acute Care Surgery and Trauma,
https://doi.org/10.1007/978-3-031-39001-2_13

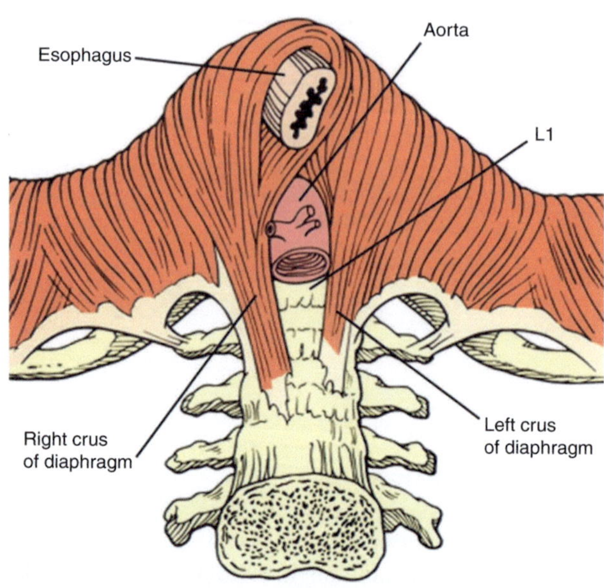

Fig. 1 The oesophageal hiatus anatomy. (Illustration by S. Rooney)

oesophageal hiatal margins, the lateral fibres of each hiatal limb join the central tendon of the diaphragm (Fig. 1). On inspiration, flattening of the diaphragm causes this muscular sling to tighten and constrict the lower oesophagus, thus acting as a functional sphincter preventing stomach contents from refluxing into oesophagus.

The oesophageal hiatus is particular vulnerable to visceral herniation due to its position traversing the thoracic and abdominal cavity. It is subjected to a pressure gradient between the thoracic and abdominal cavities. Furthermore, as the muscular oesophagus itself is designed to expand to accommodate food boli and peristalsis, therefore by natural design the oesophagus does not tightly fill the hiatus.

The phrenoesophageal ligament is an elastin-rich membrane, which inserts circumferentially to the musculature of the lower oesophagus close to the squamocolumnar junction. It acts as the main restraining structure forming the gastroesophageal junction (GOJ), anchoring the oesophagus to the diaphragm. In additional, it acts to close the potential space between the oesophagus and the diaphragm making it a key structure to consider in the pathogenesis of HH [1].

3 Aetiology

While the majority of HH are acquired, there are some familial clustering reported in the literature [2]. A number of factors have been implicated in the aetiology of HH, the prevalence of HH increases with age, elevated BMI, and chronic health conditions. Fibromuscular degeneration increases with age, this degeneration may be compounded in women by periods of increased intra-abdominal pressure in the last trimester of pregnancy or people with chronic lung conditions who experience frequent episodes of coughing. A similar mechanism is seen in people with obesity [3].

Additionally, other anatomical variations such as those with severe osteoporosis and kyphosis result in increased intra-abdominal pressure and alter the pressure gradient between the thorax and abdomen, thereby pushing the GOJ upwards to increase the risk of developing a HH [4, 5]. A similar mechanism is thought to underpin the association between occupations which involve lifting. Finally, increased gastro-esophageal reflux disease (GERD) and subsequent oesophagitis has been shown in animal models to result in oesophageal shortening because of fibrosis [6].

The prevalence of HH is difficult to accurately define, largely because the majority of HH are asymptomatic or associated with mild symptoms. Menon and his colleagues published a meta-analysis in 2011 suggesting the prevalence of HH in the general population is 27%, and as high as 73% in those >50% years of age [7].

4   Pathophysiology

The pathophysiology of HHs is not clearly understood. The widening of the oesophageal hiatus and subsequent migration of the GOJ superiorly is multifactorial, resulting from:

- Increased laxity of the phrenoesophageal membrane, and the cural muscle fibres result in widening of the diaphragmatic hiatus, facilitating migration of the GOJ into the thorax.
- The GOJ can be forced superiorly with increased intra-abdominal pressure, as seen in obesity, pregnancy, and repetitive straining.
- Oesophageal shortening can theoretically occur as a consequence of GERD and subsequent inflammation and fibrosis, which displaces the GOJ superiorly into the thorax.

5   Classification of HH

HH have been traditionally classified according to the location of the GOJ and the amount of dislocated tissue:

- *Type I: axial hernia*—The GOJ migrates above the diaphragm. While the stomach stays in its normal longitudinal alignment, with the fundus below the GOJ. Also known as a sliding hernia.
- *Type II: paraesophageal hernia*—The GOJ remains in its normal anatomical position, However a portion of the gastric fundus herniates through the diaphragmatic hiatus and lies adjacent to the oesophagus. Also known as a rolling hernia.
- *Type III: combination of I and II*—Both the GOJ and the fundus have migrated through the oesophageal hiatus. Thus, the fundus lies cephalad to the GOJ.
- *Type IV:* Large HH with migration of abdominal organs dislocated into the thorax. Type IV HH often progress from type III hernia, as the GOJ and some or all of the stomach have already migrated superiorly to the mediastinum through the hiatus as well.

Ninety-five percent of the HHs are type I and are often associated with GERD. Type II–IV HHs often grouped together and referred to as paraesophageal hernias. These are either asymptomatic or present with obstruction, strangulation or incarceration. "Giant paraesophageal hernia" is a term often attributed to type III and IV hernias, when more than half of the stomach has migrated through the hiatus.

5.1 Endoscopic Evaluation

HH are a frequently identified incidentally during a diagnostic gastroscopy. Hill et al. developed a more practical classification system to allow more precise assessment of the competence of the esophagogastric sphincter mechanism. The Hill classification inspects the gastroesophageal flap valve during endoscopic retroflexion and classifies HH into one of four categories, which can also be used to predict reflux [8].

In the Hill classification (Fig. 2), grade I is considered to be the 'normal' configuration, with a wall-like gastroesophageal flap valve, always forming a tight closure

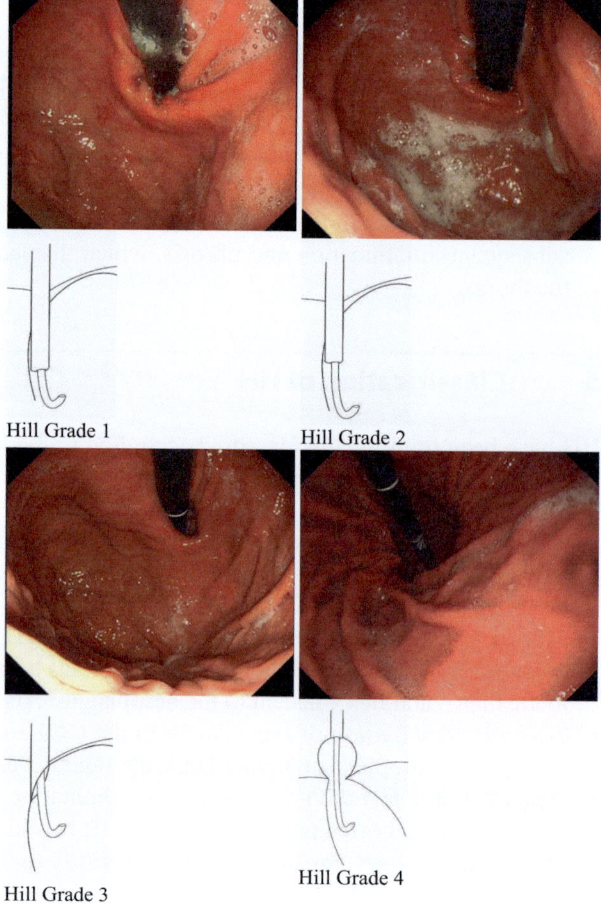

Fig. 2 Endoscopic and schematic representation of the Hill classification

round the endoscope, corresponding to the angle of His. In grade II, the GOJ adherence to the endoscope is less well-defined with some effacement of the angle of His. The gastroesophageal flap valve's competence is respiration-dependent. In grade III, the gastroesophageal flap valve does not close around the endoscope, there is complete effacement of the angle of His ridge often the oesophageal mucosa is visible. Hill grade IV is always associated with a large HH. The diaphragmatic hiatus can be seen as extrinsic compression on the gastric mucosa. In grade IV, there is no gastroesophageal flap valve adherent to the shaft of the endoscope resulting in permanent opening of the GOJ.

6   Presentation

The majority of uncomplicated or sliding HH (Hill grade 2 and 3) are asymptomatic and diagnosed incidentally. Patients can report minor symptoms of vague epigastric discomfort, reflux or retrosternal chest pain which can progress as the GOJ moves superiorly into the mediastinum (Hill grade 4/complicated HH) [9, 10]. Patients with complicated HH can develop respiratory symptoms secondary to pulmonary compression or present with episodes of recurrent aspiration pneumonia due to an incompetent lower oesophageal sphincter. Larger, complicated HH can present with gastric volvulus with vascular compromise, mucosal ischemia, ulceration, bleeding, or anaemia. In fact, iron deficiency anaemia can be seen in up to 50% of patients with a paraesophageal HH [10]. Complicated HH may also present acutely with sudden retrosternal chest pain, abdominal pain, abdominal distension, dysphagia, or intractable vomiting.

Approximately 50% of complicated hernias are symptomatic, the literature suggests that the annual risk of developing symptoms in the setting of a known paraesophageal hernias is approximately 14% [11]. Meanwhile, the risk of developing acute symptoms requiring surgical intervention is less than 2% per year.

6.1   Volvulus

Gastric volvulus is a rare but potentially life-threatening condition. A gastric volvulus can pose a diagnostic challenge due to a non-specific presentation. Gastric volvulus involves migration of the stomach superiorly to the mediastinum and rotation of the stomach either along the mesenteroaxial or organoaxial axis. Organoaxial describes the rotation of the stomach around the pylorus-cardia axis, connecting the pylorus and gastroesophageal junction. Organoaxial volvulus is the most common type of gastric volvulus and may cause obstruction at the level of the GOJ or pylorus. Gastric volvulus progresses to strangulation and necrosis in approximately 30% of cases [12]. Mesenteroaxial describes the vertical rotation of the stomach, along the lesser-greater curvature axis of the stomach. Mesenteroaxial gastric volvulus is less frequent and less likely to lead to vascular compromise. A combination of both organoaxial and mesenteroaxial rotation rarely occurs.

A rotation greater than 180° will lead to a complete gastric obstruction; a precarious presentation due to its non-specific symptoms but this high degree of rotation will result in strangulation leading to ischaemia, necrosis, and perforation in quick succession. As such, it is associated with a high mortality if it is not treated early.

Borchardt's triad of epigastric pain, retching (without vomiting), and inability to pass a nasogastric tube depicts the clinical manifestation of gastric volvulus with complete obstruction at the level of the GOJ. A patient with gastric volvulus may also present with chronic progressive symptoms of dysphagia, postprandial pain, vomiting, and breathlessness. Gastric volvulus on either axis may be chronic with vague or non-specific symptoms, thus it may be only apparent on imaging or at endoscopy.

Patients with dislocated abdominal organs and a large hiatal hernia may also be asymptomatic initially; however, eventually they may present with exertional dyspnoea and pulmonary fibrosis due to chronic recurrent silent aspiration. Dysphagia, regurgitation, postprandial fullness, atypical cardiovascular symptoms, arrhythmias, and anaemia are typical symptoms for large HH due to localized extrinsic compression. Interestingly, reflux is an infrequent symptom, many experts hypothesize that this is due to the increased tissue within the mediastinum re-enforcing the lower oesophageal sphincter.

6.2 Strangulation

Strangulation is the vascular compromise of tissues, in this case causes the hypoperfusion of the stomach and hernia contents in a catastrophic endpoint to complex HHs. Strangulation can occur due to gastric volvulus or sudden change in the position and lie of the hernia contents resulting in vascular compromise. Patients with gastric strangulation can present with a broad spectrum of symptoms; vague intermittent abdominal, atypical chest pain, or at the other end of the spectrum patients can present with constant severe retrosternal or epigastric pain radiating to the back which often leads clinicians toward searching for other diagnoses.

Frequently patients present with obstructive symptoms, respiratory distress, signs of sepsis, and evidence of inadequate end organ perfusion. Laboratory investigations may reveal a lactic acidosis and a leucocytosis or leukopenia in the elderly.

6.3 Perforation

Perforation is a much less common endpoint of an acute complicated HH, typically those presenting with symptoms of obstruction and strangulation result in an ischemic perforation (Fig. 3). Organoaxial volvulus can result in linear tears of the gastric body itself, which can further complicate surgical repair. Unfortunately, a gastric perforation is particularly prevalent in immunosuppressed patients on steroids who can have an attenuated systemic inflammatory response.

Initially perforation of hernia contents results in containment within the hernia sac; however, this can quickly extend freely into the peritoneal, mediastinum, and

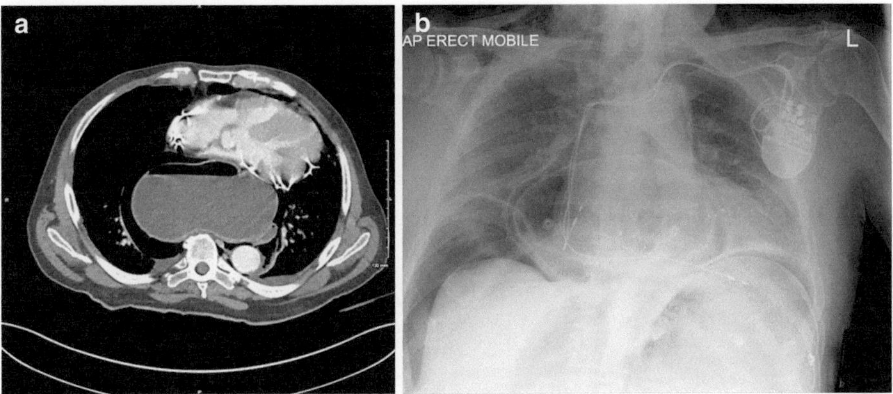

Fig. 3 (**a**) Sagittal slice of a computed tomography study illustrating a dilated, fluid-filled intra-thoracic stomach, with extensive pneumomediastinum suggesting a perforation of hernia contents. (**b**) Same patient, this plain film also illustrates extensive pneumoperitoneum

pleural cavities. These patients can rapidly develop pleural effusions and fulminant mediastinitis along with sceptic shock and respiratory failure.

6.4 Delayed Presentation

The most concerning presentation occurs in patients with delayed presentation or missed diagnosis. Given the myriad of non-specific symptom and clinical signs, obstructed or strangulated complicated hiatal hernia can often be mistake for more benign non-urgent pathologies such as gastroenteritis, reflux disease, and non-ischemic chest pain. In such incidences, patients often present with profound sepsis and organ failure requiring immediate resuscitation, stabilization, and anaesthesia involvement prior to a definitive diagnosis being reached.

7 Investigations

7.1 Computed Tomography (CT) Scan

CT scan is the gold standard initial investigation for gastrointestinal pathologies, especially in patients presenting with acute symptoms, suggestive of a complicated HH (Fig. 4). CT imaging not only delineates the upper gastrointestinal tract but allows for evaluation of hernia features and assists in surgical planning [13]. Key features which aid in management of complicated HH that are identified on CT include:

1. Volume and percentage of the stomach involved and assessment of corresponding vasculature

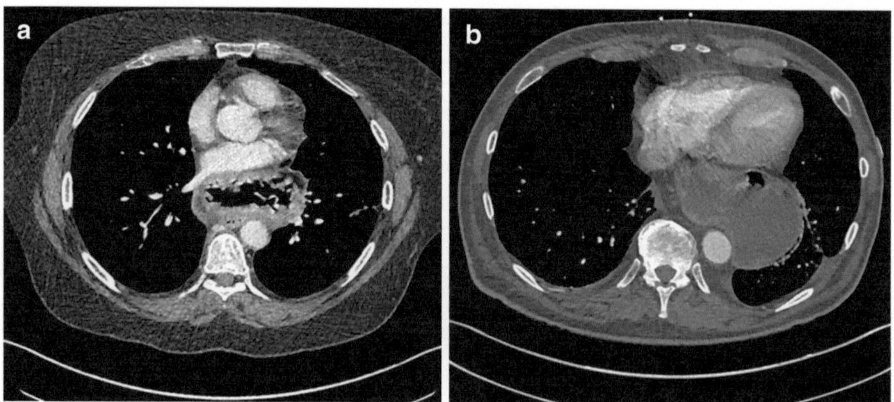

Fig. 4 Sagittal computed tomography slices showing a large paraesophageal hernia with oedematous walls suggesting inflammation and incarceration (**a**) and (**b**) shows a thin walled, fluid filled intra-thoracic stomach

2. Other peritoneal organs herniated through defect
3. Complete or partial obstruction
4. Organoaxial vs. mesenteroaxial gastric volvulus
5. Ischaemia/hypoperfusion, pneumatosis of the gastric wall
6. Identification of perforation site with free air and fluid

Ideally CT should be performed with intravenous contrast in the first instance, oral contrast can be considered in the case of diagnostic ambiguity in relation to perforation site.

7.2 Plain Chest Radiographs

Plain chest radiographs may identify opacification consistent with soft tissue within the chest, and a retrocardiac fluid level on chest radiograph is pathognomonic for a paraesophageal HH (Fig. 5a). Intraluminal gas may be within bowel loops heading upwards in a usual pattern towards the hernia sac. In cases of transverse colon herniation, upward deformity of the transverse colon may be seen (Fig. 5b).

7.3 Contrast Studies

Contrast studies such as a barium swallow can be useful in adjunct to endoscopy and CT, particularly in the detect of sliding HH in symptomatic obese patients for further definition of the anatomy of the oesophagus, GOJ level, and stomach in a stable patient in which there is low suspicion of complicating features [14]. Gastric volvulus, although best diagnosed via a CT scan, can also be identified on a barium

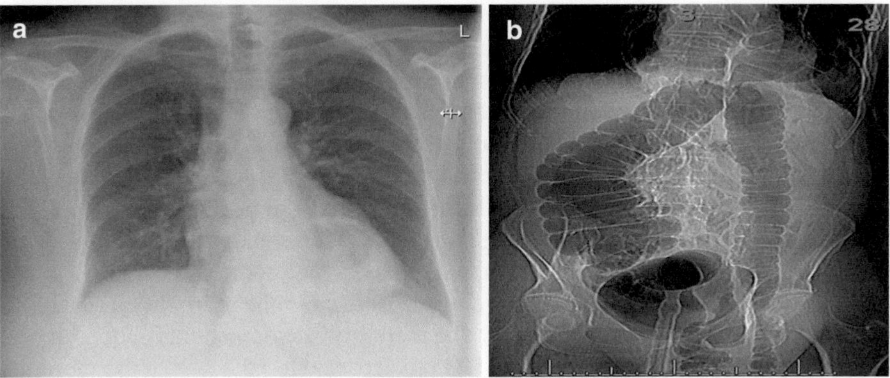

Fig. 5 (**a**) Plain film radiograph of the chest showing a large hiatus hernia. (**b**) A CT scout image showing herniation of the transverse colon through the oesophageal hiatus

study. However, they should be avoided in patients with features of complications as they serve to delay surgical intervention, and in these patients, there is an added risk of aspiration.

7.4 Oesophagogastroduodenoscopy (OGD)

OGD is a valuable adjunct in perioperative assessment of HH and classification according to the Hill classification (see section "Classification of HH"). Endoscopy provides an opportunity to evaluate the viability of the gastric mucosa, and assess for the presence of erosive esophagitis, Barrett's oesophagus, masses, and ulcers, which can guide operative planning. In an emergent setting, OGD can aid in the identification of possible perforation sites, assessment of gastric mucosa, and presence of torsion or volvulus. It may also play a therapeutic role in the decompression in an emergent gastric volvulus.

8 Treatment

In those with gastroesophageal reflux disease, sliding HH or type I HHs, laparoscopic repair with a fundoplication should be offered. Sliding HH without symptoms does not require surgical repair. There is little evidence to support elective repair of asymptomatic HH, in fact the evidence to suggests that elective laparoscopic HH repair in asymptomatic patients might actually decrease the quality-adjusted life expectancy for patients aged 65 years and older [15].

All symptomatic paraesophageal hernias (type II, II, IV, and Hill grade IV) should be considered for repair though. While the natural history of HH is poorly understood, many surgeons believe paraesophageal hernias enlarge over time, becoming more technically difficult to reduce and repair with a transabdominal approach. With time, patients' overall operative risk profile tends to increase, which furthers the argument for elective repair. The risk of paraesophageal hernia becoming acutely symptomatic is estimated to be 2% annually [11].

While patients with symptoms such as dysphagia, acid reflux, ongoing abdominal pain, and weight loss can potentially be managed non-operatively with mitigation of risk factors (weight loss, diet change, smoking cessation, medical therapy), patients with symptoms of gastric outlet obstruction, postprandial fullness, respiratory symptoms, severe gastroesophageal reflux, or anaemia should be considered for elective surgical repair in the context of patients' co-morbidities.

The underlying principle of elective repair is to avoid the morbidity and mortality associated with an emergent repair. The mortality rate for patients undergoing an emergency surgery for a complicated HH repair is about 5.5%, while the mortality rate associated with an elective repair is 0.65% [16].

8.1   Elective HH Repair

The standard elective procedure for HH is a laparoscopic repair with fundoplication (Fig. 6). An intra-operative liver retractor may be necessary to obtain adequate exposure of the oesophageal hiatus (a). Regardless of the hernia contents, the initial steps of the repair of HH are to reduce the hernia contents and completely excise the hernia sac (b), which will mobilize the lower oesophagus and gastric cardia, allowing for several centimetres of oesophagus to be intra-abdominal. The hiatal defect is

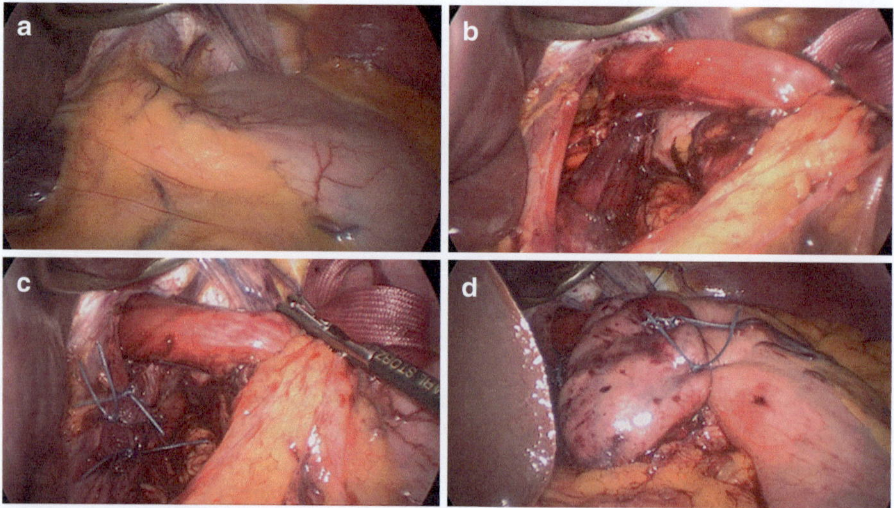

Fig. 6 Intra-operative images of a laparoscopic HH repair and Nissen fundoplication. (**a**) A liver retractor obtains adequate exposure of the oesophageal hiatus. (**b**) Reduction of the hernia contents and complete excision of the hernia sac. (**c**) Use of interrupted non-absorbable braided sutures to repair the hernia defect. (**d**) A fundoplication is formed from the cardia

then repaired with interrupted non-absorbable braided sutures (c). Finally, a fundoplication is formed from the cardia (d). It does not have to be a complete 360° fundoplication.

The traditional Nissen fundoplication (a complete 360-degree wrap) is favoured by many surgeons as the final stage of a HH repair. However, as laparoscopic surgery has progressed alternative fundoplication procedures such as the Toupet fundoplication (a 270-degree posterior fundoplication) and the Dor fundoplication (270-degree anterior fundoplication) which are used in complicated HH repairs where tissue quality and quantity of the gastric cardia may require a change in practice. This may also help to reduce post-operative dysphagia.

There remain some controversies in relation to the technical elements of HH repair. For example, it is unclear whether resection of the hernial sac with gastropexy is a valid alternative to the antireflux/fundoplication element of HH repair. Additionally, while there is a large body of evidence supporting the use of mesh in both abdominal wall and inguinal hernia repairs, there is a paucity of evidence to support the use for mesh in the repair of HH. In fact, international bodies do not support its use, due to inadequate long-term data on the topic [15].

8.2   Emergent Surgical Intervention

Acutely symptomatic patients should be resuscitated and stabilized before surgical repair. Even in an acutely symptomatic patient, a laparoscopic approach can be undertaken with a low threshold for conversion to open. Complicated HHs, those with bleeding, volvulus, perforation, or complete obstruction require urgent intervention. The surgical dilemma is how aggressive should one pursue completing a definitive repair and what techniques should be employed to enable enteral feeding.

In the cases with perforation of hernia contents, priority should be given to source control of the perforation site and septic foci, which again can be located in pleural, mediastinal, and peritoneal cavity. Limited gastric resection if mucosal necrosis is present, or suture repair if a small well-defined defect is identified, should be done. This also applies to the other herniated hollow viscus organs. Gastrointestinal continuity may be temporarily interrupted in patients who require a major oesophagogastric resection. An intra-thoracic anastomosis should be avoided in frail patients, especially if they have evidence of mediastinitis. In such cases, the stomach should be stapled off and decompressed with a gastrotomy tube, and the proximal oesophagus should be diverted with a cervical oesophagostomy.

Patients presenting with acute gastric volvulus should be decompressed, a limited resection of non -viable necrotic tissue performed if needed. Additionally for the hemodynamically unstable or severely frail patients, it may be most prudent to reduce the stomach and other herniating organs, pexy of the stomach to the anterior abdominal wall in several areas along the greater curvature, and place a G-tube to help keep the stomach in the abdomen. This again can be done laparoscopically.

After initial recovery and improvement of the patient's other medical conditions, a more formal repair with oesophageal mobilization or creation of a neo-oesophagus can be done electively.

9 In Summary

The laparoscopic approach can be applied to HH in the acute setting. Patients with HH can present in extremis or have several co-morbidities that make these patients at high risk for repair. When properly resuscitated or pre-habilitated, a laparoscopic approach can be done. Patients who present acutely should be resuscitated prior to surgery. When urgent surgical intervention is needed, reduction and pexy of the stomach is a viable option and should be considered in the hemodynamically compromised. Otherwise, a formal hernia repair should be done.

References

1. Kahrilas PJ, Kim HC, Pandolfino JE. Approaches to the diagnosis and grading of hiatal hernia. Best Pract Res Clin Gastroenterol. 2008;22:601–16. https://doi.org/10.1016/j.bpg.2007.12.007.
2. Baglaj SM, Noblett HR. Paraoesophageal hernia in children: familial occurrence and review of the literature. Pediatr Surg Int. 1999;15:85–7. https://doi.org/10.1007/s003830050522.
3. Pandolfino JE, Kwiatek MA, Kahrilas PJ. The pathophysiologic basis for epidemiological trends in gastroesophageal reflux disease. Gastroenterol Clin N Am. 2008;37:827–43. https://doi.org/10.1016/j.gtc.2008.09.009.
4. Polomsky M, Siddall KA, Salvador R, Dubecz A, Donahue LA, Raymond D, et al. Association of kyphosis and spinal skeletal abnormalities with intrathoracic stomach: a link toward understanding its pathogenesis. J Am Coll Surg. 2009;208:562–9. https://doi.org/10.1016/j.jamcollsurg.2009.01.004.
5. Yamaguchi T, Sugimoto T, Yamada H, Kanzawa M, Yano S, Yamauchi M, Chihara K. The presence and severity of vertebral fractures is associated with the presence of esophageal hiatal hernia in postmenopausal women. Osteoporos Int. 2002;13:331–6. https://doi.org/10.1007/s001980200034.
6. Eastwood GL. Histologic changes in gastroesophageal reflux. J Clin Gastroenterol. 1986;8(Suppl 1):45–51. https://doi.org/10.1097/00004836-198606001-00007.
7. Menon S, Trudgill N. Risk factors in the aetiology of hiatus hernia: a meta-analysis. Eur J Gastroenterol Hepatol. 2011;23:133–8. https://doi.org/10.1097/MEG.0b013e3283426f57.
8. Hill LD, Kozarek RA. The gastroesophageal flap valve. J Clin Gastroenterol. 1999;28:194–7. https://doi.org/10.1097/00004836-199904000-00002.
9. Awais O, Luketich JD. Management of giant paraesophageal hernia. Minerva Chir. 2009;64:159–68.
10. Low DE, Simchuk EJ. Effect of paraesophageal hernia repair on pulmonary function. Ann Thorac Surg. 2002;74:333–7. https://doi.org/10.1016/s0003-4975(02)03718-9.
11. Stylopoulos N, Gazelle GS, Rattner DW. Paraesophageal hernias: operation or observation? Ann Surg. 2002;236:492–500. https://doi.org/10.1097/00000658-200210000-00012.
12. Haas O, Rat P, Christophe M, Friedman S, Favre JP. Surgical results of intrathoracic gastric volvulus complicating hiatal hernia. Br J Surg. 1990;77:1379–81. https://doi.org/10.1002/bjs.1800771219.
13. Light D, Links D, Griffin M. The threatened stomach: management of the acute gastric volvulus. Surg Endosc. 2015;30:1847–52. https://doi.org/10.1007/s00464-015-4425-1.

14. Fornari F, Gurski RR, Navarini D, Thiesen V, Mestriner LH, Madalosso CA. Clinical utility of endoscopy and barium swallow X-ray in the diagnosis of sliding hiatal hernia in morbidly obese patients: a study before and after gastric bypass. Obes Surg. 2010;20:702–8. https://doi.org/10.1007/s11695-009-9971-y.
15. Kohn GP, Price RR, DeMeester SR, Zehetner J, Muensterer OJ, Awad Z, et al. Guidelines for the management of hiatal hernia. Surg Endosc. 2013;27:4409–28. https://doi.org/10.1007/s00464-013-3173-3.
16. Kaplan JA, Schecter S, Lin MYC, Rogers SJ, Carter JT. Morbidity and mortality associated with elective or emergency paraesophageal hernia repair. JAMA Surg. 2015;150:1094–6. https://doi.org/10.1001/jamasurg.2015.1867.

Inguinal and Incisional Hernia Emergency Management

Dario Parini, Roberta La Mendola, and Monica Zese

1 Epidemiology and Classification

Abdominal hernias can be divided into groin hernias (femoral and inguinal), and ventral hernias, classified into umbilical, epigastric, spigelian, and incisional [1]. In some cases, abdominal hernias could require emergency surgery, which is associated with higher rate of recurrence and postoperative complications [2, 3].

Classically, the emergent abdominal hernia can be classified into:

- *Incarcerated hernia*: it occurs when the abdominal content becomes irreducible due to a narrow opening in the abdominal wall or due to adhesions between the content and the hernia sac. Often, intestinal obstruction may complicate the scenario [2, 4]
- *Strangulated hernia*: it occurs when the blood supply to the contents of the incarcerated hernia (e.g., omentum, bowel) is reduced or absent [2, 5]

Strangulated hernias remain a significant challenge, as they are sometimes difficult to diagnose with only physical examination, and require always an emergent surgical intervention, which can be with laparoscopic or laparotomic access [2, 6, 7].

For choosing the best surgical technique and approach, it is important to consider the contamination of the surgical field, above all in emergency setting. According to classification of wound contamination degree (Centers for Disease Control and

D. Parini (✉) · R. La Mendola · M. Zese
General Surgery Department, Santa Maria della Misericordia Hospital, Rovigo, Italy
e-mail: roberta.lamendola@aulss5.veneto.it; monica.zese@aulss5.veneto.it

© The Author(s), under exclusive license to Springer Nature Switzerland AG 2023
F. Coccolini et al. (eds.), *Mini-invasive Approach in Acute Care Surgery*,
Hot Topics in Acute Care Surgery and Trauma,
https://doi.org/10.1007/978-3-031-39001-2_14

Table 1 Surgical field contamination classification, based on CDC wound classification [2, 8]

Class I Clean	Uninfected surgical field, without inflammation
Class II Clean- contaminated	A surgical field in which the alimentary, genital, or urinary tract is entered under controlled conditions and without unusual contamination
Class III Contaminated	A surgical field with gross spillage from the gastrointestinal tract
Class IV Dirty or infected	A surgical field with peritonitis from bowel necrosis and perforation

Prevention (CDC) wound classification and 2017 WSES Classification) [2, 8], it is possible to stratifies the surgical field contamination as follows (Table 1):

- Class I = clean wound/surgical field
- Class II = clean-contaminated wound/surgical field
- Class III = contaminated wound/surgical field
- Class IV = dirty or infected wound/surgical field

There are many risk factors correlated to higher morbidity and mortality. The most common are the following [4, 9, 10]:

- Age > 65 years
- Incarceration for more than 24 h
- Symptom duration of 3 or more days
- Prolonged symptom duration
- Delay to admission, diagnosis, and surgery or prolonged time from admission to start of surgery
- Bowel obstruction
- Associated midline laparotomy for exploration after incarcerated/strangulated hernia reduction
- Hernia-related hospitalizations in the year preceding hernia repair
- Femoral hernia, especially right-sided
- Female gender
- ASA class III and IV, BMI > 30, and recurrent hernia and anticoagulant use

2   History [11, 12]

The term Hernia comes from an ancient Greek word: kele/hernios—bud or offshoot. The first reports about hernia treatment go back to ancient Egypt. The Egyptian Papyrus of Ebers was the first document containing description of a hernia. But most of the knowledge from the ancient times until eighteenth century derives from Galen, which described it in many documents.

In eighteenth and nineteenth century, medical and surgical treatment began to change. Astley Cooper stated that no surgical disease requires to the surgeon so broad knowledge and skills as hernia and its many variants. The treatment improved with the introduction of anesthesia and antiseptic procedures and new techniques repair slowly appeared (nineteenth–twentieth century). Three important elements changed the approach to surgery: antiseptic and aseptic procedures, high ligation of hernia sac, and narrowing of the internal inguinal ring. In that period, recurrence rate at 4–5 years was about 100% and postoperative mortality gained even 7%.

In 1898, Bassini introduced a new reconstruction of the posterior wall of inguinal canal. He can be considered the inventor of the modern treatment of hernia. In 1945, the Canadian surgeon E. Shouldice proposed (plicature) plication of the transverse fascia and strengthening of the posterior wall of inguinal canal by four layers of fasciae and aponeuroses of oblique muscles. These modifications decreased recurrence rate to 3%.

The next step in hernia treatment has been introduced by Lichtenstein in 1987. He described the first tensionless technique, based on strengthening of the posterior wall of inguinal canal with prosthetic material. Lichtenstein published the data on 1000 operations with Marlex mesh without any recurrence in 5 years after surgery. Another treatment method was introduced some years before by Rene Stoppa, who used Dacron mesh situated in preperitoneal space without fixing sutures. First operation was performed in 1975 and reported a recurrence rate quite low (1.4%).

Another step was introduction of a Prolene Hernia System, which enabled repair of the tissue defect in three spaces: preperitoneal, above transverse fascia, and inside inguinal canal.

The last important step was introduced by laparoscopic treatment of groin and ventral hernias, which began in twentieth century. The first laparoscopic procedure was performed by P. Fletcher in 1979. In 1990, Schultz plugged inguinal canal with polypropylene mesh. Later new procedures, trans-abdominal preperitoneal (TAPP) technique and totally extra-peritoneal (TEP) approach, were introduced for groin hernias repair.

3   Inguinal Hernia Laparoscopic Repair

Inguinal hernia lifetime incidence is between 27 and 43% in men and only 3–6% in women [4]. In general, inguinal hernias are symptomatic and are requiring surgery, nowadays, as only curative treatment. The natural history of inguinal hernia shows that 0.29–2.9% of cases become complicated, and 10–15% of these become strangulated, with a mortality rate of up to 5% in older patients [13].

3.1   Indications (Table 2)

Laparoscopic approach for elective inguinal hernia repair has been demonstrated to be at least equivalent to open technique [17, 18]. In emergency setting, as incarcerated or strangulated hernia, since the 90s, literature demonstrated the feasibility of

Table 2 Indications and contraindications to laparoscopic emergency repair of inguinal hernia [2, 7, 14–16]

Indications	Contraindications
Hemodynamic stability	Hemodynamic instability (absolute)
Inguinal defect <4 cm	Pneumoperitoneum contraindicated (absolute)
No bowel ischemia	Peritonitis - CDC class III-IV (absolute)
No bowel distension	Abdominal wall defect >4–5 cm (relative)
No peritonitis—CDC class I–II	Bowel distension (relative)
Abdominal cavity exploration	Need of bowel resection (relative)
Inguinal-scrotal hernia reduction	

mini-invasive approach [19] and, more recently, a systematic review confirmed these findings [20], but comparative studies are lacking in this field.

The role of laparoscopy in complicated inguinal hernia surgery is of two types: a simple exploration of abdominal cavity in support to anterior hernia approach or a total or partial laparoscopic hernia repair.

Laparoscopic exploration is indicated to verify bowel viability after spontaneous reduction of strangulated hernia during anterior approach, demonstrating an important reduction of unnecessary laparotomy and bowel resection [2, 7, 14]. When mini-invasive approach has this only aim, it is possible to enter the abdominal cavity by hernia sac (so-called hernioscopy) [21].

According to the literature, laparoscopic approach is feasible for both incarcerated or strangulated hernia, with a clean (CDC class I) and a clean-contaminated (CDC class II) surgical field, but it is contraindicated in case of peritonitis and if abdominal wall is infected (CDC class III–IV) [15, 16].

A total extra-peritoneal (TEP) or trans-abdominal preperitoneal (TAPP) mini-invasive approach for large and difficult inguinal-scrotal hernias could help to perform preperitoneal dissection and to remove hernia content, in order to facilitate and complete hernia sac reduction, before classic anterior repair and mesh placement [16, 22].

Hemodynamic instability and heart or respiratory failure are absolute contraindications to laparoscopy, as well as bowel perforation evidence at radiologic images. Bowel distension, often present in case of strangulated hernia, is a relative contraindication and depends on surgeon laparoscopic experience, because the intestinal manipulation is more dangerous.

The need for bowel resection is not an absolute contraindication to laparoscopic approach, but literature suggest to perform it extra-corporeally after defect repair, in order to reduce surgical time and to avoid spillage of bowel content in abdominal cavity or in the extra-peritoneal inguinal space [6, 15, 16].

Large size defect (>4–5 cm) is not a contraindication to laparoscopic repair, but in this case, larger mesh use is suggested, in order to reduce the risk of recurrence [15, 16].

3.2   Technique

The surgical steps sequence in laparoscopic approach is different from classic anterior technique. This aspect contributes to the benefit of mini-invasive approach [6]. In fact, as first surgical time, after pneumoperitoneum induction and trocars placement, in the same way and position than elective procedure, the strangulated bowel in the sac is reduced and a first assessment of its viability is performed. If there is not a bowel perforation, next step will be the hernia repair. During this surgical time, which lasts more or less 45–60 min, the previously strangulated bowel is visible and surgeon can constantly reassess it. This observational time is longer than that available with anterior approach, where decision of bowel resection should be taken before hernia repair. In this way, laparoscopic approach reduces bowel resection rate, because bowel has more time to recover. Furthermore, in case of spontaneous reduction of sac content during hernia dissection with inguinal approach, surgeon should subsequently explore the abdominal cavity with a laparotomy or laparoscopy, with lengthening of total surgical time [14].

In this last case, a mixed laparoscopic-open technique has been proposed, in order to explore peritoneal cavity through inguinotomy by an "hernioscopy" [21]. A 12-mm trocar is positioned in the deep inguinal ring, and pneumoperitoneum is induced. If necessary, a second 5-mm trocar can be inserted through the abdominal wall, to better explore the whole bowel [23].

Once mini-invasive approach has been decided, the choice is between a totally laparoscopic intervention or a hybrid technique. In the second case, laparoscopic time is used to explore bowel viability and to reduce strangulated sac content, before to repair hernia defect with mesh with classic inguinal incision. The intervention ends with a new laparoscopic exploration to reassess bowel aspect.

For reduction of the strangulated content, it will be very useful to combine an external inguinal-scrotal compression. Under laparoscopic view, the direction of external compression can be accurately determined. Furthermore, this compression can reduce the edema of the strangulated content. This aspect, together with the effect of pneumoperitoneum, which strength the abdominal wall, and the relaxation due to general anesthesia, facilitates hernia reduction. If laparoscopic grasping of sac content is needed, it is recommended to grasp the less important structures, like omentum or peritoneal fat first. If it is required to directly manage the bowel, it is suggested to grasp the distal collapsed bowel loop. If, even with these maneuvers, the sac content cannot be reduced, the surgeon has two different options: he can sacrifice the strangulated bowel segment by using an endoscopic GIA to transect it completely and then remove the strangulated stump, performing bowel anastomosis as last surgical time, or convert to laparotomy [6].

In the full laparoscopic technique, even hernia repair is performed laparoscopically. Both mini-invasive techniques, TEP and TAPP, are valid in the emergency setting, and literature didn't demonstrate the superiority of one of them [13, 15, 16]. Nevertheless, each of the 2 techniques shows some advantages and disadvantages. TAPP approach allows to constantly reassess bowel aspect, without need to change surgical field between intra- and extra-peritoneal. Moreover, during sac reduction step, it is possible to grasp hernia content, in order to facilitate this maneuver. On the other hand, if there is an important bowel distension, this could be an operative problem, with reduction of the operating field and augmented risk of intestinal lesions. Conversely, TEP approach doesn't have problem with intestinal distension because the peritoneum separates surgical field from intra-abdominal content. Furthermore, in case of large and difficult inguinal-scrotal hernia, requiring conversion to an open anterior approach, the dissection of preperitoneal space can facilitate sac complete reduction and subsequent mesh placement [16]. The limit of extra-peritoneal approach is that it doesn't consent to check the bowel viability, for this reason it is always necessary to explore the peritoneal cavity, as first and last step of the intervention [6].

If bowel resection is necessary, literature recommends to perform it extra-corporally, through a small extended sub-umbilical incision, after hernia repair [6, 15, 16]. In fact, intracorporeal anastomosis, even if feasible in surgical expert hands, has major risk of enteric spillage during enterotomy time because often bowel is distended and under tension.

3.3 Results

Since early 90s, literature demonstrated the feasibility of laparoscopic approach for inguinal hernia repair, before in elective setting and after even in complicated presentation, as incarcerated or strangulated hernia [17–19].

Deeba et al. [20], in a systematic review, calculated an average operative time of 61 min, average length of hospital stay (LOS) of 3.8 days, mortality rate at 0.28%, and complication rate of 10.3%. Conversion rate was 1.8%, with a bowel resection rate of 5.1%, and reoperation rate was 0.9%. Major complications were two colonic lesions and one section of deferens. Others were infected mesh (0.6%), wound infection (0.3%), deep venous thrombosis (0.3%). The recurrence rate at 7 years was 5.8%. Finally, the overall complication rate, recurrence rate, and LOS are very similar to those documented in open emergent repair for incarcerated or strangulated hernias.

Yang et al. [14], in a retrospective comparative study on open versus laparoscopic treatment for strangulated hernia, reported a bowel resection rate in laparoscopic group of 1.75% vs 7.63% in the open group. Surgical site infection was higher in the open group (12 pts. vs 0). The wound infection rate in open group was 6% in inguinotomy and 21% in laparotomy. The LOS was longer in the open group, although it was not statically significant.

3.4 Conclusions

Laparoscopic inguinal hernia repair in emergency setting is feasible, safe, and effective, but requests an expertise in both laparoscopic emergency surgery and mini-invasive inguinal hernia repair.

The major benefits of laparoscopic approach in emergency setting are an accurate diagnostic ability, to establish bowel viability; the avoidance of unnecessary laparotomy; lower rate of bowel resection compared to open approach; lower wound infection rate.

4   Incisional Hernia Laparoscopic Repair

Incisional hernia is a common disease surgeons have to deal with, affecting 10% of patients who underwent laparotomy [24]. Although it may be asymptomatic for a long time, in about 15% of cases it can give rise to complications, including incarceration and strangulation, requiring emergency surgery [25] that is characterized by up to 15-fold higher mortality, reoperation, and readmission rates than elective repair [3].

In elective setting, laparoscopy showed to be safe and effective in selected patients, with less frequent complications compared to open approach and similar recurrence rate [26, 27]. As regards incisional hernia needing emergency surgery, open repair still represents the standard procedure in clinical practice of most of surgeons. Nevertheless, guidelines recommend a minimally invasive approach if surgical experience and patient characteristics allow it, since results are comparable to that of elective cases [7, 28].

4.1   Indications (Table 3)

The indications for laparoscopic incisional hernia repair are almost the same in elective and emergent surgery, although it is known that in emergency context, patient selection is even more important in order to minimize complications rate and mortality. Patients have to be evaluated concerning theirs past medical and surgical history, comorbidities, timing and modality of clinical onset, physical examination, lab tests results, and preoperative imaging. In complex urgent cases, contrast-enhanced CT scan represents the gold standard to study incisional hernia, due to its

Table 3 Indications and contraindications to laparoscopic emergency repair of incisional hernia [7, 26–32]

Indications	Contraindications
Hemodynamic stability	Hemodynamic instability (absolute)
Abdominal wall defect <15 cm	Abdominal wall defect >15 cm with loss of domain (absolute)
No bowel ischemia	Peritonitis—CDC class III–IV (absolute)
No bowel distension	Mesh positioning not allowed (absolute)
No peritonitis—CDC class I–II	Pneumoperitoneum contraindicated (absolute)
	Need of bowel resection (relative)
	Bowel ischemia (relative)
	Bowel distension (relative)

accuracy in the definition of visceral involvement, eventual gangrene signs, and size of the abdominal wall defect [33].

The principal indications to mini-invasive approach are as follows:

- *Hemodynamic stability*: an impaired hemodynamic status, such as severe sepsis or septic shock, requires open approach [7, 26–28]
- *Absence of general contraindications to pneumoperitoneum* (e.g., severe heart or pulmonary diseases) [7, 26–28]
- *Abdominal wall defect < 15 cm without loss of domain of hernia content:* wall defect larger than 15 cm doesn't represent an absolute contraindication, but it is better managed performing an open component separation and an additional fascia closure, because the reduced intra-abdominal space can make more difficult to place trocars and to insert a large mesh [29, 30]
- *Absence of peritonitis and inflammatory status of bowel (CDC class I–II):* in CDC class III-IV, handle the intestinal loops laparoscopically can be dangerous, for the high risk of unintentional iatrogenic bowel lesions due to edema and frailty of intestinal wall [7, 26–28];
- *Absence of gangrene and need of bowel resection:* presence of bowel necrosis, requiring a resection, is not an absolute contraindication, but guidelines state that this condition is better managed with conversion to open laparotomy [7, 26–28];
- *Absence of significant bowel distension:* bowel diameter is related to the occlusive status, so indirectly to the timing of diagnosis and treatment, and literature shows that a small bowel diameter > 4 cm predicts a high rate of visceral injury and conversion [31, 32]
- *Absence of contraindications to mesh positioning:* conditions as enterocutaneous fistulae, infected wounds, and concomitant dirty-contaminated abdominal procedures represent indications to open defect repair without synthetic mesh (direct repair if defect <3 cm, otherwise prosthetic repair by a biological mesh) [7, 26–28].

Advanced age, Child A–B compensated cirrhosis, obesity, recurrent incisional hernia and etiology, type, and number of previous operations do not represent contraindications to minimally invasive approach, if surgeon has adequate laparoscopic skills. In particular regarding obesity, some evidence on ventral and incisional hernia shows that laparoscopy gives some advantages in reducing postoperative infections rate and in facilitating detection of wall defects that should be unrecognized due to abdominal fat [27].

4.2 Technique

The surgical steps of incisional hernia repair in elective and emergency setting are pneumoperitoneum induction, trocars insertion, adhesiolysis, hernia content reduction, careful bowel exploration, and mesh positioning and fixing [7, 26–28, 30, 34].

Pneumoperitoneum is usually inducted by a Veress needle, inserted at a safe distance from the wall defect and the surgical scars, in order to avoid visceral injuries. Left upper quadrant (Palmer's point) is the most frequently chosen site, but it can vary according to previous laparotomies. An open access can be also performed, and it is considered safer by many surgeons. After insufflation, the abdominal cavity exploration is performed by a 10 mm–30° scope, in order to identify any conditions requiring a conversion (e.g., bowel ischemia). In case of extensive adhesions, a first step of blunt dissection can be performed by the scope before the insertion of the other two trocars (generally at least one of 12 mm). They are placed under direct vision as far away as possible from the hernia, creating a triangle converging toward the wall defect. In case of large hernia, an additional 5 mm trocar can be placed at the opposite site of the abdomen to achieve a better mesh fixation.

Adhesiolysis is the crucial step of laparoscopic incisional hernia repair, because of the risk of iatrogenic enterotomies, that could be missed during operation and lead to postoperative peritonitis, the most serious complication for this intervention. It should preferably be performed by cold dissection (e.g., by scissors), minimizing the use of electrified instruments (e.g., monopolar and bipolar coagulation, ultrasound, and radiofrequency), that should be kept at a safe distance from intestinal loops and always with the inert blade closer to the bowel and the other organs, in order to avoid direct damage. Bowel should be carefully handled only by atraumatic graspers and touched as little as possible with operative instruments. Accidental enterotomies have to be immediately repaired by intracorporeal sutures, to avoid surgical field contamination. Adhesiolysis should include the whole area of the defect and the surrounding peritoneal surface, in order to detect even minor covert defects and to allow an adequate mesh overlap.

Once peritoneal adhesion is dissected and all intestinal contents are reduced into the abdominal cavity and inspected for viability, the wall defect has to be measured to choose the appropriate mesh, that should overlap the defect by at least 5 cm, according to evidence of literature. An intraperitoneal mesh (polypropylene or polytetrafluoroethylene [PTFE]) is introduced through a 12 mm trocar and then unrolled inside the abdominal cavity. The mesh can be firstly suspended and held in place with four-corner transcutaneous stitches. After an accurate positioning is achieved, it is fixed to the abdominal wall. The most commonly used fixation method is with spiral tacks (absorbable or permanent, without significant differences [35]), set in a double crown configuration and about 2 cm apart from each other, sometimes combined with transfixed sutures, according to the personal technique and experience, but apparently without any advantage [36]. Some authors reported good results with the use of fibrin glue alone for prosthesis fixation [37], but no significant conclusions can be drawn as further evidence is needed [38]. Then, the omentum is usually placed over the bowel to separate it from the mesh and a final abdominal exploration is performed. The accesses greater than 5 mm are closed with resorbable sutures under direct vision with an appropriate port-closure needle or in the traditional way after pneumoperitoneum desufflation. A compressive dressing is applied for 5–7 days.

The use of biological mesh, that is suggested by some authors to reduce infections rate in potentially contaminated fields, is a controversial topic in current literature [39]. A recent multinational, randomized, controlled, and double-blind trial comparing synthetic and biological mesh in laparoscopic and open ventral hernia repair (LAPSIS trial) was prematurely stopped due to an unacceptable high recurrence rate in the biological mesh arms (both open and laparoscopic) [40]. Results from some other trials investigating this field are expected in order to update guidelines.

4.3 Results

Over the last years, literature has shown that laparoscopic incisional hernia emergency repair is feasible and safe in selected patients [34, 41]. Several authors reported lower length of stay, postoperative pain, wound-related, and infectious complications compared to open approach in emergency [42–44]. Some evidence show also a reduction of 30-day morbidity (including major complications), 30-day mortality and reoperation rate are comparable to open repair [45] and recurrence rate is acceptable [34, 41].

Rate of conversion after a laparoscopic emergency approach is reported to be around 4–9% [34, 41]. The most frequent reasons for conversion are bowel distension with subsequent reduced working space, dense adhesions, bowel necrosis, and laparoscopically unmanageable iatrogenic perforations [31, 32, 34].

The incidence of accidental enterotomies varies from 5 to 15%. Some authors state the feasibility of laparoscopic repair of the bowel injuries if they are not associated with enteric spillage in abdominal cavity [32, 46]. For this reason, enterotomies represent a relative contraindication to continue operation by a minimally invasive approach. By the way, in case of colon perforation with fecal contamination or extensive enteric spillage, conversion to laparotomy is recommended, with subsequent suture of lesions and accurate toilette of peritoneal cavity. As regards the mesh placing, a biological type should be preferred, otherwise a two-steps operation with a deferred mesh positioning should be performed [7, 26–28, 34].

Since peritonitis is the most feared and impacting complication (incidence 6%, mortality 0.3%) [47], surgeon has to explore the bowel after adhesiolysis, to check any missed enterotomy, whose incidence is reported to be 0.9% in elective laparoscopic operations for incisional hernia [34]. Some comparative analysis in literature shows that laparoscopic emergent repair is associated with a higher rate of missed enterotomies than open technique, but the reported rate is low (0.7%) and comparable to the incidence in election [42]. So it is important to highlight the importance of a careful abdominal exploration during laparoscopic hernia repair, before mesh placing, to consent an immediate identification of eventual lesions to repair and to evaluate if conversion is necessary.

4.4   Conclusions

Laparoscopic incisional hernia repair is safe and effective even in emergency setting and surgeon with good laparoscopic skills can use it as standard approach in selected patients. More research is needed to evaluate long-terms outcomes and to better define the selection criteria of patients with incarcerated hernias suitable for a minimally invasive approach, in order to reduce conversion rate and risk of complications.

References

1. Di Saverio S, et al., editors. Acute care surgery handbook. https://doi.org/10.1007/978-3-319-15362-9_21.
2. Birindelli A, et al. 2017 update of the WSES guidelines for emergency repair of complicated abdominal wall hernias. World J Emerg Surg. 2017;12:37. https://doi.org/10.1186/s13017-017-0149-y.
3. Helgstrand F, Rosenberg J, Kehlet H, Bisgaard T. Outcomes after emergency versus elective ventral hernia repair: a prospective nationwide study. World J Surg. 2013;37(10):2273–9. https://doi.org/10.1007/s00268-013-2123-5.
4. Hernia Surg Group. International guidelines for groin hernia management. Hernia. 2018;22(1):1–165. Published online 2018 Jan 12. https://doi.org/10.1007/s10029-017-1668-x.
5. Miserez M, Alexandre JH, Campanelli G, et al. The European hernia society groin hernia classification: simple and easy to remember. Hernia. 2007;11(2):113–6. https://doi.org/10.1007/s10029-007-0198-3.
6. Yang GP. Laparoscopy in emergency hernia repair. Ann Laparosc Endosc Surg. 2017;2:107.
7. De Simone B, Birindelli A, Ansaloni L, et al. Emergency repair of complicated abdominal wall hernias: WSES guidelines. Hernia. 2020;24(2):359–68.
8. Garner J. CDC guideline for prevention of surgical wound infections, 1985. Infect Control. 1986;7(3):193–200.
9. Özkan E, et al. Incarcerated abdominal wall hernia surgery: relationship between risk factors and morbidity and mortality rates (a single center emergency surgery experience). Turk J Trauma Emerg Surg. 2012;18(5):389–96. https://doi.org/10.5505/tjtes.2012.48827.
10. Surek A, Gemici E, Ferahman S, Karli M, Bozkurt MA, Dural AC, Donmez T, Karabulut M, Alis H. Emergency surgery of the abdominal wall hernias: risk factors that increase morbidity and mortality—a single-center experience. Hernia. 2021;25(3):679–88. https://doi.org/10.1007/s10029-020-02293-5. Epub 2020 Sep 10. PMID: 32914294.
11. Brown CVR, et al., editors. Emergency general surgery. https://doi.org/10.1007/978-3-319-96286-3_33.
12. Legutko J, Pach R, Solecki R, Matyja A, Kulig J. Rys historyczny leczenia chirurgicznego przepuklin [The history of treatment of groin hernia]. Folia Med Cracov. 2008;49(1–2):57–74. Polish. PMID: 19140492.
13. Agresta F, Ansaloni L, Baiocchi GL, et al. Laparoscopic approach to acute abdomen from the consensus development conference of the Società Italiana di Chirurgia Endoscopica e nuove tecnologie (SICE), Associazione Chirurghi Ospedalieri Italiani (ACOI), Società Italiana di Chirurgia (SIC), Società Italiana di Chirurgia d'Urgenza e del Trauma (SICUT), Società Italiana di Chirurgia nell'Ospedalità Privata (SICOP), and the European Association for Endoscopic Surgery (EAES). Surg Endosc. 2012;26:2134–64. https://doi.org/10.1007/s00464-012-2331-3.
14. Yang GP, Chan CT, Lai EC, et al. Laparoscopic versus open repair for strangulated groin hernias: 188 cases over 4 years. Asian J Endosc Surg. 2012;5:131–7.

15. Bittner R, Arregui ME, Bisgaard T, et al. Guidelines for laparoscopic (TAPP) and endoscopic (TEP) treatment of inguinal hernia [International Endohernia Society (IEHS)]. Surg Endosc. 2011;25:2773–843. https://doi.org/10.1007/s00464-011-1799-6.

16. Bittner R, Montgomery MA, Arregui E, et al. Update of guidelines on laparoscopic (TAPP) and endoscopic (TEP) treatment of inguinal hernia (International Endohernia Society). Surg Endosc. 2015;29:289–321. https://doi.org/10.1007/s00464-014-3917-8.

17. McCormack K, Scott NW, Go PM, et al.; Hernia Trialists Collaboration. Laparoscopic techniques versus open techniques for inguinal hernia repair. Cochrane Database Syst Rev. 2003;(1):CD001785.

18. Dedemadi G, Sgourakis G, Radtke A, et al. Laparoscopic versus open mesh repair for recurrent inguinal hernia: a meta-analysis of outcomes. Am J Surg. 2010;200(2):291–7.

19. Watson SD, Saye W, Hollier PA. Combined laparoscopic incarcerated herniorrhaphy and small bowel resection. Surg Laparosc Endosc. 1993;3(2):106–8.

20. Deeba S, Purkayastha S, Paraskevas P, et al. Laparoscopic approach to incarcerated and strangulated inguinal hernias. JSLS. 2009;13(3):327–31.

21. Sgourakis G, Radtke A, Sotiropoulos GC, et al. Assessment of strangulated content of the spontaneously reduced inguinal hernia via hernia sac laparoscopy: preliminary results of a prospective randomized study. Surg Laparosc Endosc Percutan Tech. 2009;19(2):133–7.

22. Palanivelu C, Rangarajan M, John SJ. Modified technique of laparoscopic intraperitoneal hernioplasty for irreducible scrotal hernias (omentoceles): how to remove the hernial contents. World J Surg. 2007;31(9):1889–91. https://doi.org/10.1007/s00268-007-9157-5.

23. White-Gittens IC, Kalabin A, Mani VR, et al. Hernioscopy in incarcerated inguinal hernia spontaneously reduced after general anesthesia induction. Cureus. 2017;9(11):e1849. https://doi.org/10.7759/cureus.1849.

24. Le Huu Nho R, Mege D, Ouaissi M, et al. Incidence and prevention of ventral incisional hernia. J Visc Surg. 2012;149(5 Suppl):e3–e14.

25. Beadles CA, Meagher AD, Charles AG. Trends in emergent hernia repair in the United States. JAMA Surg. 2015;150(3):194–200.

26. Cuccurullo D, Piccoli M, Agresta F, et al. Laparoscopic ventral incisional hernia repair: evidence-based guidelines of the first Italian consensus conference. Hernia. 2013;17(5):557–66.

27. Silecchia G, Campanile FC, Sanchez L, et al. Laparoscopic ventral/incisional hernia repair: updated guidelines from the EAES and EHS endorsed consensus development conference. Surg Endosc. 2015;29:2463–84.

28. Sauerland S, Agresta F, Bergamaschi R, et al. Laparoscopy for abdominal emergencies: evidence-based guidelines of the European Association for Endoscopic Surgery. Surg Endosc. 2006;20:14–29.

29. Dumanian GA, Denham W. Comparison of repair techniques for major incisional hernias. Am J Surg. 2003;185:61–5.

30. Olmi S, Cesana G, Erba L, et al. Emergency laparoscopic treatment of acute incarcerated incisional hernia. Hernia. 2009;13(6):605–8.

31. Franklin ME, Gonzalez JJ, Miter DB, et al. Laparoscopic diagnosis and treatment of intestinal obstruction. Surg Endosc. 2004;18:26–30.

32. Kirshtein B, Roy-Shapira A, Lantsberg L, et al. Laparoscopic management of acute small bowel obstruction. Surg Endosc. 2005;19:464–7.

33. Reinke CE, Matthews BD. What's new in the management of incarcerated hernia. J Gastrointest Surg. 2020;24(1):221–30.

34. Shah RH, Sharma A, Khullar R, et al. Laparoscopic repair of incarcerated ventral abdominal wall hernias. Hernia. 2008;12:457–63.

35. Smith AM, Faulkner JD, Chase N, et al. The effect of tack fixation methods on outcomes in laparoscopic ventral hernia repair. J Laparoendosc Adv Surg Tech A. 2021;31(7):779–82.

36. Baker JJ, Öberg S, Andresen K, et al. Adding sutures to tack fixation of mesh does not lower the re-operation rate after laparoscopic ventral hernia repair: a nationwide cohort study. Langenbecks Arch Surg. 2018;403(4):521–7.

37. Olmi S, Scaini A, Erba L, et al. Use of fibrin glue (Tissucol®) in laparoscopic repair of abdominal wall defects: preliminary experience. Surg Endosc. 2007;21:409–13.
38. Mathes T, Prediger B, Walgenbach M, et al. Mesh fixation techniques in primary ventral or incisional hernia repair. Cochrane Database Syst Rev. 2021;5(5):CD011563.
39. Campanelli G, Catena F, Ansaloni L. Prosthetic abdominal wall hernia repair in emergency surgery: from polypropylene to biological meshes. World J Emerg Surg. 2008;3:33.
40. Miserez M, Lefering R, Famiglietti F, et al. Synthetic versus biological mesh in laparoscopic and open ventral hernia repair (LAPSIS): results of a multinational, randomized, controlled, and double-blind trial. Ann Surg. 2021;273(1):57–65.
41. Landau O, Kyzer S. Emergent laparoscopic repair of incarcerated incisional and ventral hernia. Surg Endosc. 2004;18:1374–6.
42. Azin A, Hirpara D, Jackson T, et al. Emergency laparoscopic and open repair of incarcerated ventral hernias: a multi-institutional comparative analysis with coarsened exact matching. Surg Endosc. 2019;33(9):2812–20.
43. Kao AM, Huntington CR, Otero J, et al. Emergent laparoscopic ventral hernia repairs. J Surg Res. 2018;232:497–502.
44. Pechman DM, Cao L, Fong C, et al. Laparoscopic versus open emergent ventral hernia repair: utilization and outcomes analysis using the ACSNSQIP database. Surg Endosc. 2018;32(12):4999–5005.
45. Elnahas A, Kim SHH, Okrainec A, et al. Is laparoscopic repair of incarcerated abdominal hernias safe? Analysis of short-term outcomes. Surg Endosc. 2016;30(8):3262–6.
46. Grafen FC, Neuhaus V, Schob O, et al. Management of acute small bowel obstruction from intestinal adhesions: indications for laparoscopic surgery in a community teaching hospital. Langenbecks Arch Surg. 2010;395:57–63.
47. Piccoli M, Ferronato M, Morici R, et al. Emergency laparoscopic repair of complicated ventral and incisional hernias. Updates Surg. 2008;2:227–35.

Internal and Congenital Hernias

Giovanni D. Tebala, Emanuela Ceriati, Roshneen Ali,
Sonia Battaglia, Francesco De Peppo, Frances Dixon,
Mahul Patel, Amanda Shabana, and Valerio Voglino

1   Introduction

Hernias are a common cause for hospitalisation, both as elective and emergency cases. Each year, about one million hernia operations are performed in the United States [1] and about 100,000 in England [2], but due to issues around the classification of hernias, particularly those that do not involve the anterior abdominal wall, these numbers are likely an underestimate.

There are two main types of hernias: external hernias which involve protrusion of intestinal loops through an abdominal wall defect and internal hernias which refer to the protrusion of abdominal viscera through an aperture within the peritoneal cavity, whether the normal anatomical apertures or a pathologically abnormal aperture. Other types of hernias are far less common, such as musculofascial

---

Giovanni D. Tebala and Emanuela Ceriati contributed equally to this work.

G. D. Tebala (✉) · R. Ali · F. Dixon · A. Shabana
Department of General Surgery, Surgical Emergency Unit, Oxford University Hospitals NHS Foundation Trust, Oxford, UK
e-mail: giovanni.tebala@ouh.nhs.uk; roshneen.ali@ouh.nhs.uk; frances.dixon@ouh.nhs.uk; amanda.shabana@ouh.nhs.uk

E. Ceriatie.ceriati@opbg.net

S. Battaglia · F. De Peppo · V. Voglino
Department of Paediatric Surgery, IRCCS "Bambino Gesù" Children's Hospital, Rome, Italy
e-mail: francesco.depeppo@opbg.net; v.voglino@opbg.net

M. Patel
Department of General Surgery, Albany Medical Centre, Albany, NY, USA
e-mail: patelm7@amc.edu

© The Author(s), under exclusive license to Springer Nature Switzerland AG 2023
F. Coccolini et al. (eds.), *Mini-invasive Approach in Acute Care Surgery*,
Hot Topics in Acute Care Surgery and Trauma,
https://doi.org/10.1007/978-3-031-39001-2_15

hernias, or are of no interest to the general surgeon, such as intervertebral disc hernias and cerebral hernias.

Some hernias are congenital, i.e. present at birth, whereas others are acquired during life. They usually present with symptoms due to the protrusion of tissue (either fat or bowel) through a rigid ring. In this chapter, we will analyse internal and congenital hernias in detail and will try to delineate some guidance for their diagnosis, prevention and treatment.

2 Internal Hernias

2.1 Definition

The real incidence of internal hernias and of their subtypes is not known, mostly due to classification issues. In fact, many internal hernias are still described as obstruction due to adhesions or simply 'bowel obstruction'.

Internal hernias can occur through a number of intra-abdominal orifices, whether pre-existing apertures or acquired defects of the peritoneal folds due to trauma, inflammation or previous surgery. Possible apertures include normal anatomical structures like the foramen of Winslow but also abnormal ones such as those that occur with intestinal malrotation. Herniation of bowel or omentum through any of these orifices can lead to obstruction or strangulation. Congenital and acquired diaphragmatic hernias are also considered internal abdominal hernias even though the protrusion is intra-thoracic and therefore technically extra-abdominal.

Internal hernias are also recognised complications occurring after upper and lower gastrointestinal procedures. Their incidence after upper oesophagogastric surgery has been reported at between 0.5 and 11% [3]. They are less commonly reported following laparoscopic colorectal surgery, with the majority of those occurring after left-sided colonic anastomoses [4].

Laparoscopic surgery has been considered a risk factor for internal hernias when compared to open surgery, mostly due to the reduced formation of adhesions tethering mobile structures and preventing herniation. Other risk factors following upper gastrointestinal and bariatric surgery include non-closure of the mesenteric defects, low BMI, excessive weight loss and female sex [5]. Risk factors following colorectal surgery are less clear, but left-sided resections and early post-operative mobilisation of the patient may be contributing factors [4, 6]. Large mesenteric defects, full mobilisation of the splenic flexure and high ligation of the mesenteric vessels performed in oncological resections may also contribute to higher rates [7].

Internal hernias can be classified according to their location and pathophysiology (Table 1). Understanding the exact anatomy of the hernial sac is crucial in order to reduce the risk of complications. In fact, in most cases, at least one of the boundaries of the neck incorporates a significant vessel that must be identified and preserved during mobilisation of the hernia (Figs. 1, 2, 3, and 4). The risk of bowel ischaemia is increased when any of the major vessels of the abdomen are in close proximity to the hernia.

Table 1 Summary of types of internal hernias

Hernia	Pathophysiology	Anatomy of the hernia ring	Subtype
Left para-duodenal	Bowel prolapses through Landzert's fossa (present in 2% of the population) (Fig. 1)	The inferior mesenteric vein runs at its anterior and lateral edge along with the left colic artery. The medial and superior borders are formed by the duodenojejunal junction and the aorta	Congenital
Right para-duodenal	Bowel herniates through Waldeyer's fossa (defect in first part of jejunal mesentery seen in <1% of population) (Fig. 1)	The right paraduodenal recess is behind the superior mesenteric pedicle or the ileocolic pedicle which forms the anterior border of the hernia sac. The posterior and superior borders are usually formed by the third part of the duodenum	Congenital
Pericaecal	Four subtypes (ileocolic, retrocecal, ileocecal and paracaecal) which often consist of an ileal segment protruding through a defect in the caecal mesentery or one of the paracaecal recesses (Fig. 2)	Depends on the site of the hernia. One of the edges of the ring is usually the caecal wall. In the paracaecal and retrocaecal types, the posterior edge is the posterior abdominal wall. The hernia sac is usually within the right mesocolon or below the ascending colon	Congenital
Lesser sac	Bowel herniates through the foramen of Winslow, which is a normal communication located beneath the hepatogastroduodenal ligament, also known as lesser omentum (Fig. 1)	Hepatic pedicle and hepatoduodenal ligament anteriorly, duodenum and stomach inferiorly, caudate lobe of the liver superiorly, posterior peritoneum covering the inferior vena cava posteriorly	Congenital
Intersigmoid	Herniated bowel, usually ileum protrudes into the intersigmoid fossa (or recess) (Fig. 3)	The hernia ring is formed by mesosigmoid for the most and the posterior edge is the posterior abdominal peritoneum and the ureter	Congenital

(continued)

Table 1 (continued)

Hernia	Pathophysiology	Anatomy of the hernia ring	Subtype
Transomental	Small and, less frequently, large bowel loops can herniate through defects of the greater omentum	The hernia ring is formed entirely by the greater omentum	Congenital or acquired
Transmesenteric	In children, it can arise from a defect in the small bowel mesentery, near the ileocaecal region or ligament of Treitz, or through a congenital defect of the mesosigmoid at the level of the sigmoid recess. In adults, it is usually secondary to abdominal surgery, especially gastrojejunal anastomosis, trauma or inflammation. There are four types: (1) transmesocolic, after transmesocolic gastrojejunal anastomosis; (2) transmesosigmoid, through a defect of the mesosigmoid; (3) transmesenteric, the bowel protrudes through a defect in the small bowel mesentery; (4) transfalciform, when bowel herniates through a defect of the falciform ligament anteriorly or anterocaudally to the liver	The hernia ring is composed by mesentery but at least one of the sides of the ring contains a vascular pedicle	Congenital or acquired
Retroanastomotic	Small bowel loops herniate posteriorly through defect related to a surgical anastomosis, commonly with gastrojejunal or bilioenteric anastomosis. The most common herniated loop consists of the efferent jejunal segment. The Petersen's hernia occurs posteriorly to a gastric bypass (Fig. 4)	Small bowel anteriorly, colon or duodenum posteriorly	Acquired
Retrocolic	Small bowel loops herniate below the transposed transverse colon after a distal colectomy with mobilisation of the splenic flexure	Transverse colon anteriorly, Gerota fascia posteriorly	Acquired

(continued)

Table 1 (continued)

Hernia	Pathophysiology	Anatomy of the hernia ring	Subtype
Diaphragmatic[a]	Occurs when any abdominal organ, including stomach, pancreas, liver, large and small bowel, spleen, herniate towards the chest through a defect of the diaphragm. The Bochdalek hernia happens through a posterolateral defect of the diaphragm, usually on the left side. The Morgagni hernia occurs through an anterior retrosternal defect of the diaphragm. Post-traumatic hernias are more frequent on the left side	The hernia ring is formed by the diaphragm, either the tendineal or the muscular part	Congenital or acquired
Hiatal[a]	Any abdominal organ, mostly the stomach, herniates towards the mediastinum, and sometimes also the pleural cavity, through an enlarged hiatus	The hernia ring is constituted by the oesophageal hiatus, that is, two diaphragmatic crura laterally, diaphragm and phreno-oesophageal membrane anteriorly	Congenital or acquired

[a] Some authors do not consider diaphragmatic and hiatal hernias as internal hernias as they are not contained within the abdominal cavity. Hiatal hernias will be described in another chapter

Fig. 1 Paraduodenal and lesser sac hernias

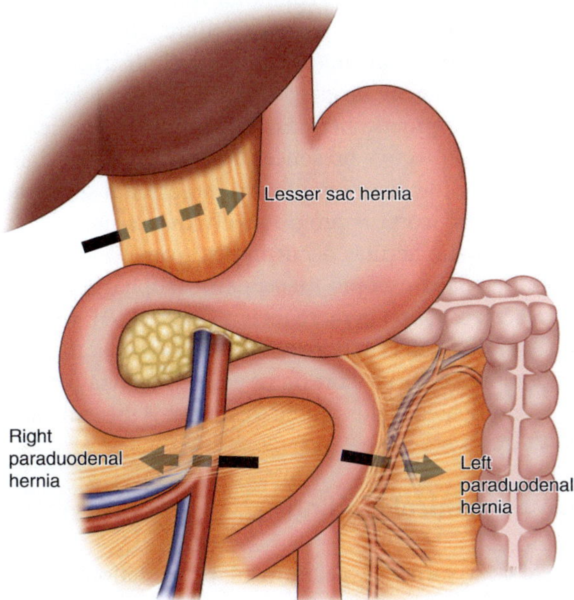

Fig. 2 Pericaecal hernias

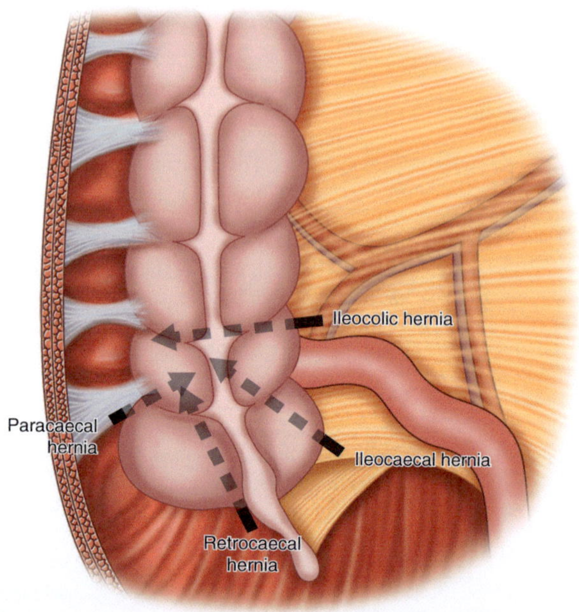

Post-traumatic hernias of the diaphragm can happen at any time after a blunt (5%) or penetrating (19%) trauma of the torso. A diaphragmatic defect can be diagnosed at the time of the trauma laparotomy (about 50% of cases) or subsequently, even as late as several years after the trauma, usually after a clinical presentation with thoracic pain, respiratory failure, dysphagia due to stomach inlet or outlet obstruction or small and/or large bowel obstruction. Sometimes they are discovered incidentally during investigations done for other reasons in asymptomatic patients. Most diaphragmatic hernias occur through the left hemidiaphragm (about 90%), due to the protective presence of the liver on the right, but right diaphragmatic hernias may follow liver resectional surgery if a small diaphragmatic lesion goes undiagnosed and worsens progressively over a number of years. Post-oesophagectomy diaphragmatic hernias occur in just over 2% of cases and appear to be more common after laparoscopic than open oesophagectomy [8, 9]. However, higher rates have been reported in more recent studies [10], which beg the question as to whether the complication is under-reported, or whether the increased incidence can be attributed to the larger proportion of cases done via the minimally invasive approach.

Complicated hiatus hernia treatment is the subject of another chapter of this book.

2.2 Clinical Findings

There is a variable spectrum of presentation ranging from hours to years postoperatively, and symptoms may be acute or chronic. Sixty-nine percent of patients who developed internal hernia following colorectal resection presented within

Fig. 3 Intersigmoid hernias

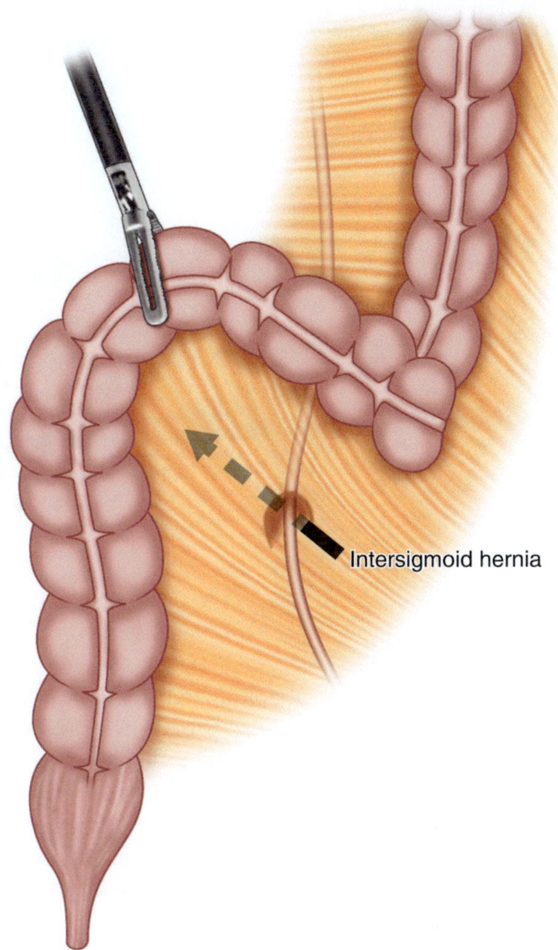

10 days of the initial operation [4], whereas for bariatric surgery patients, the highest incidence happens at around 1–2 years post-surgery, which corresponds to the greatest period of weight loss [11]. While the incidence of acute presentations is low, the true incidence of post-operative internal hernias is likely to be far greater than that quoted in literature. Small bowel herniating behind the neo-descending colon has been identified radiologically in 21% of asymptomatic patients following laparoscopic anterior resection [12]. Additionally, in a non-acute context, internal hernias have been found in patients with unexplained intermittent abdominal pain following bariatric procedures [3]. Therefore, a high index of suspicion must be maintained.

Clinically, the range of symptoms from internal hernias ranges from no symptoms to acute abdominal pain, often vague epigastric pain or intermittent colicky periumbilical pain. This pain is often associated with non-specific symptoms such

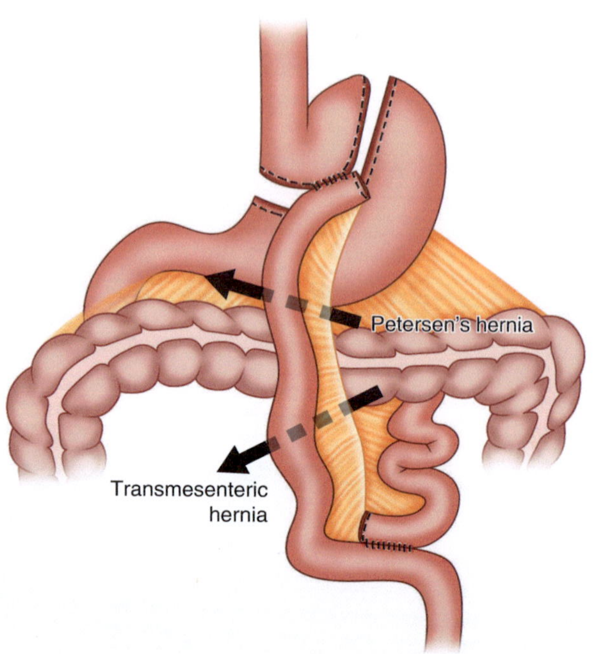

Fig. 4 Petersen's hernia and transmesenteric hernia

as nausea, vomiting or abdominal distention, which can complicate diagnosis. Diaphragmatic hernias may also present with acute respiratory distress. Symptom severity relates to the duration and reducibility of the hernia and the presence or absence of incarceration and strangulation. Examination findings may demonstrate a palpable intra-abdominal mass of herniated loops with localised tenderness. It is important to highlight that the clinical presentation of an internal hernia is often that of an acute bowel obstruction, and symptoms and initial assessment overlap those of bowel obstruction.

Post-traumatic and post-surgical diaphragmatic hernias can present with symptoms of chest pain, gastric inlet or outlet obstruction (nausea, vomiting, dysphagia) and progressive or acute respiratory failure due to compression of the lung or the inferior vena cava.

Every patient presenting with acute bowel obstruction or acute abdomen must be thoroughly assessed for comorbidities and acute complications such as bowel ischaemia. It is crucial to collect a thorough clinical history, in particular regarding recurrent and vague symptoms of abdominal pain, with or without vomiting and nausea, weight loss, reduction of appetite and any prior history of abdominal operations or traumas. A complete set of blood tests must be sent including haemoglobin, inflammatory markers, renal and liver function tests, coagulation, lactate and blood gases, bearing in mind that in most non-hyperacute cases, blood tests may be normal.

Due to the generally vague and non-specific nature of typical clinical findings, diagnosis is often delayed, and therefore the risk of complications is high, which highlights the importance of prompt and thorough investigation.

2.3 Investigations

Although the final diagnosis of internal hernia can be done only with direct exploration, contrast-enhanced CT scan is the first-line investigation and can demonstrate features of small or large bowel obstruction, with or without a clear transition point (Figs. 5 and 6). However, CT scan can be falsely negative in up to 50% of cases [13].

The usual radiological appearance is of crowded and often encapsulated dilated small bowel loops. Other commonly observed radiological signs include the 'swirl sign' described as the swirling appearance of mesenteric fat and vessels found in 95% [14], superior mesenteric vein 'beaking' in 81% (where the vein appears to taper off), and the 'mushroom' shape of herniated bowel which is present in 62% of patients with internal hernia [15].

In hernias of the foramen of Winslow, a loop of bowel can be seen in the lesser sac, posteriorly and cephalically to the stomach and anteriorly and cephalically to the pancreas. The transition point is usually posterior to the hepatic pedicle (Fig. 5). It is not unusual that the herniated loop pushes posteriorly on the common bile duct, causing mild dilatation of the intra-hepatic ducts.

In diaphragmatic hernias, the typical CT finding is of bowel (or any other abdominal organ) transposed into the chest, usually dilated and with air-fluid level (Fig. 6).

Following bariatric procedures, bowel loops behind the superior mesenteric artery were only observed in 29% but had a very high positive predictive value [16].

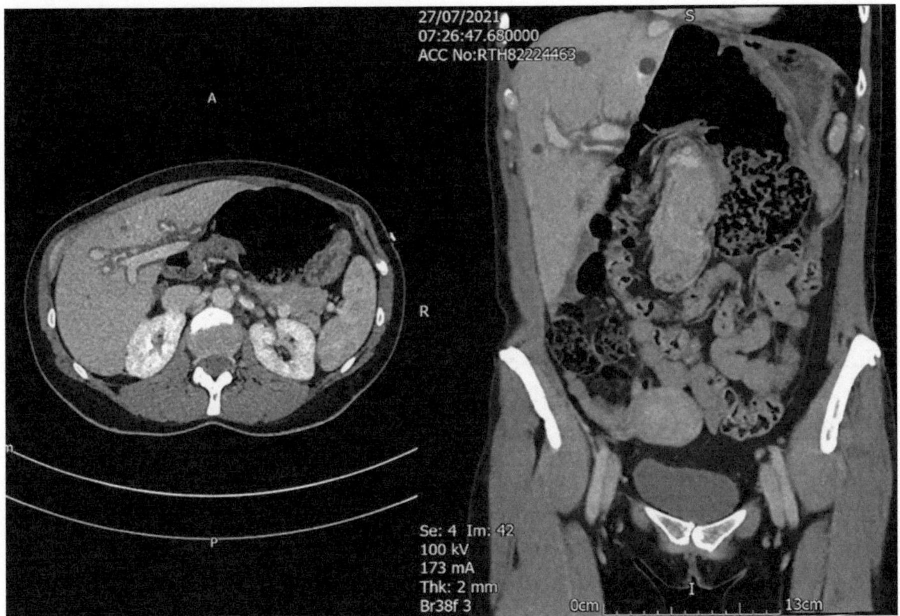

Fig. 5 Hernia of the foramen of Winslow, CT scan. Whole ascending colon with terminal ileum and proximal transverse colon migrated into the lesser sac through the foramen of Winslow

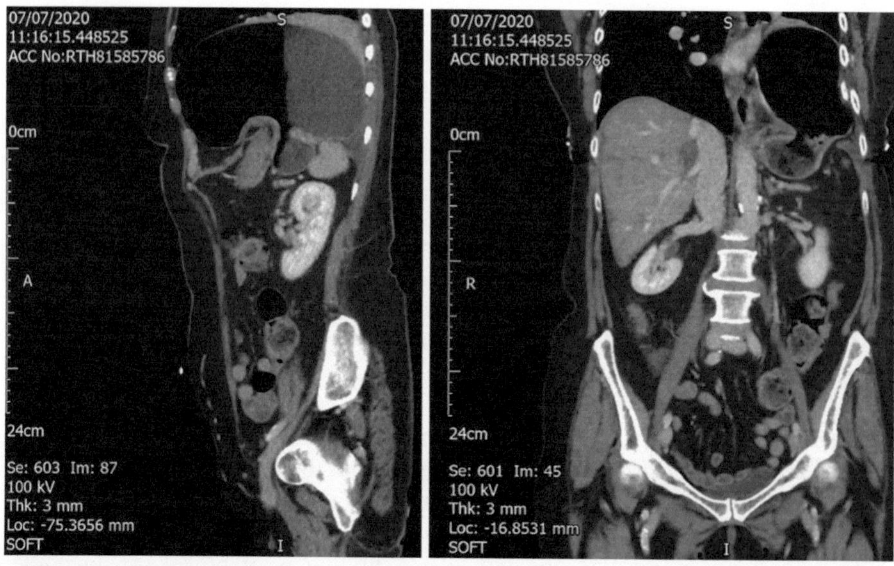

Fig. 6 Post-traumatic diaphragmatic hernia, CT scan. Dilated bowel transposed into the left chest cavity with air-fluid level

However, it must be observed that positive CT findings can be seen only in 74% of patients with Petersen's hernia [17] which tends to occur post Roux-en-Y gastric bypass, and diagnostic laparoscopy is much more reliable than CT scan in evaluating abdominal pain for possible internal hernia in these patients [13].

After colonic resections, U- or C-shaped small bowel loops can be apparent on CT postero-laterally to transposed transverse colon or left neo-descending colon and anterior to the retroperitoneum [6, 18, 19].

CT signs of bowel ischaemia include reduced enhancement of the bowel wall, thickening of the bowel wall, small bowel dilatation, the presence of peritoneal fluid, congestion of small veins, ascites, pneumatosis of the bowel wall and porto-mesenteric venous gas [20, 21]. Although plain chest X-rays can show large diaphragmatic and hiatal hernias, the reliability of plain abdominal films is generally quite low, and we do not suggest performing any plain film before or after the CT scan. Similarly, the diagnostic value of barium or water-soluble contrast studies is minimal, unless in the context of an attempted conservative management with water-soluble oral contrast where the progression of the contrast medium within the gastrointestinal tract may be a useful diagnostic aid as well as a therapeutic one. In experienced hands, an abdominal ultrasound scan can show features of bowel obstruction and even rule out intestinal ischaemia, but nowadays a quick and complete contrast-enhanced abdominopelvic CT scan remains the investigation of choice.

2.4   Prevention

Generally, the traditional rule has always been to close every mesenteric defect that can potentially give rise to an internal hernia. This is mandatory in small bowel resections and in small segmental resections of the large bowel where the mesenteric defect is small, and therefore any internal hernia would have a high likelihood of strangulation. There has been much debate on the necessity of closing large defects, such as the posterior space behind a gastrojejunostomy or the mesocolic defect after a right or left colectomy, in particular after the introduction of laparoscopic surgery where closure of the peritoneal defects may not be easy.

There are clear recommendations for reduction of internal hernias following laparoscopic upper gastrointestinal procedures and bariatric surgery. Closure of the mesenteric defects is widely recommended following Roux-en-Y gastric bypass. Closure of one defect has been reported to reduce the incidence from 3.5% to 1.7% [22], and closure of both defects may further halve the incidence in comparison to only closing one defect [23]. A recent meta-analysis of more than 10,000 pooled patients who underwent Roux-en-Y gastric bypass revealed that closing the defects reduces the risk of internal hernias, in both observational and randomised studies (odds ratio 0.28 and 0.29, respectively) [24]. Numerous methods of closure have been trialled, including sutures, staples and glue with no conclusive recommendation. Closure of mesenteric defects is commonly performed with continuous non-absorbable sutures with the first stitch placed at the transition between small bowel serosa and mesentery [11]. Care should be taken not to cause kinking of the jejuno-jejunal anastomosis [25]. An antecolic, antegastric approach for Roux-en-Y gastric bypass has been suggested to prevent formation of a potential space in the transverse mesocolon and has been reported to have a fourfold reduced risk in comparison to a retrocolic approach [26].

Hiatoplasty does not appear to prevent trans-hiatal post-oesophagectomy hernias [9], but many surgeons would tend to reduce the hiatus anyway and may also suture the transposed gastric tubule to the crura before or after the oesophageal anastomosis.

There is no clear evidence whether the large mesenteric defects created by colorectal surgery should be closed routinely [27]. A recent cohort study on 198 patients showed that 21% of patients who underwent an anterior resection develop an asymptomatic internal hernia, but only a small percentage (0.5%) present with small bowel obstruction [12]. That study proposes that a routine closure of the defect should be considered, but they did not explore the risks related to this manoeuvre, such as closing or kinking the ureter with a stich or injuring the left colic pedicle. Similarly, there is no consensus as to whether the splenic flexure should be fully mobilised or not. Full mobilisation creates a larger defect for potential herniation, whereas incomplete mobilisation may increase the risk of incarceration should herniation occur [9]. Some studies suggest repositioning the small bowel to the contralateral side from the resection to prevent immediate post-operative internal herniation [9], but we suggest that, after the anastomosis, the surgeon routinely checks if any small bowel loop has remained trapped behind the transposed colon. The large mesocolic defect in distal colectomies can be safely closed with glue [28], but sutures increase the risk of vascular injuries and subsequent distal ischaemia [27]. However, routine closure of the defect may be justified by the high mortality associated with postoperative internal hernia.

2.5   Treatment

The treatment of these patients follows the evidence and guidelines for small bowel obstruction [29], with some adaptation. In stable patients with no signs of peritonitis, strangulation or bowel ischaemia, initial non-operative management can potentially be attempted. However, having a precise diagnosis is mandatory as an excessive delay may lead to extremely severe complications such as bowel ischaemia. Delayed surgery may increase mortality and morbidity [30], but emergency laparotomies also carry a high burden of risk, and therefore an initial non-operative treatment plan is justified. Early laparoscopic exploration may be a good option in some selected patients where the CT scan cannot definitively rule out ischaemia of the bowel. However, some internal hernias should be immediately referred for surgery as they are particularly high risk for ischaemia and recurrence.

Non-operative management should not extend beyond 3 days [30] and would entail fasting and gastric decompression through a nasogastric tube. The administration of water-soluble contrast may facilitate the early resolution of obstruction and also has diagnostic value as it may demonstrate a complete obstruction which would prompt an early operation. The patient should concurrently be maintained on intravenous fluids or total parenteral nutrition. However, it is worth emphasising that non-operative management is a risky strategy in patients with suspected internal hernia, and its choice must be based on clear criteria and convincing the absence of ischaemia or perforation on the CT scan.

If conservative management fails or if there are signs of ischaemia at CT or at blood tests (lactate), surgical exploration is mandatory. A laparoscopic exploration has the dual purpose of both diagnosis and treatment. The vast majority of internal hernias after laparoscopic operation can be treated laparoscopically, in particular those that occur after gastric bypass [31]. This is the case, for instance, with a Petersen's hernia or obstruction of the small bowel loops entrapped below the transposed transverse colon after distal colectomy. Many cases have been reported in the literature, but no large series. A recent comparatively small cohort study from Japan [32] showed that laparoscopic repair of Petersen's hernia has some advantages with respect to open surgery in terms of quicker recovery but demonstrated no difference in operative time, mortality and morbidity.

However, the laparoscopic approach is not easy and is further complicated by two factors due to the underlying pathology; the distension of the obstructed bowel may reduce the operative field in the abdomen, and oedema of the bowel loops may hamper reduction of the hernia sac. Furthermore, the laparoscopic approach needs a skilled surgeon who has experience in surgery for obstructed bowel, as the risk of bowel injury is extraordinarily high in those conditions.

Clearly the surgical technique changes according to the site of the hernia. We suggest putting the patient in a Lloyd-Davies position, with legs on stirrups so that the surgeon can stand between the legs of the patient, if needed. This is particularly important in diaphragmatic hernias as it gives good laparoscopic access to the upper abdomen.

The operation should start with an exploration of the abdomen through a port located as centrally as possible. For the first trocar, the use of the blunt 'Hasson' technique is highly recommended, in particular for patients who have had multiple abdominal operations and certainly in those with a massively distended abdomen. Clearly, the classical laparoscopic rules still apply on where to obtain the initial access. The umbilical position provides good access to all abdominal quadrants but may be complicated by a midline scar, and the right upper quadrant (Palmer's point) should be considered for these patients.

The position of the other ports depends on the planned operation while also taking into account the correct triangulation of the ports. Three ports including the one for the laparoscope guarantee good access and good manoeuvrability within the abdomen but may not be enough. Overtly distended bowel or diffuse faecal or enteric contamination as well as complications or other difficulties in carrying out a laparoscopic operation may require a prompt conversion to open surgery. In the case of an unstable patient or in the absence of a suitably skilled laparoscopic surgeon, it is still perfectly acceptable to approach these conditions with a routine midline laparotomy.

The initial inspection of the abdominal cavity is aimed at ruling out ischaemia or perforation of the bowel. In case of perforation, free gas would escape as soon as the first trocar is inserted. The surgeon should look for free intestinal content and/or pus in the abdomen, as well as any localised collections of pus or bile, before following the bowel to find the transition point of the obstruction. Where there is a strangulated closed loop, the bowel may be ischaemic or frankly necrotic. In hernias of the lesser sac, it is possible to see the herniated loop of bowel bulging through the hepato-gastric ligament (Fig. 7).

Mobilisation of the herniated bowel should happen with delicate traction on the bowel or omentum but avoiding traction on the mesentery wherever possible (Figs. 8 and 9). If this is not feasible, it may be necessary to incise the neck of the hernia. The

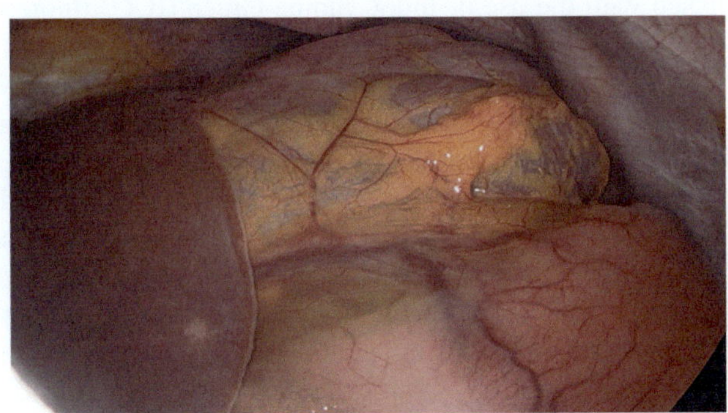

Fig. 7 Hernia of the foramen of Winslow, same clinical case as Fig. 5. The dilated caecum can be seen through the hepatogastric ligament

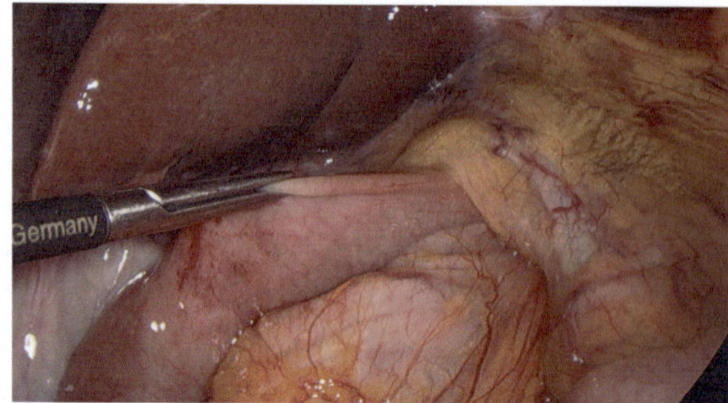

Fig. 8 Hernia of the foramen of Winslow, same clinical case as Fig. 5. Afferent and efferent loops passing below the hepatic pedicle

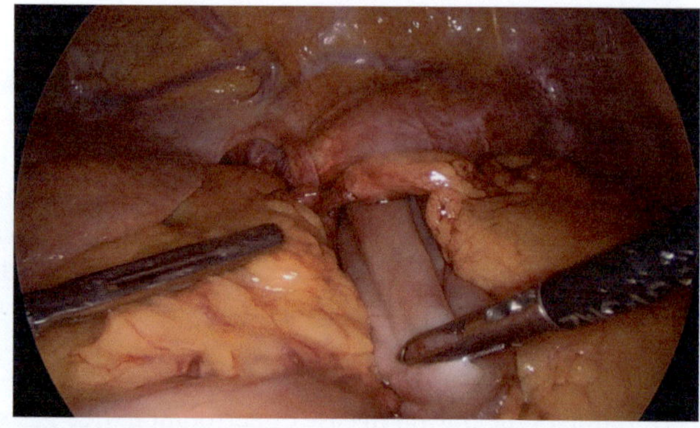

Fig. 9 Post-traumatic diaphragmatic hernia, same clinical case as Fig. 6, intraoperative view. The herniated bowel is cautiously pulled back into the abdomen

surgeon must fully consider the anatomy of the internal hernia when deciding where to make the incision rather than making it randomly. As previously mentioned, very often at least one of the sides of the neck of the hernia contains a major vessel (see Table 1), and therefore the incision must be made as far as possible from it. After mobilising the hernia, the viability of the bowel must be fully established with immediate inspection of the serosal surface and review again after re-warming (either using wet hot swabs or simply immersion in warm water). If the bowel is frankly necrotic or its appearance does not improve after several minutes of re-warming, then resection and anastomosis are indicated. The viability of the bowel can also be established with the use of IndoCyanine Green (ICG) fluorescence using a near-infrared light [33]. The aim of the next steps of the operation is to reduce the risk of recurrent internal hernia. If possible, the defect should be closed with suture, glue or mesh.

Left and right paraduodenal, paracaecal and intersigmoid recesses and mesenteric or mesocolic defects should either be closed with glue or with sutures involving only the peritoneal layers, to avoid damaging the underlying vascular structures. Defects of the transverse mesocolon at the point of passage of a jejunal limb heading to or from a supramesocolic anastomosis must be reduced by suturing the edges of the defect to the bowel going through it and its mesentery directly or with the interposition of greater omentum. The retrocolic space created after transposition of the transverse colon towards the pelvis is usually a wide space, and obstructions of a herniated loop of small bowel happen only when the latter is compressed by the large bowel and fixed by adhesions. After mobilising the herniated bowel, it may be advisable to glue or suture the transverse mesocolon to the fascia of Gerota from the duodenojejunal angle to the pelvis. However, this suture may reduce the space behind the colon without closing it completely, thus predisposing to the risk of a recurrence of the hernia through a much tighter space. When fixing these hernias, consider that in these cases, the herniation of the small bowel does not usually happen spontaneously but rather during the original colectomy and that the transposed transverse mesocolon tends to attach spontaneously to the fascia of Gerota, and therefore the simple extraction of the small bowel from behind the transverse colon without any other manoeuvre may well suffice, provided that the bowel is still viable.

In case of hernia of the lesser sac, the foramen of Winslow must be closed, possibly with a running suture, making sure that only the peritoneum is taken with the stitches and that the elements of the hepatic pedicle (mostly, the common bile duct) are not kinked or sutured.

Retroanastomotic hernias such as Petersen's hernias also require the closure of the defect. This can be accomplished with a running suture with a slowly absorbable material or with glue. Another option would be to open up the defect completely in order to allow easy passage of small bowel in and out the defect, for example, with right paraduodenal hernias. To reduce a right paraduodenal hernia and prevent recurrence, it may be necessary to completely mobilise the right colon with a Cattell's manoeuvre, either laparoscopically or via laparotomy. The whole right colon and proximal transverse must be repositioned into the left abdomen so to open the right paraduodenal recess wide and prevent further herniation. This is in contrast to the repair of left paraduodenal hernias where the hernia sac is opened along the base of the descending mesocolon.

Acute post-traumatic diaphragmatic hernias are often treated with open surgery due to as yet unresolved concerns on the use of laparoscopy in the acute trauma setting, unless it is an isolated diaphragmatic injury, bearing in mind that acute laparoscopy may miss associated injuries in up to 40% of cases. However, acute cases are often easier than chronic ones as the defect is well defined, and there has not yet been time for adhesions to form [34]. More commonly, diaphragmatic hernias do not present until months or years after the trauma and are usually approached laparoscopically (Figs. 9, 10, and 11).

The repair of a hiatus or diaphragmatic hernia is better standardised than intraperitoneal hernias, usually because CT scan is more reliable for diagnosis. However, it is important to have a degree of flexibility in the position of the trocars. A post-traumatic diaphragmatic hernia can be approached with only three trocars. We tend to put the first port on the parasternal line, about 5–10 cm above the umbilicus, in line with the stomach and the oesophagus, although a more central position is an acceptable alternative position. The two operating ports are usually inserted about 10 cm to the left and right of the main port and slightly cephalad, below the costal margin. An additional port for the liver retractor can be inserted in the epigastrium or in the right flank, while a port to help with the traction on the herniated viscera may be useful if inserted on the patient's left side.

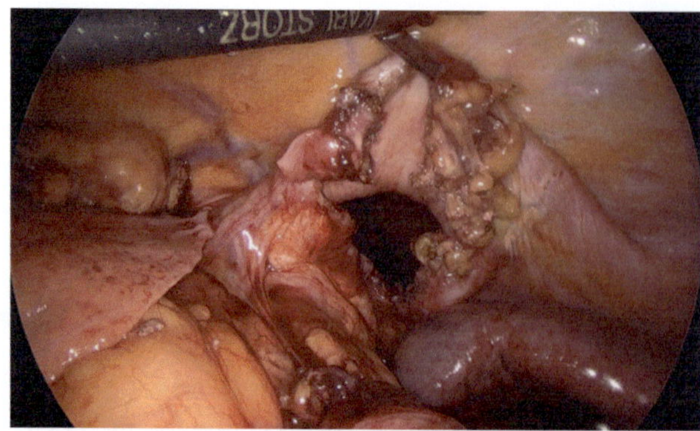

Fig. 10 Post-traumatic diaphragmatic hernia, same clinical case as Fig. 6, intraoperative view. Diaphragmatic defect

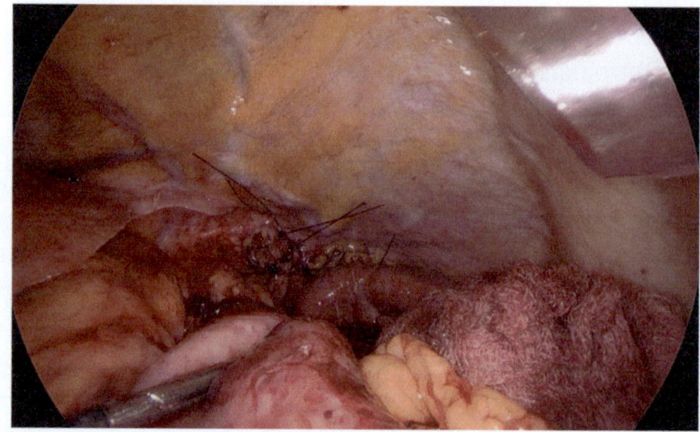

Fig. 11 Post-traumatic diaphragmatic hernia, same clinical case as Fig. 6, intraoperative view. Defect closed with suture

The initial step of the operation is to conduct a thorough examination of the abdominal cavity and an exploration of the site of the hernia. Once the diagnosis and site have been confirmed, the herniated viscera are slowly and carefully reduced into the abdomen. All adhesions within the sac and to the diaphragm must be divided. The closure of the diaphragmatic defect is usually carried out with single stitches or a running suture with a non-absorbable or slowly absorbable material (such as polydioxanone). Before closing the diaphragm, the defect must be inspected to ensure that the pleura is not damaged. In case of a pneumothorax, it is advisable to ask the anaesthetist to increase the tidal volume and expand the lung before finishing the suture. A chest tube should be placed either at this stage or later on in the operation but must be in place before extubating the patient.

Large hernias may require the use of a mesh to bridge the defect or to reinforce the suture if the edges can be approximated. Obviously, the mesh must be centred on the defect. Some authors suggest suturing the mesh to the previous diaphragmatic suture and gluing the edges of the mesh to the diaphragm [35]. An alternative technique is to suture the four corners of the mesh to the diaphragm and glue the rest, but it is important to be flexible and adapt your operative technique based on the location and features of the diaphragmatic hernia. The use of tacks to fix the mesh to the diaphragm is not advisable, particularly medially, due to the risk of cardiac injury. A systematic review identified 23 cases of cardiac injury due to diaphragmatic tacks, with a mortality of 48% [36]. Reducing the abdominal pression during the suture and positioning of the mesh may be of great help to decrease the tension on the surface of the diaphragm and allow an easy closure of the defect.

The use of mesh to reinforce diaphragmatic defects has always been a controversial question, and there remains wide disagreement. A recent RCT published in 2020 on the use of suture vs. absorbable vs. non-absorbable mesh did not show any advantage with the use of mesh to repair large hiatus hernias [37], but the sample size was not very large. A meta-analysis published in the same year on more than 300 pooled patients yielded similar results [38]. It is not clear if these results can be extended to the repair of diaphragmatic non-hiatus hernias.

The treatment of trans-hiatal post-oesophagectomy hernias can be performed laparoscopically with great efficacy and low risk [39]. Some studies suggest placing a chest tube prior to induction of pneumoperitoneum [39], but in our experience, a chest drain can be inserted at any time during or after the procedure, particularly if the anaesthetist reports high respiratory pressure and low compliance. The first step of the operation is an adhesiolysis, to mobilise the contents of the hernia, while being very careful not to injure the gastroepiploic vessels as they represent the only source of vascular supply to the gastric tubule. For the same reasons, the dissection of the herniated bowel must be performed close to the crura [40]. After reducing the hernia, the repair of the hiatus is achieved through an anterior and posterior cruroplasty with non-absorbable or slowly absorbable sutures, possibly with the use of non-absorbable pledgets to avoid muscular tears [9]. Some studies advocate the use of a biological mesh to plug the enlarged hiatus [41] or to reinforce a weak diaphragmatic suture or residual defect [39]. Most of these repairs can be done laparoscopically or robotically, but with a low threshold for conversion [39].

3　　Congenital Hernias

3.1　　Introduction

Abdominal wall defects represent a broad spectrum of congenital anomalies, varying from benign umbilical cord hernias to lethal conditions.

The two most common anomalies included in this group are omphalocele and gastroschisis [42–44]. Both are usually diagnosed during pregnancy via foetal ultrasound, and their treatment requires assistance in a high-volume tertiary centre with immediate access to high-risk obstetric services, neonatology and paediatric surgery [43, 44].

Although both conditions affect the umbilical area, the underlying pathology, outcomes and associated abnormalities are different, and therefore treatment of the two disorders is distinct (Table 2).

Table 2 Congenital abdominal wall defects' characteristics

Characteristic	Omphalocele	Gastroschisis
Location of the defect	Umbilicus	Right of umbilicus
Sac	Present	Absent
Extraintestinal-associated anomalies	Common (40–80%)	Uncommon (5–15%)
Bowel atresia	Uncommon	6–28%
Bowel motility	Typically preserved	Impaired

3.2 Omphalocele

3.2.1 Anatomical Definition and Epidemiology

Omphalocele (exomphalos) is a herniation of viscera through a midline abdominal wall defect [45]. This anomaly occurs at the umbilical ring, and typically, the herniated viscera are covered by a three-layer sac composted by an inner peritoneal layer, Wharton's jelly and an external amniotic layer [43, 46]. The presence of the sac is the main feature differentiating omphalocele from gastroschisis. With omphalocele, the herniated organs are protected from the irritant effect of the amniotic fluid, and intestinal motility is therefore typically preserved, while in gastroschisis, bowel exposure to the amniotic fluid results in gastrointestinal dysmotility and functional impairment [46]. Omphalocele most commonly contains the small bowel, but it can include other abdominal organs, such as liver, colon, stomach, bladder, spleen and gonads, and its size can range from 2 to 10 cm. The term *giant omphalocele* is used for defects larger than 5 cm. Association with other anomalies is frequent, varying from 40 to 80%. The anomalies can include cardiac (7–47%), respiratory (17–60%), musculoskeletal (4–25%), genitourinary (6–20%), gastrointestinal (3–20%) and central nervous system (4–30%). Sometimes omphalocele may be present as part of a genetic disorder or syndrome (3–20%) such as Beckwith-Wiedemann syndrome (macroglossia, gigantism, hypoglycaemia, omphalocele, increased risk of childhood cancer), pentalogy of Cantrell (defects to the midline abdominal wall, lower sternum, anterior diaphragm, diaphragmatic pericardium and some form of intracardiac defect), OEIS complex (omphalocele, exstrophy of the bladder, imperforate anus and spinal anomaly) and trisomy 12, 18 and 21 [42, 44–53]. Morbidity in children with omphalocele is mostly due to associated congenital anomalies, and the long-term outcomes are directly related to these rather than to the abdominal defect itself, although the size of the defect has recently been demonstrated to be an independent predictor of neonatal morbidity and mortality [47–49]. The incidence rate of omphalocele is approximately 1–2 per 10.000 live births, although this number is higher if elective abortions and foetal deaths are taken into account (1 in 1.000–4.000) [52]. An association has been observed with advanced or young maternal age, black infants, maternal obesity and maternal glycaemic control disorders. The estimated survival rate for isolated omphalocele is 50–90%; however, it significantly decreases when concurrent anomalies are present [45].

3.2.2 Diagnosis

The diagnosis is usually made prenatally, most commonly in the late first or second trimester. Since the midgut undergoes physiologic herniation during the sixth week of gestation and normally does not fully return into the abdomen before the 11th or 12th week, definitive diagnosis of omphalocele should not be made before the 12th week of gestation [42, 46, 55]. Elevated maternal serum α-fetoprotein should raise suspicion, and prenatal ultrasonography (US) is the gold standard imaging modality for detecting ventral abdominal wall defects [55]. When an omphalocele is diagnosed, prenatal evaluation should focus on detecting potential associated anomalies, as these are the major determinants of outcome. Foetal magnetic resonance imaging (MRI) is a valid method to assess these anomalies and allow prediction of postnatal morbidity, and it can particularly be useful in cases where the diagnosis is not evident on prenatal US [55]. Karyotype analysis is also indicated when an omphalocele is suspected to rule out numerical chromosomal aberrations [45].

3.2.3 Management

After diagnosis of omphalocele, delivery should be carried out at a tertiary centre where neonatological and pediatric surgical support is available. Full-term delivery is recommended unless otherwise indicated for obstetric reasons or foetal distress [43, 44]. No studies have demonstrated a clear benefit of one route of delivery over another, and this continues to be a topic of debate. Vaginal delivery has been demonstrated to be safe and feasible in children with small defects, while some advocate for caesarean section in cases of giant omphalocele, due to the risk of sac rupture during vaginal delivery, or when the liver is herniated, to avoid hepatic trauma [52]. Further prospective studies are needed to cast light on this issue in order to make valid recommendations. As associated cardiopulmonary anomalies are the principal source of morbidity, the initial management of newborns with omphalocele should be focused on evaluating cardiorespiratory function, and support provided if necessary. Fluid loss is common in these children (although less so compared to gastroschisis), and fluid balance status must be assessed, and fluid resuscitation provided where necessary. An oro- or nasogastric tube should be placed for gastric decompression, and the sac should be kept moist and protected with saline-soaked gauze [56]. Antibiotics are typically administered for the first 48 h after birth in newborns with surgical issues to rule out sepsis and should be discontinued if cultures are negative after that period. Antibiotic treatment may not be necessary in infants with intact omphalocele, and course duration should be as short as possible in all cases [46]. Definitive surgical correction is not an emergency in children with omphalocele with an intact sac, and so the first step after initial stabilisation is thorough evaluation in order to detect and assess potential associated anomalies. This includes almost invariably renal ultrasound, echocardiography, blood glucose level and karyotype analysis [57, 58]. Surgical evaluation is mandatory to establish the appropriate management in order to reduce the herniated viscera and repairing the abdominal defect. Intra-abdominal pressure levels should guide the surgical repair strategy in order to avoid abdominal compartment syndrome, which is the most threatening complication in omphalocele correction, causing impaired venous return, decreased pulmonary compliance, renal failure and bowel ischaemia [59].

Surgical management is dictated by the size of the defect, the degree of visceraabdominal disproportion, the presence or absence of an intact sac and the cardiopulmonary status of the infant. In children with small defects, primary reduction and closure may be attempted. This is performed by excising the sac at the skin and fascia edge, with careful identification and ligation of the umbilical vessels. Then, after reduction of the herniated viscera, and separation of the skin from the deep fascia layers, the fascial edges are closed transversely with running or interrupted absorbable sutures, and the overlying skin can be closed with a purse-string suture, reconstructing the umbilicus [56, 58]. Although some surgeons advocate leaving the sac intact and repairing the fascia and skin over it, in most cases, sac excision is preferred to allow complete abdominal exploration. If primary closure is not achievable while also maintaining appropriately low intra-abdominal pressure levels, a staged repair can be undertaken. In staged repair, the gradual reduction of the herniated viscera allows the abdominal wall to stretch in order to accommodate the content of the sac avoiding excessive intra-abdominal pressures. As gastrointestinal function and motility are not impaired in children with omphalocele, unlike those with gastroschisis, enteral feeding can be administered while awaiting definitive closure of the ventral abdominal wall. The Schuster technique is the main staged repair strategy currently in use. It is made using a prosthetic 'silo' to gradually reduce the herniated viscera into the abdomen. After excising the sac, the silo is then sewn to the fascia or to the muscular and fascial layers of the whole abdominal wall using a running non-absorbable suture. Alternatively, the silo can be sewn over the sac, or the sac itself can be used as a silo if it is free from the underlying viscera (amnion inversion technique). The silo is sequentially and progressively tightened over the course of days and weeks, typically at the bedside, without anaesthesia, to gradually reduce its content into the abdomen with the goal of fascial closure [43, 46, 56, 57, 60, 61]. The silo can be hung over the patient's bed to allow gravity to enhance visceral reduction.

In some cases, significant cardiopulmonary alterations or giant defects may lead the caregivers to prefer initial non-operative management. Topical escharotic therapy, also known as the 'paint and wait' technique is a non-surgical strategy, described for giant omphaloceles, that can postpone surgical repair for months, providing time to let the child's body and lungs grow. In this case, a thin layer of escharotic agent (a corrosive paste that promotes eschar formation) [58] is applied over the sac and wrapped with sterile gauze, and this procedure is repeated daily until the sac is replaced by granulation tissue (usually 3–4 weeks), which will then be gradually covered by intact skin leaving a ventral hernia that will likely need repair at a later stage [52]. Different topical agents have been described and might be considered. These include silver sulfadiazine and other silver-based solutions, povidone-iodine solution, neomycin and polymyxin/bacitracin ointments [61–64]. Each of these agents promotes the formation of granulation tissue over the omphalocele membrane [61]. The escharotic agent can be applied also by the parents at home, allowing the infant to be discharged from the hospital when appropriate, until ready for delayed abdominal wall closure. Other techniques described for giant omphalocele treatment include the use of a biologic or synthetic bridging mesh to cover the defect (Gross technique) or a temporary vacuum dressing (negative pressure wound therapy) [65, 66]. No single method is universally applicable to all cases, which has led to the wide variety of techniques that are performed [58, 61].

Abdominal wall defects derive embryologically from an interruption of the physiological rotation of the intestines during foetal development, and infants with omphalocele will therefore have abnormal bowel rotation and fixation. As a result, patients with abdominal wall defects are at risk of developing midgut volvulus. The risk is higher in children with omphalocele, particularly in those born with an intact sac. This may be due to fewer adhesions being formed after reduction, which would normally prevent the intestines from rotating. Therefore, some surgeons recommend performing a prophylactic Ladd procedure during or after closure to decrease the risk, although other studies do not support this practice [43, 54, 58, 67].

Infants with omphalocele may suffer from complications associated with the disease itself or with the method of repair. The most frequent complication is sepsis [68]. Primary repair can lead to hernia, particularly if under tension. Separation of the abdominal wall layers can lead to seroma or haematoma development in the subcutaneous space, and damage to perforating vessels can lead to skin necrosis. The use of a silo or a bridging mesh can damage fascial edges and lead to infection. With regard to topical therapies, the chronic use of iodine can lead to hypothyroidism, and in general, escharotic agents can lead to ruptured omphalocele [62].

3.2.4 Ruptured Omphalocele

Omphaloceles can have a ruptured membrane. These ruptures can be defined as primary (prenatal) or secondary (postnatal) [51]. Tears or rupture result in exposure of the herniated viscera to the irritating effect of amniotic fluid or environmental stimuli as in gastroschisis, and postnatal management of the defect in these two conditions is therefore similar. Both small and giant omphaloceles may have a ruptured membrane, although the risk of rupture is greater in giant defects. Differential diagnosis between prenatal ruptured omphalocele and gastroschisis may be challenging, but it is of vital importance to determine the correct diagnosis in order to identify potential associated anomalies. The method of delivery has not been associated with a change in rate of rupture, and therefore caesarean section is not routinely recommended [68]. Postnatal rupture can occur during medical or surgical treatment of omphalocele, including during escharotic therapy. The rate of rupture has been estimated at between 7 and 15% [51, 68].

In omphalocele, rupture represents an emergency and necessitates immediate intervention. After initial cardiopulmonary stabilisation, management of the neonate with ruptured omphalocele should focus on maintaining euvolemia and normothermia. As in children with gastroschisis, these patients suffer from significant third-space and evaporative fluid losses, meaning intravenous access should be obtained, and fluid resuscitation must be promptly started. The abdominal defect should be covered with moist sterile gauze, or the lower half of the infant should be placed in a sterile plastic bag during initial stabilisation, and an oro- or nasogastric tube should be placed for gastric decompression [56, 57]. Care should be taken in avoiding injuries to the liver and spleen when the membrane is ruptured. Broad-spectrum antibiotic prophylaxis should be started in infants with ruptured omphalocele [69].

Primary closure is appropriate when the abdominal wall defect is small to moderate in size and it obviates the morbidity of the multiple procedures required by staged or delayed repair. When primary closure is not feasible, the use of a synthetic or biological mesh bridge (Gross technique) or a prosthetic silo (Schuster technique) allows the gradual reduction of the herniated viscera serving also as a barrier against external agents. In large defects, vacuum-assisted repair has also been described as an appropriate method to progressively gain abdominal domain. In case of ruptured omphaloceles with minimal loss of membrane, topical escharotic therapy has been described after re-approximation of the membrane with absorbable sutures [51].

3.3 Gastroschisis

3.3.1 Anatomical Definition and Epidemiology

Gastroschisis is a herniation of the bowel, and in some cases, other abdominal organs through a ventral abdominal wall defect normally located 1–2 cm right to the umbilicus, and it does not have a membranous covering [56] (Fig. 12). Typically, gastroschisis is an isolated finding and lacks congenital associated anomalies. The absence of a sac exposes the herniated viscera to the irritant effect of amniotic fluid during gestation, resulting in gastrointestinal dysmotility, which is the main cause of morbidity in gastroschisis.

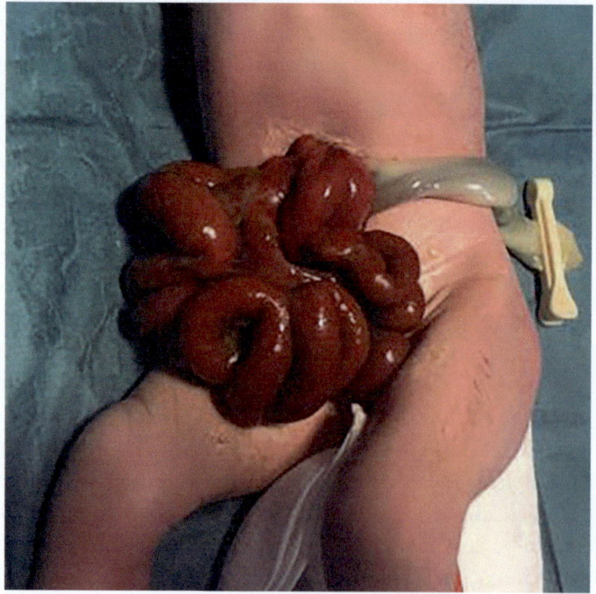

Fig. 12 Infant with simple gastroschisis. The abdominal wall defect is located to the right side of the umbilical cord insertion

Intestinal atresia is the most common associated anomaly in infants with gastroschisis (6–28% of the children), and it is probably secondary to trauma of the bowel against the abdominal wall or vascular compromise due to segmental volvulus [42, 46].

The incidence of gastroschisis is approximately 1–5 per 10.000 live births [43]. The most significant risk factor seems to be young maternal age; others include tobacco, alcohol, recreational drug and some decongestant use [70–72]. These agents (smoke, cocaine, amphetamines, decongestants) are thought to have sympathomimetic effects during embryogenesis, promoting the vascular accident hypothesis. Other theories around embryogenesis of gastroschisis include failure of lateral body wall folding, regression of the right umbilical vein with associated localised paraumbilical tissue weakness and vascular accidents of the vitelline artery [73].

In gastroschisis, the proximal intestine is typically dilated and suffers from dysmotility. In severe cases, a large portion of bowel is compromised, which can lead to short bowel syndrome, partly due to the corrective surgery required [73]. In some cases, the abdominal wall defect closes before birth, strangulating the bowel passing through it. This phenomenon can lead to ischaemia, necrosis and, potentially, amputation of the bowel and is referred to as 'vanishing gastroschisis' [74]. Gastroschisis is classified into simple and complex based on the presence of associated bowel conditions (atresia, matting, necrosis, perforation, ischaemia, volvulus, vanishing gastroschisis) [75]. Complex gastroschisis (17% of cases) has been associated with higher rates of morbidity and mortality and with longer duration of total parenteral nutrition and time to full enteral feeding [76].

3.3.2 Diagnosis

Unlike omphalocele, infants with gastroschisis tend not to be born at term but rather at an average gestational age of 35–36 weeks, and intrauterine foetal death rate is approximately 5% [77, 78]. Gastroschisis is associated with higher maternal α-fetoprotein levels than omphalocele (seven times normal vs. four times normal) [79]. Prenatal US is a sensitive test that can detect the free-floating bowel with no covering membrane outside of the foetal abdomen; the umbilical cord insertion site appears paraumbilical [55].

Although gastroschisis is typically an isolated finding, approximately 5–15% of the newborns affected will have associated extraintestinal congenital anomalies; therefore, it is important to run tests to rule out additional malformations [55, 73]. Serial prenatal US is vital to monitor bowel development and viability, as intestinal loops may appear progressively thickened as a result from irritation caused by exposure to amniotic fluid. Intra-abdominal bowel dilation and polyhydramnios have been associated with underlying intestinal atresia and gastric dilation with neonatal death [80]. Increasing dilation and echogenicity of the bowel may be a sign of impending ischaemia of the bowel. A contrast enema should be performed, when intestinal atresia is suspected or confirmed, to determine the level of the lesion [46].

3.3.3 Management

Vaginal delivery is preferred in gastroschisis, as in omphaloceles, unless caesarean section is indicated for foetal distress or obstetric reasons. The current literature shows no differences in outcomes between vaginal and caesarean delivery in children with gastroschisis [73]. A recent meta-analysis demonstrated no difference in terms of overall mortality, feasibility of primary repair, incidence of necrotising enterocolitis, sepsis, time to full feeding or duration of hospital stay [81]. Currently, there is debate over the appropriate time of delivery in gastroschisis. Although the policy in most centres consists of waiting until the natural onset of labour, some groups recommend preterm delivery as it is associated with shorter duration of exposure to amniotic fluid and, therefore, lower degree of intestinal dysmotility, shorter time to first enteral feed and decreased risk of neonatal sepsis [82, 83].

Immediately after birth, the herniated viscera must be protected from the external environment, so humidity and temperature can be kept constant. The most common option for achieving this is to use a Lahey bag (or 'bowel bag'). This is a sterile bag into which the lower half of the newborn is placed; the bag is then loosely tied around the chest. The bowel must be positioned in a way that protects the mesentery, and the vessels therein contained from twisting or kinking against the abdominal wall to preserve the intestinal blood flow. Intravenous access should be obtained in order to stabilise the newborn with fluids when necessary and in anticipation of starting total parenteral nutrition soon after birth. Fluid resuscitation must be judicious, to prevent pulmonary oedema and the subsequent need for mechanical ventilation, and should be guided by vital parameters, capillary refill time, urine output and acid-base status [73]. Primary surgical closure of the defect is the strategy of choice if achievable without causing abdominal compartment syndrome. Normally, it is obtained suturing the fascia after reduction of the viscera in the abdomen. More recently a 'sutureless' method has gained popularity. This approach consists of coiling or hanging the umbilical cord remnant over the abdominal wall defect and placing a tight adhesive dressing over it, and the dressing is then changed every few days until the fascial defect has closed (Fig. 13). This method can be performed at the bedside, and it does not require general anaesthesia. Some infants may initially develop an umbilical hernia, but most of these will close over time [84]. If the herniated bowel mass is too large or too oedematous to perform primary reduction and closure, a prosthetic silo can be placed over the viscera. The infant should then be transferred into a NICU, where the silo can be tightened once or twice daily at the bedside, with a small amount of sedation, to progressively reduce its contents into the abdomen. During reductions, constant attention must be given to the haemodynamics of the newborn [56, 73]. Once completely reduced, the infant can then undergo primary surgical closure or 'sutureless' repair. Regardless of the method chosen, the herniated bowel should be inspected before reduction to check for the presence of atretic segments before attempting reduction. In children with gastroschisis complicated by atresia, perforation or necrosis, a bowel resection or creation of stoma may be necessary. At birth, the bowel is usually too oedematous to safely undergo resection and immediate anastomosis to repair intestinal atresia. Therefore, these are treated after 4–6 weeks, when anastomoses are thought to be more secure

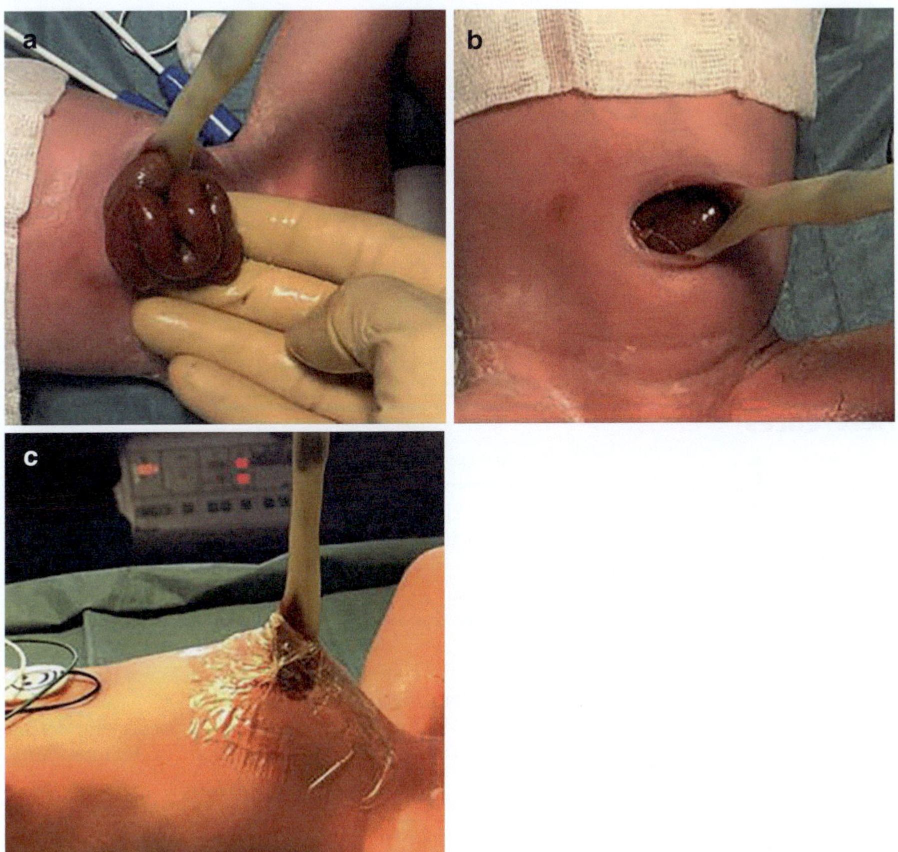

Fig. 13 Primary reduction of gastroschisis. The bowel loops are carefully and progressively reduced into the abdomen (**a**, **b**), the umbilical cord remnant is then hung above the defect, and a tight adhesive dressing is placed over it (**c**)

[43, 46]. The bowel is typically malrotated in infants with gastroschisis. However, the presence of intestinal adhesions is significant enough that volvulus is a rare event [85]. Mortality from gastroschisis and its associated complications has decreased to less than 10% in most series due to recent advances in prenatal diagnostic accuracy, neonatal critical care and surgical management [86]. Bowel dysmotility and ileus affect these children long after surgical correction, resulting in hospitalisation for weeks to months. Total parenteral nutrition must be started soon after birth, anticipating intestinal failure and preventing malnutrition. Enteral feeding is then slowly and progressively initiated, and the infant is monitored to evaluate tolerance. The Gastroschisis Prognostic Score (GPS) is a validated scale performed at the bedside shortly after birth that evaluates the presence and severity of bowel necrosis, matting, atresia and perforation in order to predict the duration of hospitalisation and total parenteral nutrition [87] (Table 3). To optimise care for these

Table 3 Gastroschisis Prognostic Score (GPS). Bowel appearance must be evaluated within 6 h from birth

Matting	None (0)	Mild (1)	Severe (4)
Atresia	Absent (0)	Suspected (1)	Present (2)
Perforation	Absent (0)	–	Present (2)
Necrosis	Absent (0)	–	Present (4)

patients, they should be referred to tertiary centres, and multidisciplinary intestinal failure teams should be created and involved in the long-term management of dysmotility.

References

1. Rutkow IM. Demographics and socioeconomic aspects of hernia repair in the United States in 2003. Surg Clin North Am. 2003;83:1045–51.
2. Pawlak M, Tulloh B, de Beaux A. Current trends in hernia surgery in NHS England. Ann R Coll Surg Engl. 2020;102:25–7.
3. Iannelli A, Buratti MS, Novellas S, Dahman M, Amor IB, Sejor E, Facchiano E, Addeo P, Gugenheim J. Internal hernia as a complication of laparoscopic Roux-en-Y gastric bypass. Obes Surg. 2007;17(10):1283–6.
4. Toh J, Lim R, Keshava A, Rickard M. The risk of internal hernia or volvulus after laparoscopic colorectal surgery: a systematic review. Colorect Dis. 2016;18(12):1133–41.
5. Stenberg E, Ottosson J, Szabo E, Näslund I. Comparing techniques for mesenteric defects closure in laparoscopic gastric bypass surgery—a register-based cohort study. Obes Surg. 2019;29(4):1229–35.
6. Portale G, Popescu G, Parotto M, Cavallin F. Internal hernia after laparoscopic colorectal surgery: an under-reported potentially severe complication. A systematic review and meta-analysis. Surg Endosc. 2019;33(4):1066–74.
7. Lee S, Kim C, Kim Y, Kim H. Internal hernia following laparoscopic colorectal surgery: a rare but fatal complication. Hernia. 2016;21(2):299–304.
8. Benjamin G, Ashfaq A, Chang YH, Harold K, Jaroszewski D. Diaphragmatic hernia post-minimally invasive esophagectomy: a discussion and review of literature. Hernia. 2015;19:635–43.
9. Gooszen JAH, Slaman AE, van Dieren S, Gisbertz SS, van Berge Henegouwen MI. Incidence and treatment of symptomatic diaphragmatic hernia after esophagectomy for cancer. Ann Thorac Surg. 2018;106:199–206.
10. Hanna AN, Guajardo I, Williams N, Kucharczuk J, Dempsey DT. Hiatal hernia after esophagectomy: an underappreciated complication? J Am Coll Surg. 2020;230:700–7.
11. Stenberg E, Szabo E, Ågren G, Ottosson J, Marsk R, Lönroth H, et al. Closure of mesenteric defects in laparoscopic gastric bypass: a multicentre, randomised, parallel, open-label trial. Lancet. 2016;387(10026):1397–404.
12. Däster S, Xiang H, Yang J, Rowe D, Keshava A, Rickard M. High prevalence of asymptomatic internal hernias after laparoscopic anterior resection in a retrospective analysis of postoperative computed tomography. Int J Colorect Dis. 2020;35(5):929–32.
13. Altinoz A, Maasher A, Jouhar F, Babikir A, Ibrahim M, Al Shaban T, et al. Diagnostic laparoscopy is more accurate than computerized tomography for internal hernia after Roux-en-Y gastric bypass. Am J Surg. 2020;220(1):214–6.
14. Farukhi M, Mattingly M, Clapp B, Tyroch A. CT scan reliability in detecting internal hernia after gastric bypass. JSLS. 2017;21(4):e2017.00054.

15. Riaz R, Myers D, Williams T. Multidetector CT imaging of bariatric surgical complications: a pictorial review. Abdom Radiol. 2015;41(1):174–88.
16. Bordonaro V, Brizi M, Lanza F, Gallucci P, Infante A, Giustacchini P, et al. Role of CT imaging in discriminating internal hernia from aspecific abdominal pain following Roux-en-Y gastric bypass: a single high-volume Centre experience. Upd Surg. 2020;72(4):1115–24.
17. de Bakker JK, van Namen YWB, Bruin SC, de Brauw LM. Gastric bypass and abdominal pain: think of Petersen hernia. JSLS. 2012;16:311–3.
18. Jain A, Ng SC, Savage N, Lamanna D, Warrier S, Smart P. Heterogeneity of internal hernia post anterior resection: a missed diagnosis. ANZ Surg. 2020;91:E350. https://doi.org/10.1111/ans.16376.
19. Sereno Trabaldo S, Anvari M, Leroy J, Marescaux J. Prevalence of internal hernias after laparoscopic colonic surgery. J Gastrointest Surg. 2009;13(6):1107–10.
20. Olson MC, Fletcher JG, Nagpal P, Froemming AT, Khandelwal A. Mesenteric ischemia: what the radiologist needs to know. Cardiovasc Diagn Ther. 2019;9(S1):S74–87.
21. Zalcman M, Sy M, Donckier V, Closset J, Van Gansbeke D. Helical CT signs in the diagnosis of intestinal ischaemia in small-bowel obstruction. Am J Roentgenol. 2000;175:1601–7.
22. Chowbey P, Baijal M, Kantharia N, Khullar R, Sharma A, Soni V. Mesenteric defect closure decreases the incidence of internal hernias following laparoscopic Roux-En-Y gastric bypass: a retrospective cohort study. Obes Surg. 2016;26(9):2029–34.
23. Blockhuys M, Gypen B, Heyman S, Valk J, van Sprundel F, Hendrickx L. Internal hernia after laparoscopic gastric bypass: effect of closure of the Petersen defect—single-center study. Obes Surg. 2018;29(1):70–5.
24. Hajibandeh S, Hajibandeh S, Abdelkarim M, Shehadeh A, Mohsin M, Khan KA, Morgan R. Closure versus non-closure of mesenteric defects in laparoscopic Roux-en-Y gastric bypass: a systematic review and meta-analysis. Surg Endosc. 2020;34:3306. https://doi.org/10.1007/s00464-020-07544-1.
25. Magouliotis D, Tzovaras G, Tasiopoulou V, Christodoulidis G, Zacharoulis D. Closure of mesenteric defects in laparoscopic gastric bypass: a meta-analysis. Obes Surg. 2020;30(5):1935–43.
26. Ahmed A, Rickards G, Husain S, Johnson J, Boss T, O'Malley W. Trends in internal hernia incidence after laparoscopic Roux-en-Y gastric bypass. Obes Surg. 2007;17(12):1563–6.
27. Causey MW, Oguntoye M, Steele SR. Incidence of complications following colectomy with mesenteric closure versus no mesenteric closure: does it really matter? J Surg Res. 2011;171:571–5.
28. Angelini P, Sciuto A, Cuccurullo D, Pirozzi F, Reggio S, Corcione F. Prevention of internal hernias and pelvic adhesions following laparoscopic left-sided colorectal resection: the role of fibrin sealant. Surg Endosc. 2017;31:3048–51.
29. ten Broek RPG, Krielen P, Di Saverio S, et al. Bologna guidelines for diagnosis and management of adhesive sall bowel obstruction (ASBO): 2017 update of the evidence-based guidelines from the world society of emergency surgery ASBO working group. World J Emerg Surg. 2018;13:24.
30. Keenan JE, Turley RS, McCoy CC, Migaly J, Shapiro L, Scarborough JE. Trials of nonoperative management exceeding 3 days are associated with increased morbidity in patient undergoing surgery for uncomplicated adhesive small bowel obstruction. J Trauma Acute Care Surg. 2014;76:1367–72.
31. Petrucciani N, Martini F, Kassir R, Juglard G, Hamid C, Boudrie H, Van Haverbeke O, Liagre A. Internal hernia after one anastomosis gastric bypass (OAGB): lessons learned from a retrospective series of 3368 consecutive patients undergoing OAGB with a biliopancreatic limb of 150 cm. Obes Surg. 2021;31:2537–44.
32. Min JS, Seo KW, Jeong SH, et al. A comparison of postoperative outcomes after an open and laparoscopic reduction of Petersen's hernia: a multicenter observational cohort study. BMC Surg. 2021;21:195.
33. Guerra F, Coletta D, Greco PA, Eugeni E, Patriti A. The use of indocyanine green fluorescence to define bowel microcirculation during laparoscopic surgery for acute small bowel obstruction. Colorectal Dis. 2021;23:2189. https://doi.org/10.1111/codi.15680.

34. Frazzetta G, Lanaia A, Luppi D, Bonilauri S. Emergency laparoscopic surgery for post-traumatic incarcerated diaphragmatic hernia: defect closure and intraperitoneal mesh manual fixation. Asian J Surg. 2020;43:864. https://doi.org/10.1016/j.asjsur.2020.05.003.

35. Shao G, Wu L, Li J, Dai C. Laparoscopic diaphragmatic hernia repair with mesh reinforcement. Am Surg. 2020;86:476–9.

36. Kockerling F, Schug-Pass C, Bittner R. A word of caution: never use tacks for mesh fixation to the diaphragm! Surg Endosc. 2018;32:3295–302.

37. Watson DI, Thompson SK, Devitt PG, Aly A, Irvine T, Woods SD, Gan S, Game PA, Jamieson GG. Five years follow-up of a randomized controlled trial of laparoscopic repair of very large hiatus hernia with sutures versus absorbable versus nonabsorbable mesh. Ann Surg. 2020;272:241–7.

38. Campos VAP, Palacio DS, Glina FPA, Tustumi F, Bernardo WM, Sousa AV. Laparoscopic treatment of giant hiatal hernia with or without mesh reinforcement: a systematic review and meta-analysis. Int J Surg. 2020;77:97–104.

39. Puccetti F, Cossu A, Parise P, Barbieri L, Elmore U, Carresi A, De Pascale S, Fumagalli Romario U, Rosati R. Diaphragmatic hernia after Ivor Lewis esophagectomy for cancer: a retrospective analysis of risk factors and post-repair outcomes. J Thorac Dis. 2021;13:160–8.

40. Takeda FR, Tustumi F, Filho MAS, Silva MO, Junior UR, Sallum RAA, Cecconello I. Diaphragmatic hernia repair after esophagectomy: technical report and lessons after a series of cases. J Laparoendosc Adv Surg Tech. 2020;30:433–7.

41. Narayanan S, Sanders RL, Herlitz G, Langenfeld J, August DA. Treatment of diaphragmatic hernia occurring after transhiatal esophagectomy. Ann Surg Oncol. 2015;22:3681–6.

42. Christison-Lagay ER, Kelleher CM, Langer JC. Neonatal abdominal wall defects. Semin Fetal Neonatal Med. 2011;16:164–72.

43. Gamba P, Midrio P. Abdominal wall defects: prenatal diagnosis, newborn management, and long-term outcomes. Semin Pediatr Surg. 2014;23:283–90.

44. Slater BJ, Pimpalwar A. Abdominal wall defects. Neoreviews. 2020;21:e383–91.

45. Verla MA, Style CC, Olutoye OO. Prenatal diagnosis and management of omphalocele. Semin Pediatr Surg. 2019;28:84–8.

46. Mansfield SA, Jancelewicz T. Ventral abdominal wall defects. Pediatr Rev. 2019;40:627–35.

47. Ayub SS, Taylor JA. Cardiac anomalies associated with omphalocele. Semin Pediatr Surg. 2019;28:111–4.

48. Baerg JE, Munoz AN. Long term complications and outcomes in omphalocele. Semin Pediatr Surg. 2019;28:118–21.

49. Duggan E, Puligandla PS. Respiratory disorders in patients with omphalocele. Semin Pediatr Surg. 2019;28:115–7.

50. Raymond SL, Downard CD, St. Peter SD, Baerg J, Qureshi FG, Bruch SW, Danielson PD, Renaud E, Islam S. Outcomes in omphalocele correlate with size of defect. J Pediatr Surg. 2019;54:1546–50.

51. Gonzalez KW, Chandler N. Ruptured omphalocele: diagnosis and management. Semin Pediatr Surg. 2019;28:101–5.

52. Islam S. Advances in surgery for abdominal wall defects. Gastroschisis and omphalocele. Clin Perinatol. 2012;39:375–86.

53. Williams AP, Marayati R, Beierle EA. Pentalogy of Cantrell. Semin Pediatr Surg. 2019;28:106–10.

54. Lauriti G, Miscia ME, Cascini V, Chiesa PL, Pierro A, Zani A. Intestinal malrotation in infants with omphalocele: a systematic review and meta-analysis. J Pediatr Surg. 2019;54:378–82.

55. Torres US, Portela-Oliveira E, Braga FDCB, Werner H, Daltro PAN, Souza AS. When closure fails: what the radiologist needs to know about the embryology, anatomy, and prenatal imaging of ventral body wall defects. Semin Ultrasound CT MRI. 2015;36:522–36.

56. Kelly KB, Ponsky TA. Pediatric abdominal wall defects. Surg Clin North Am. 2013;93:1255–67.

57. Roux N, Jakubowicz D, Salomon L, Grangé G, Giuseppi A, Rousseau V, Khen-Dunlop N, Beaudoin S. Early surgical management for giant omphalocele: results and prognostic factors. J Pediatr Surg. 2018;53:1908–13.

58. Skarsgard ED. Immediate versus staged repair of omphaloceles. Semin Pediatr Surg. 2019;28:89–94.

59. Divarci E, Karapinar B, Yalaz M, Ergun O, Celik A. Incidence and prognosis of intraabdominal hypertension and abdominal compartment syndrome in children. J Pediatr Surg. 2016;51:503–7.

60. Schuster SR. A new method for the staged repair of large omphaloceles. Surg Gynecol Obs. 1967;125:837–50.

61. Mortellaro VE, Peter SDS, Fike FB, Islam S. Review of the evidence on the closure of abdominal wall defects. Pediatr Surg Int. 2011;27:391–7.

62. Whitehouse JS, Gourlay DM, Masonbrink AR, Aiken JJ, Calkins CM, Sato TT, Arca MJ. Conservative management of giant omphalocele with topical povidone-iodine and its effect on thyroid function. J Pediatr Surg. 2010;45:1192–7.

63. Lee SL, Beyer TD, Kim SS, Waldhausen JHT, Healey PJ, Sawin RS, Ledbetter DJ. Initial nonoperative management and delayed closure for treatment of giant omphaloceles. J Pediatr Surg. 2006;41:1846–9.

64. Lewis N, Kolimarala V, Lander A. Conservative management of exomphalos major with silver dressings: are they safe? J Pediatr Surg. 2010;45:2438–9.

65. Gross RE. A new method for surgical treatment of large omphaloceles. Surgery. 1948;24:277–92.

66. Aldridge B, Ladd AP, Kepple J, Wingle T, Ring C, Kokoska ER. Negative pressure wound therapy for initial management of giant omphalocele. Am J Surg. 2016;211:605–9.

67. Sinha CK, Kader M, Dykes E, Said AJ. An 18 years' review of exomphalos highlighting the association with malrotation. Pediatr Surg Int. 2011;27:1151–4.

68. Saxena AK, Raicevic M. Predictors of mortality in neonates with giant omphaloceles. Minerva Pediatr. 2018;70:289–95.

69. Travassos D, van Eerde A, Kramer W. Management of a Giant Omphalocele with non–cross-linked intact porcine-derived acellular dermal matrix (Strattice) combined with vacuum therapy. Eur J Pediatr Surg Rep. 2015;03:061–3.

70. Siega-Riz AM, Herring AH, Olshan AF, Smith J, Moore C. The joint effects of maternal pre-pregnancy body mass index and age on the risk of gastroschisis. Paediatr Perinat Epidemiol. 2009;23:51–7.

71. Baldacci S, Santoro M, Coi A, Mezzasalma L, Bianchi F, Pierini A. Lifestyle and sociodemographic risk factors for gastroschisis: a systematic review and meta-analysis. Arch Dis Child. 2020;105:756–64.

72. Lausman AY, Langer JC, Tai M, Seaward PGR, Windrim RC, Kelly EN, Ryan G. Gastroschisis: what is the average gestational age of spontaneous delivery? J Pediatr Surg. 2007;42: 1816–21.

73. Bhat V, Moront M, Bhandari V. Gastroschisis: a state-of-the-art review. Children. 2020;7:302.

74. Kimble RM, Blakelock R, Cass D. Vanishing gut in infants with gastroschisis. Pediatr Surg Int. 1999;15:483–5.

75. Molik KA, Gingalewski CA, West KW, Rescorla FJ, Scherer LR, Engum SA, Grosfeld JL. Gastroschisis: a plea for risk categorization. J Pediatr Surg. 2001;36:51–5.

76. Bergholz R, Boettcher M, Reinshagen K, Wenke K. Complex gastroschisis is a different entity to simple gastroschisis affecting morbidity and mortality—a systematic review and meta-analysis. J Pediatr Surg. 2014;49:1527–32.

77. Barseghyan K, Aghajanian P, Miller DA. The prevalence of preterm births in pregnancies complicated with fetal gastroschisis. Arch Gynecol Obstet. 2012;286:889–92.

78. South AP, Stutey KM, Meinzen-Derr J. Metaanalysis of the prevalence of intrauterine fetal death in gastroschisis. Am J Obstet Gynecol. 2013;209:114.e1–e13.

79. Palomaki G, Hill L, Knight G, Haddow J, Carpenter M. Second-trimester maternal serum alpha-fetoprotein levels in pregnancies associated with gastroschisis and omphalocele. Obstet Gynecol. 1988;71:906–9.

80. D'Antonio F, Virgone C, Rizzo G, et al. Prenatal risk factors and outcomes in gastroschisis: a meta-analysis. Pediatrics. 2015;136:e159–69.

81. Kirollos DW, Abdel-Latif ME. Mode of delivery and outcomes of infants with gastroschisis: a meta-analysis of observational studies. Arch Dis Child Fetal Neonatal Ed. 2018;103:F355–63.
82. Landisch RM, Yin Z, Christensen M, Szabo A, Wagner AJ. Outcomes of gastroschisis early delivery: a systematic review and meta-analysis. J Pediatr Surg. 2017;52:1962–71.
83. Shamshirsaz AA, Lee TC, Hair AB, et al. Elective delivery at 34 weeks vs routine obstetric care in fetal gastroschisis: randomized controlled trial. Ultrasound Obstet Gynecol. 2020;55:15–9.
84. Sandler A, Lawrence J, Meehan J, Phearman L, Soper R. A "plastic" sutureless abdominal wall closure in gastroschisis. J Pediatr Surg. 2004;39:738–41.
85. Fawley JA, Abdelhafeez AH, Schultz JA, Ertl A, Cassidy LD, Peter SS, Wagner AJ. The risk of midgut volvulus in patients with abdominal wall defects: a multi-institutional study. J Pediatr Surg. 2017;52:26–9.
86. Raymond SL, Hawkins RB, St Peter SD, Downard CD, Qureshi FG, Renaud E, Danielson PD, Islam S. Predicting morbidity and mortality in neonates born with gastroschisis. J Surg Res. 2020;245:217–24.
87. Cowan KN, Puligandla PS, Laberge JM, Skarsgard ED, Bouchard S, Yanchar N, Kim P, Lee S, McMillan D, Von Dadelszen P. The gastroschisis prognostic score: reliable outcome prediction in gastroschisis. J Pediatr Surg. 2012;47:1111–7.

Post-traumatic Diaphragmatic Hernia

Camilla Cremonini, Enrico Cicuttin, Dario Tartaglia,
Silvia Strambi, Serena Musetti, Massimo Chiarugi,
and Federico Coccolini

1 Introduction

1.1 Surgical Anatomy

The diaphragm (from Greek: «dia» between, through; «phragma» fence) is a dome-shaped skeletal muscle, formed by a central aponeurotic segment (attached to the pericardium) and a peripheral muscular part, and it separates the thorax from the abdomen. The muscle is attached to the lower sternum anteriorly, to the six lower costal ribs laterally, and to the lumbar spine posteriorly. Other than separating the thoracic and abdominal cavities, it also plays a key role in the respiratory function: during expiration, the diaphragm reaches the nipple line or, more precisely, the level of the fourth-fifth intercostal spaces (usually the fourth on the right and the fifth on the left [1]).

The diaphragm has three openings, also called hiatuses, that offers the passage of the aorta (along with the azygos vein and the thoracic duct, through the aortic hiatus posteriorly); the esophagus (along with the vagus nerve through the esophageal foramen); and the inferior vena cava (through the vena cava foramen).

The diaphragm is highly perfused, making necrosis an extremely rare event [2]; main arterial blood supply is ensured by the phrenic arteries, direct branches of the aorta, whereas the IVC warrants the venous drainage. The innervation is provided by the two phrenic nerves that from their cervical origin (C3–C5 nerve routes) descend into the mediastinum, along with the pericardium, and finally spread into several branches on the thoracic surface of the two hemidiaphragms.

C. Cremonini (✉) · E. Cicuttin · D. Tartaglia · S. Strambi · S. Musetti · M. Chiarugi ·
F. Coccolini
General, Emergency and Trauma Surgery Department, Pisa University Hospital, Pisa, Italy
e-mail: camilla.cremonini@phd.unipi.it; enrico.cicuttin@phd.unipi.it; dario.tartaglia@unipi.it; silvia.strambi@phd.unipi.it; serena.musetti@phd.unipi.it; massimo.chiarugi@med.unipi.it; federico.coccolini@unipi.com

F. Coccolini et al. (eds.), *Mini-invasive Approach in Acute Care Surgery*,
Hot Topics in Acute Care Surgery and Trauma,
https://doi.org/10.1007/978-3-031-39001-2_16

## 1.2	Epidemiology and Etiopathogenesis of Traumatic Injuries

Due to its particular shape and to its nature of boundary between the thorax and the abdomen, the diaphragm can be injured in either lower chest or upper abdominal trauma, other than in combined thoraco-abdominal trauma (both blunt and penetrating) [3, 4]. Diaphragmatic injuries (DI) occur in around 0.4% of all trauma cases [1, 5]. Penetrating trauma is known to be more common as mechanism of injury when compared to blunt trauma: 63% of DI are caused by penetrating trauma [5, 6]. The literature reports an incidence of DI after blunt and penetrating trauma that ranges between 1–7% and 10–15%, respectively [7, 8]. More specifically, the reported incidence of DI after penetrating trauma that occurs to the thoraco-abdominal area is even higher (Fig. 1), reaching rates of 42% according to the series [9]. Overall, DI are more commonly described on the left side (in 57% of cases; 40% on the right hemidiaphragm and 3% bilateral) [10].

Injuries to the diaphragm usually have different aspects and characteristics in relation to different mechanisms:

- In case of *blunt trauma*, the diaphragm can be injured by the displacement of fractured ribs or by massive application of a blunt force to the abdomen [4]. In this latter case, a sudden and intense increase of the intra-abdominal pressure can result in a diaphragmatic rupture due to the excessive tension applied to the muscle itself. Considered the etiology, blunt injuries are typically large tears in the diaphragm with associated herniation of intra-abdominal organs into the chest [11]. They occur more frequently on the left side, condition likely related to the protective effect that the liver plays on the right hemidiaphragm: this organ, in fact, may mitigate the damage caused by the kinetic energy applied to the abdomen during a blunt trauma [1].
- Penetrating trauma can cause lacerations of the diaphragmatic muscle. Any stab wound of the thoracoabdominal area should raise suspicion of a DI, while GSWs could damage the diaphragm occurring anywhere in the trunk [1]. Generally, penetrating DI consist in small tears (2–5 cm according to the weapon); hence, they are rarely associated with herniation of intra-abdominal organs into the

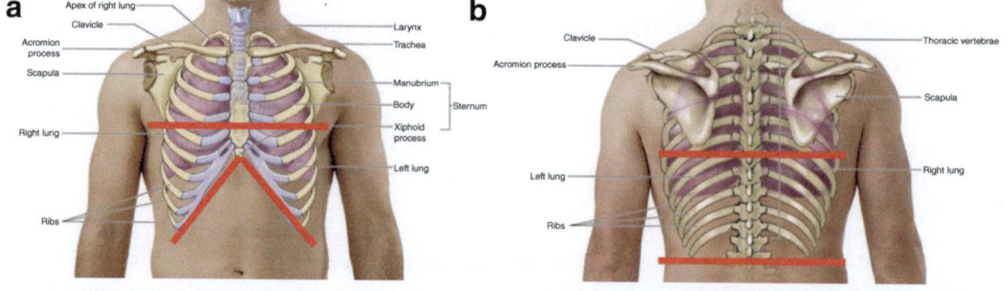

Fig. 1 Thoracoabdominal region (between the red lines). Any asymptomatic penetrating trauma of this region, especially on the left, should raise high level of suspicion for DI and should be evaluated with diagnostic laparoscopy. anterior (**a**) and posterior (**b**) view

thorax, at least in the acute setting. Similarly to blunt injuries, the incidence of penetrating DI is prevalent on the left side of the diaphragm [12], likely due to the related prevalence of right-handed assailants [1].

1.3   Post-traumatic Diaphragmatic Hernia: Etiology

Injuries to the diaphragm may range from contusion to tears (usually due to penetrating trauma) up to diaphragmatic hernias. Post-traumatic diaphragmatic hernias (PTDH) can be divided in two categories, according to the time of their presentation:

- Acute PTDH, usually due to blunt trauma, are a less common presentation than smaller tears (30% vs. 48%) [13].
- Late PTDH: Small tears of the diaphragm (usually due to penetrating trauma) can be challenging to be diagnosed and may be missed [14, 15], especially when isolated (not associated with other organ's injuries) penetrating DI are unlikely to have visceral organ herniation into the thoracic cavity; hence, they are really subtle in presentation, being asymptomatic on physical examination, and resulting in the absence of significant findings on radiographic studies [12, 16]. Consequently, DI that are not diagnosed in the acute setting and are left untreated may enlarge over time and eventually result in late diaphragmatic hernias, with associated high morbidity and mortality due to potential adverse conditions like organ obstruction and strangulation [15]. Firstly, the constant respiratory movement of the diaphragm prevents its tears to spontaneously heal. Secondary, the positive pressure gradient that exists between the abdomen and the chest may be the leading cause of the progressive growth of the diaphragmatic defect and of the subsequent herniation of abdominal organs into the chest [3].

Abdominal organs that may herniate into the thorax in case of a diaphragmatic rupture are the stomach, the spleen, the colon (either transverse or descending), the small bowel, the omentum, and the left liver lobe [1, 17]. These differ depending to the hemidiaphragm that has been injured: spleen, bowel, and stomach are more common on the left side, while the liver (or more precisely, a portion of it) is the organ that may herniate most commonly on the right side [11].

2   Presentation

2.1   Clinical Presentation

Diaphragmatic injuries may be completely asymptomatic, especially when small and not associated to other organs injuries, even though this is a rare event. Symptoms related to PTDH can be divided into three phases according to Grimes [18]:

1. *Acute phase*: during the first time period, that goes from the trauma itself until the recovery from the injuries. Symptoms of this phase are usually related to concomitant injuries (see below). Patients may experience a wide range of clinical signs varying from severe shock and/or respiratory dysfunction (that may be or may be not related to the DI itself) to mild symptoms, like shoulder pain or vomiting. Other symptoms may be epigastric or chest pain, dyspnea, absent breath sounds, or bowel sounds at chest auscultation [1]. The majority of diaphragmatic hernias are diagnosed during this phase.
2. *Latent phase*: this time frame may go from days to months up to several years. During this phase, the diaphragm defect is increasing in dimension, and intra-abdominal organs may start to herniate. Patients are often asymptomatic, and the diagnosis may be occasionally made during imaging performed for other reasons. Mild symptoms such as gastrointestinal complaints or epigastric pain may be present [3].
3. *Obstructive phase*: the herniation of abdominal organs into the chest and the consequent mechanical compression may result in severe respiratory compromise on one hand, and in visceral obstruction and strangulation on the other. The following visceral ischemia may lead to perforation and septic shock. Dyspnea, intense chest and abdominal pain, vomiting, and nausea are some of the symptoms that can be present before these final phases [1, 3]. The morbidity and mortality rates related to these life-threatening complications are quite high [14].

2.2 Associated Injuries

In both blunt and penetrating trauma, diaphragmatic injuries are rarely isolated and are more frequently associated with other organ injuries. Blunt DI occur in the context of a high energy trauma that makes easy to understand the high chance to have associated injuries (i.e., brain injuries, pelvic or long bones fractures, etc.). Traumatic brain injuries may be present in up to 50% of cases, and it also represents a predictor of mortality [7]. Other organs that may be injured are either thoracic or intra-abdominal: lung contusions or laceration, pneumo- or hemo-thorax, aortic injuries, rib fractures, and abdominal solid organs injuries are common [5, 15].

Similarly, penetrating trauma carries a high rate of concomitant injuries, especially of intra-abdominal organs. Other than presenting with hemo- or pneumothorax, penetrating DI are often associated with intra-abdominal organ injuries such as hollow viscous injuries (HVI) and liver and spleen lacerations [5]. SW are a more common cause of isolated, DI while DI associated with concomitant abdominal injuries are more frequently cause by GSWs [12, 16].

3 Diagnosis

The initial diagnostic workup and management of a traumatized patient follow the principles of Advanced Trauma Life Support (ATLS) in order to recognize and treat potential life-threatening conditions. A diaphragmatic hernia may be diagnosed in

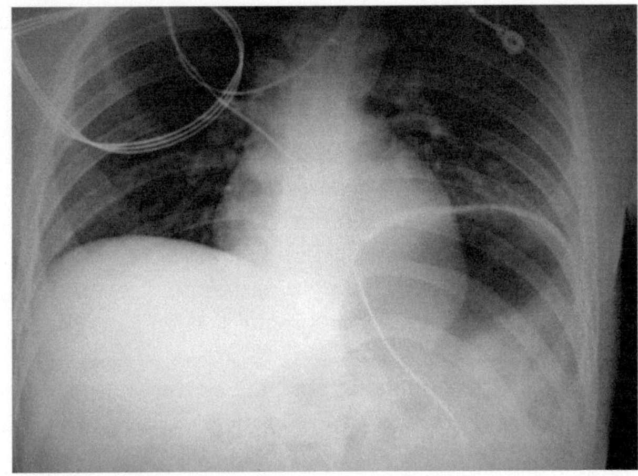

Fig. 2 Chest X-ray evidence of a left diaphragmatic hernia after blunt trauma: the stomach is herniated into the chest

this phase, for example, through a chest X-ray when the defect is large and the organs are already herniated into the chest (Fig. 2). Otherwise, being frequently associated with other organs injuries, DI are often diagnosed intraoperatively during the abdominal examination. These patients may undergo a trauma laparotomy for other reasons such as hemodynamic instability, signs of peritonitis, or to surgically treat other injuries detected at the imaging [15].

Chest X-ray (CXR) is the first imaging modality usually used in trauma patients. Its sensitivity in diagnosing DI is low, especially for right-sided injuries or for penetrating injuries that are usually small. Reported rates of normal CXR in patients with penetrating diaphragmatic injuries range between 11 and 62% [12, 14, 15]. Chest plain films are able to diagnose an injury to the right hemidiaphragm in 18–33%; the sensitivity rises to 27–62% in case of left-sided injuries [19]. Pathognomonic findings of PTDH detectable at CXR are:

- Visualization of a hollow viscous (i.e., colon, small bowel, or stomach) above the diaphragm
- Identification of a radiopaque naso- or orogastric tube abnormally located in the chest

Nonspecific findings associated with diaphragmatic herniation are:

- Elevation of the hemidiaphragm
- Hemo- or pneumothorax

In hemodynamically stable patients, **computed tomography (CT) scan** has proven itself to be a reliable and effective imaging method to diagnose diaphragmatic rupture with or without herniation. In case of a PTDH, CT scan imaging is the gold standard not only to diagnose it but also to evaluate size, exact locations, and contents of the hernia itself [11, 20]. CT scan findings may differ in case of blunt or penetrating due to different etiopathology and injury characteristics as already described.

Reported rates of sensitivity and specificity of this imaging method in diagnosing blunt diaphragmatic rupture are 70–100% and 80–100%, respectively [1]. The following are direct signs of a diaphragmatic injury [11]:

- Visualization of a visceral herniation through a diaphragmatic defect: in this case, radiologists may describe the so called "collar sign," representing the constriction point of the herniated organ that passes through the defect (Fig. 3).
- Visualization of the diaphragmatic defect: this may appear differently, ranging from a small discontinuity of the diaphragm profile up to a large displacement of torn ends ("dangling diaphragm").

In case of penetrating trauma, the abovementioned findings are uncommon, especially the visualization of organ displacement. The diaphragmatic defect may be detected or suspected at the CT scan (44–65% of cases [12]). In case of penetrating trauma, CT scan has reported sensitivity and specificity that range between 14–78% and 76–100%, respectively [20]. Higher sensitivities, up to 82 and 94% according to the series, were reached, thanks to the improved quality of images obtained with multidetector CT scan (MDCT): this technique, processing multi-slice sections, allows multiple reconstructions (axial, coronal, sagittal) and the visualization of the entire muscle dome [20]. Other than the direct identification of the defect, some indirect signs may help the diagnosis of penetrating DI: contiguous injuries on either sides of the diaphragm (i.e., left hemothorax and splenic injury) rise the suspect of a lesion of the muscle itself [4, 20]. The visualization of the bullet path or of the tract of the stab wound (also called "trajectography"), reconstructing the trajectory, is another important feature that may help excluding or suspecting a DI [11].

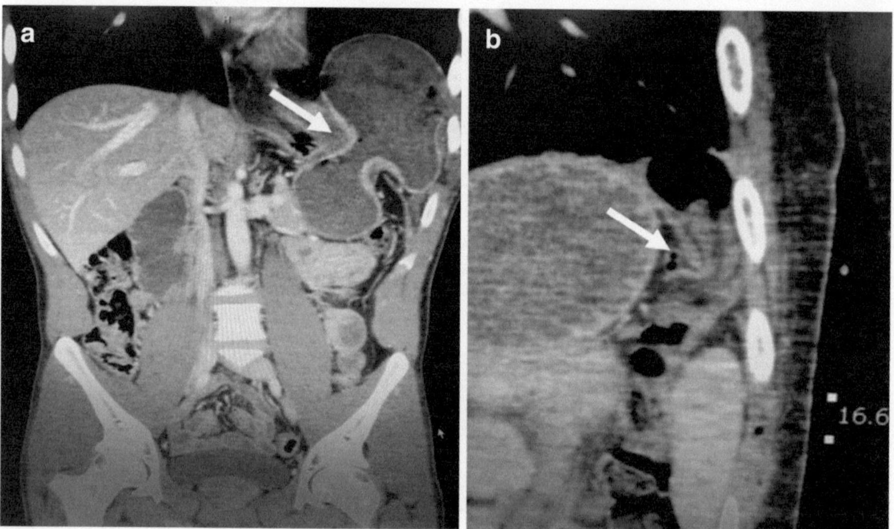

Fig. 3 CT scan images of herniation into the chest of the stomach (**a**) and of the left colon (**b**) through the diaphragmatic injury for left penetrating trauma (white arrows)

Other imaging modalities, such as contrast studies and magnetic resonance (MRI), have been described and used for the diagnosis of DI, but their use, especially in the acute setting, is limited [1].

Some penetrating DI, especially when isolated, may be challenging to diagnose due to the lack of clinical and radiographic findings. The importance of early diagnosis of even small DI lies in the possible life-threatening consequences of a delayed diaphragmatic hernia.

These aspects explain why, in the last decades, **diagnostic laparoscopy** has gained more and more consent among trauma surgeons both as a diagnostic and therapeutic tool [16]. Laparoscopy, in fact, is the most accurate and safe method to completely evaluate the entire diaphragmatic dome, allowing not only for DI diagnosis but also for definitive repair of the injury with minimal morbidity and good outcomes [21]. Hemodynamically stable patients that have sustained a penetrating trauma of the thoracoabdominal region (especially on the left side) with no signs of peritonitis or other organs injuries are the perfect candidates that may benefit from this minimally invasive option. Hence, when a DI is suspected on the basis of the mechanism but not detected, a diagnostic laparoscopy should always be considered.

Alternatively, a thoracoscopy may be used to evaluate the diaphragm from above. This is most commonly used when evacuation of retained hemothorax or empyema is needed [1, 7], although some elect this surgical strategy anyway.

4   Management

The Organ Injury Scaling Committee of the American Association for the Surgery of Trauma (AAST) classified diaphragmatic injuries into five grade, as shown in Table 1 [22]. Intraoperative findings are usually needed to accurately determine the grade and help the surgeon in choosing the most appropriate method of repair.

4.1   Surgical Principles and Technique of Repair

The two principal steps to follow when treating a PTDH are:

Table 1 AAST-OIS diaphragm injury scale

Grade	Injury description
I	Contusion
II	Laceration <2 cm
III	Laceration 2–10 cm
IV	Laceration >10 cm with tissue loss <25 cm^2
V	Laceration with tissue loss >25 cm^2

Adapted from Moore EE, Malangoni MA, Cogbill TH, Shackford SR, Champion HR, Jurkovich GJ, et al. Organ injury scaling IV: Thoracic vascular, lung, cardiac, and diaphragm. J Trauma. 1994;36(3):299–300

- Reduction of herniated organs back into the abdominal cavity
- Watertight suture of the diaphragm

The entire diaphragm must be visualized in order to detect even small lacerations. To perform a complete inspection of the muscle, it may be necessary to take down the falciform ligament (to accurately see the right hemidiaphragm) or to gently retract spleen and stomach (to evaluate the left hemidiaphragm).

Organs reduction should be done carefully, but it is rarely difficult in the acute setting. It may be complicated in delayed hernias due to the adherence (see below).

Once the dimension of the defect has been addressed, the edges should be pulled with the aid of Allis clamps and approximated. Consider **debridement**: in case of necrotic tissue on the margins of the defect, these should be debrided in order to obtain viable edges.

Prior to suture the diaphragmatic injury, attention should be posed to **inspecting and irrigating the ipsilateral pleural cavity** in order to address eventual bleeding from the chest cavity or to reduce the contamination in case of hollow viscous injury. In fact, the high incidence of empyema in case of DI associated with bowel injuries makes accurate irrigation essential [6].

As regards the **type of repair**, in case the defect is small, usually as a consequence of penetrating trauma, an interrupted vertical suture may be performed. Otherwise, in case of large blunt injuries, several types of suture can be considered according to the surgeons preference like interrupted figure of eight suture, horizontal mattress suture, running suture, or double-layer repair [1, 23]. A 1- or 0-slowly absorbable or nonabsorbable monofilament (i.e., Prolene or PDS) may be used.

Finally, consider positioning of an **ipsilateral chest tube**: different factors such as degree of contamination, eventual chest or lung injuries, and size of the defect should be taken into account.

Sometimes, in the presence of large defect (usually >8 cm), a prosthetic mesh may be considered for the repair [24]. In case of peripheral defects or avulsion of the diaphragm, secure the muscle around the ribs with horizontal mattress suture may be indicated. Different methods of reconstruction, translated from congenital DH treatment, have been described (i.e., latissimus dorsi flap), when extensive defects with diaphragm disruption are encountered [24].

4.2 Different Approaches

Several approaches may be used to surgically treat PTDH, through either the thoracic or the abdominal cavity, with both open and minimally invasive surgery. The choice of the approach should be done depending on the hemodynamic status of the patient and on the surgical skills or preference of the surgeon. Already described repair techniques are similar for all types of approaches.

Repair of the diaphragm is feasible using **minimally invasive techniques** such as laparoscopy or thoracoscopy [6, 25]. In case of laparoscopy, three to five ports may be used: one umbilical for the camera; two additional ports, one subxiphoid, and one below the costal margin (on the left or on the right depending on the injury side) for liver and stomach retraction; finally, two operative ports in the bilateral midclavicular lines.

During laparoscopy for DI, surgical and anesthesiologist team should be aware of the risk of developing tension pneumothorax due to abdominal insufflation [14, 21]. This complication may occur in up to 20% of cases [12] and usually require insertion/repositioning of a chest tube or even conversion to open surgery. Thoracoscopy may be considered especially when evacuation of residual hemothorax is needed or in case of multiple previous abdominals surgeries.

In the acute setting, almost 30% of patients will undergo **exploratory laparotomy** for management of associated injuries that mandate emergent treatment. In this scenario, DI are intraoperatively diagnosed and treat at the same time, after managing life-threatening injuries.

4.3   Acute vs. Chronic Hernia

Some differences between acute and delayed post-traumatic DH have been described. Usually, reduction of the herniated organs back into the abdomen is not difficult in the acute setting; conversely, in case of chronic hernia, reduction may be complicated due to intrathoracic adhesions. In this case, surgeons should consider enlargement of the defect or extension for the phrenotomy (with attention not to damage the phrenic nerve) to facilitate reduction.

In the acute setting, even large defects usually are amenable to primary repair. On the opposite, in late hernias, due to the retraction and atrophy of the muscle, approximation and suture of diaphragmatic edges may be impossible. Synthetic prosthetic mesh, rarely necessary in the acute setting, may be crucial to fill this gap [25]. Anyway, defects up to 8 cm of diameter may be closed primarily [24]. Biological or absorbable mesh can be considered in case of field contamination due to HVI.

Chronic diaphragmatic hernia can be repaired either transthoracically or transabdominally, depending on the surgeon preference. In some cases, a combined approach may be required. Laparoscopy has been described for the reduction and repair of delayed PTDH but usually is not recommended for defect greater than 10 cm [25].

5   Outcomes

Diaphragmatic injuries and hernia outcomes are directly dependent on associated injuries severity and pattern. Reported mortality and morbidity rates range between 18–40% and 40–60%, respectively (depending also on the mechanism) [1]. Complications directly related to diaphragmatic repair are empyema and subphrenic abscess, suture dehiscence, and hemidiaphragm paralysis (due to phrenic nerve damage).

As regards to chronic DH, literature reports rates of morbidity and mortality of 30% and 20%, respectively [26]. In case of dramatic complications such as strangulation, ischemia, and perforation of herniated viscera, the mortality rate may reach 80%.

References

1. Schuster K, Davis KA. Diaphragm. In: Moore EE, Feliciano DV, Mattox KL, editors. Trauma. 8th ed. McGraw-Hill Education; 2017. p. 539–49.
2. Anraku M, Shargall Y. Surgical conditions of the diaphragm: anatomy and physiology. Thorac Surg Clin. 2009;19:419–29. https://pubmed.ncbi.nlm.nih.gov/20112625/.
3. Furák J, Athanassiadi K. Diaphragm and transdiaphragmatic injuries. J Thorac Dis. 2019;11:S152–7. https://pubmed.ncbi.nlm.nih.gov/30906579/.
4. Leichtle SW, Aboutanos MB. Diaphragm. In: Galante JM, Coimbra R, editors. Thoracic surgery for the acute care surgeon. 1st ed. Springer Nature Switzerland AG; 2021. p. 253–60.
5. Fair KA, Gordon NT, Barbosa RR, Rowell SE, Watters JM, Schreiber MA. Traumatic diaphragmatic injury in the American College of Surgeons National Trauma Data Bank: a new examination of a rare diagnosis. Am J Surg. 2015;209(5):864–9. https://pubmed.ncbi.nlm.nih.gov/25952278/.
6. Hanna WC, Ferri LE, Fata P, Razek T, Mulder DS. The current status of traumatic diaphragmatic injury: lessons learned from 105 patients over 13 years. Ann Thorac Surg. 2008;85(3):1044–8. https://pubmed.ncbi.nlm.nih.gov/18291194/.
7. Hanna WC, Ferri LE. Acute traumatic diaphragmatic injury. Thorac Surg Clin. 2009;19:485–9. https://pubmed.ncbi.nlm.nih.gov/20112631/.
8. Scharff JR, Naunheim KS. Traumatic diaphragmatic injuries. Thorac Surg Clin. 2007;17:81–5. https://pubmed.ncbi.nlm.nih.gov/17650700/.
9. Murray JA, Demetriades D, Cornwell EE, Asensio JA, Velmahos G, Belzberg H, et al. Penetrating left thoracoabdominal trauma: the incidence and clinical presentation of diaphragm injuries. J Trauma - Inj Infect Crit Care. 1997;43(4):624–6. https://pubmed.ncbi.nlm.nih.gov/9356058/.
10. Zarour AM, El-Menyar A, Al-Thani H, Scalea TM, Chiu WC. Presentations and outcomes in patients with traumatic diaphragmatic injury: a 15-year experience. J Trauma Acute Care Surg. 2013;74(6):1392–8. https://pubmed.ncbi.nlm.nih.gov/23694863/.
11. Hammer MM, Raptis DA, Mellnick VM, Bhalla S, Raptis CA. Traumatic injuries of the diaphragm: overview of imaging findings and diagnosis. Abdom Radiol. 2017;42(4):1020–7. https://pubmed.ncbi.nlm.nih.gov/27641159/.
12. Cremonini C, Lewis MR, Jakob D, Benjamin ER, Chiarugi M, Demetriades D. Diagnosing penetrating diaphragmatic injuries: CT scan is valuable but not reliable: penetrating diaphragmatic injuries diagnosis. Injury. 2022;53(1):116–21. https://pubmed.ncbi.nlm.nih.gov/34607700/.
13. Lim BL, Teo LT, Chiu MT, Asinas-Tan ML, Seow E. Traumatic diaphragmatic injuries: a retrospective review of a 12-year experience at a tertiary trauma centre. Singap Med J. 2017;58:595–600. https://pubmed.ncbi.nlm.nih.gov/27933327/.
14. Murray JA, Demetriades D, Asensio JA, Cornwell EE, Velmahos GC, Belzberg H, et al. Occult injuries to the diaphragm: prospective evaluation of laparoscopy in penetrating injuries to the left lower chest. J Am Coll Surg. 1998;187(6):626–30. https://pubmed.ncbi.nlm.nih.gov/9849737/.
15. Demetriades D, Kakoyiannis S, Parekh D, Hatzitheofilou C. Penetrating injuries of the diaphragm. Br J Surg. 1988;75(8):824–6. https://pubmed.ncbi.nlm.nih.gov/3167540/.
16. Powell BS, Magnotti LJ, Schroeppel TJ, Finnell CW, Savage SA, Fischer PE, et al. Diagnostic laparoscopy for the evaluation of occult diaphragmatic injury following penetrating thoracoabdominal trauma. Injury. 2008;39(5):530–4. https://pubmed.ncbi.nlm.nih.gov/18336818/.

17. Testini M, Girardi A, Isernia RM, De Palma A, Catalano G, Pezzolla A, et al. Emergency surgery due to diaphragmatic hernia: case series and review. World J Emerg Surg. 2017;12:23. https://pubmed.ncbi.nlm.nih.gov/28529538/.

18. Grimes OF. Traumatic injuries of the diaphragm. Diaphragmatic hernia Am J Surg. 1974;128(2):175–81. https://pubmed.ncbi.nlm.nih.gov/4843862/.

19. Mirvis SE, Shanmuganagthan K. Imaging hemidiaphragmatic injury. Eur Radiol. 2007;17(6):1411–21. https://pubmed.ncbi.nlm.nih.gov/17308925/.

20. Stein DM, York GB, Boswell S, Shanmuganathan K, Haan JM, Scalea TM. Accuracy of computed tomography (CT) scan in the detection of penetrating diaphragm injury. J Trauma. 2007;63(3):538–43. https://pubmed.ncbi.nlm.nih.gov/18073598/.

21. Mjoli M, Oosthuizen G, Clarke D, Madiba T. Laparoscopy in the diagnosis and repair of diaphragmatic injuries in left-sided penetrating thoracoabdominal trauma: laparoscopy in trauma. Surg Endosc. 2015;29(3):747–52. https://pubmed.ncbi.nlm.nih.gov/25125096/.

22. Moore EE, Malangoni MA, Cogbill TH, Shackford SR, Champion HR, Jurkovich GJ, et al. Organ injury scaling IV: thoracic vascular, lung, cardiac, and diaphragm. J Trauma - Inj Infect Crit Care. 1994;36(3):299–300.

23. Lam L, Tadlock MD. Diaphragm injury. In: Demetriades D, Inaba K, Velmahos GC, editors. Atlas of surgical techniques in trauma. Cambridge University Press; 2015. p. 162–4.

24. Finley DJ, Abu-Rustum NR, Chi DS, Flores R. Reconstructive techniques after diaphragm resection. Thorac Surg Clin. 2009;19:531–5. https://pubmed.ncbi.nlm.nih.gov/20112636/.

25. Matthews BD, Bui H, Harold KL, Kercher KW, Adrales G, Park A, et al. Laparoscopic repair of traumatic diaphragmatic injuries. Surg Endosc Other Interv Tech. 2003;17(2):254–8. https://pubmed.ncbi.nlm.nih.gov/12399834/.

26. Hegarty MM, Bryer JV, Angorn IB, Baker LW. Delayed presentation of traumatic diaphragmatic hernia. Ann Surg. 1978;188(2):229–33. https://pubmed.ncbi.nlm.nih.gov/686890/.

Minimally Invasive Approach to Intestinal Bleeding

Aditi M. Kapil and Kimberly A. Davis

GI bleeding is classified as per the location of the bleed: upper (proximal to the ligament of Treitz), small bowel, or lower (colonic). More commonly bleeding results from upper or lower GI tract and rarely from the small bowel. After resuscitation of the patient, identifying the location of the bleed is the mainstay of treatment.

Upper GI bleeding is more common than lower GI bleeding, the incidence being about 65 out of 10,000 patients admitted yearly. Peptic ulcer disease is the most common cause of upper GI bleeding. Bleeding from peptic ulcer disease typically presents with melena or hematemesis, yet if the bleeding is particularly brisk, it can also present as hematochezia. Up to 50% of patients who present with GI bleeding do so without prior symptoms. Lower GI bleeding is most commonly caused by diverticulosis; however, other causes are arteriovenous malformations (AVM), hemorrhoids, or inflammatory bowel disease. Small bowel bleeding has multiple causes that can be in part distinguished by the age of the patient. In patients younger than 40, possible bleeding sources include inflammatory bowel disease and a Meckel's diverticulum. A Dieulafoy lesion, or dilated artery in the wall of the small bowel, is uncommon. Older patients with small bowel hemorrhage are more commonly caused by AVMs or tumors.

Resuscitation should be the first priority in the bleeding patient, including hemodynamic monitoring and volume resuscitation with crystalloid, blood, and blood products as indicated by lab values and thromboelastography. Coagulopathies should be aggressively corrected. Diagnostic studies to localize the bleed may occur concurrently as tolerated. A nasogastric tube may assist in determining an upper vs. lower source, as it may demonstrate active bleeding. Although not foolproof, bilious aspirate in an NG tube suggests that the bleeding source may be distal to the ligament of Treitz. Since an UGI bleed is the most common and up to 15% of UGI

A. M. Kapil · K. A. Davis (✉)
Department of Surgery, Yale School of Medicine, New Haven, CT, USA
e-mail: aditi.kapil@yale.edu; kimberly.davis@yale.edu

F. Coccolini et al. (eds.), *Mini-invasive Approach in Acute Care Surgery*,
Hot Topics in Acute Care Surgery and Trauma,
https://doi.org/10.1007/978-3-031-39001-2_17

bleeds can present with hematochezia, it should be excluded first. The gold standard for identification is an EGD (esophagogastroduodenoscopy) at the time of presentation.

1   Upper GI Bleeds

As stated above, an upper GI bleed is the most common type of intestinal bleed requiring hospitalization and an intervention. There are many scoring systems that evaluate the need for endoscopy and intervention. The most studied of those systems is the Glasgow Blatchford score (see Table 1), which is calculated pre-endoscopy and predicts mortality and need for treatment.

A solitary predictor of mortality is an increase in the blood urea nitrogen (BUN) level at 24 h. A study of 357 patients with acute nonvariceal upper GI bleeding found that an increase in the BUN at 24 h was a predictor of a composite outcome that included rebleeding and mortality [1].

Medical therapies with proton pump inhibitors (PPI) are the mainstay in the management of an UGI bleed. Bleeding usually resolves without any endoscopic or operative intervention.. PPIs should be started empirically prior to the EGD with either 12-h dosing or a continuous drip. Studies have shown that acid suppression with a PPI, in comparison to a H2 blocker, has reduced the rate of bleeding and the risk of rebleed [2]. PPIs also may reduce the bleeding with lesions other than ulceration due to their mechanism of neutralization of gastric acid. Other agents can be

Table 1 Glasgow Blatchford score. From: Blatchford O, Murray WR, Blatchford M. A risk score to predict need for treatment for upper-gastrointestinal hemorrhage. Lancet 2000. 356(9238):1318–1321, with permission

Admission risk marker	Score component value
Blood urea (mmol/L)	
≥6-5 <8-0	2
≥8-0 <10-0	3
≥10-0 <25-0	4
≥25	6
Haemoglobin (g/L) for men	
≥120 <130	1
≥100 <120	3
<10-0	6
Haemoglobin (g/L) for women	
≥100 <120	1
<100	6
Systolic blood pressure (mm Hg)	
100–109	1
90–99	2
<90	3
Other markers	
Pulse ≥100 (per min)	
Presentation with melaena	1
Presentation with syncope	2
Hepatic disease	2
Cardiac failure	2

used as well including prokinetics, like erythromycin, and vasoactive medication to aid in hemostasis and improve visualization for endoscopy. Finally, tranexamic acid (TXA) may be administered in the actively hemorrhaging patient requiring blood transfusion as its antifibrinolytic properties promote clotting.

Some patients may be taking antiplatelet and anticoagulation medication, for instance, in the management of cardiovascular disease. Although these medications are recognized risk factors for GI bleeding, no clear evidence has been shown to indicate their use worsens the outcomes after the bleed. A 2016 guideline suggested platelet transfusion for patients on antiplatelet therapy for clinically significant GI bleeding; however, observational studies afterward show no clinical benefit and possible higher mortality in some cohort studies. An alternate therapy for drug-induced platelet dysfunction is desmopressin which enhances the ability to form procoagulant platelets and increases platelet-dependent thrombin generation [3].

For patients on oral anticoagulants, reversal agents are available. Patients on coumadin should be reversed using vitamin K alone or in combination with fresh frozen plasma (FFP) or prothrombin complex concentrate (PCC) to decrease potential for ongoing bleeding. In patients with underlying heart failure, PCC is preferred due to smaller volume and rapid onset. Direct oral anticoagulants (DOACs) have short half-lives and are renally cleared—thus may not need to be reversed in patients with normal renal function. If reversal is needed, idarucizumab, andexanet alfa, or PCC may be used.

Cirrhotic patients represent a unique challenge when they present with UGI bleeding due to the complex clotting abnormalities, with both decreases in proco-agulation and anticoagulation factors inherent in end-stage liver disease. PTT and INR are not reliable markers of coagulation in a cirrhotic patient. FFP is often given to reverse INR in patients with portal hypertensive bleeding; however, recent guide-lines recommend against correcting INR. Thrombocytopenia is also often seen in cirrhotic patients, but studies have shown limited benefits of platelet transfusion in this population [4].

Upper endoscopy of gold standard for both diagnosis and treatment of upper GI bleeds. Guidelines recommend endoscopy within 24 h (see Table 2) after appropri-ate resuscitation, and this includes patients that are admitted after hours and on the weekends. The European Society of Gastroenterology and the Asia-Pacific non-variceal upper GI bleeding working group's consensus statements both recommend that high-risk patients and continuously unstable patients despite resuscitation ben-efit from EGD within 12 h from admission.

Endoscopic treatment is recommended when active bleeding or high-risk stig-mata of bleeding such as a visible vessel or adherent clot are visible. The ESGE also recommends removal of the clot in order to control the underlying vessel. The cur-rent recommended treatment for ulcer bleeding includes injection of epinephrine, thermal coagulation, or the placement of clips. Injection therapy results in local tamponade and vasospasm. This method is inexpensive and effective for temporary hemostasis. Aliquots of diluted epinephrine are injected in the four quadrants within 3 mm of the bleeding site. Epinephrine injection should not be used as a single modality, and studies have shown decreased rates of rebleeds with epinephrine in

Table 2 Summary of the management of upper gastrointestinal bleeding. From Stanley A J, Laine L. Management of acute upper gastrointestinal bleeding *BMJ* 2019; 364:l536 doi:10.1136/bmj. l536, with permission

Pre-endoscopic management
- Hemodynamic assessment and resuscitation as needed
- Blood transfusion at a hemoglobin threshold of 70–80 g/L; higher threshold if severe bleeding with hypotension
- Risk assessment:
  - If Glasgow-Blatchford score ≤1 consider outpatient endoscopy and management
- Erythromycin (as a prokinetic agent) and proton pump inhibitor may be considered
- Patients with cirrhosis should receive vasoactive drugs and antibiotics

Endoscopic
- Endoscopy is generally recommended within 24 h in patients admitted to hospital—If the patient has severe bleeding with hemodynamic instability, urgent endoscopy should be performed after resuscitation
- Ulcers with active bleeding and non-bleeding visible vessels should receive endoscopic therapy; endoscopic therapy may also be used for ulcers with adherent clots
- Injection therapy (e.g., epinephrine), thermal probes (eg, bipolar electrocoagulation, heater probe), or clips should be used
- Epinephrine injection should always be followed by a second modality
- Recurrent bleeding should be treated with repeat endoscopic therapy but subsequent bleeding by transarterial embolization or surgery
- Esophageal variceal bleeding should be treated with ligation and gastric varices with the injection of tissue adhesive
- Refractory variceal bleeding should be treated with transjugular portosystemic shunt
- For massive refractory esophageal variceal bleeding a removable covered metal stent is preferred to balloon tamponade as a temporizing measure

Post-endoscopic management
- Patients who have ulcers with high risk lesions (active bleeding, visible vessel, adherent clot) should receive high dose proton pump inhibitors for 72 h
- Patients with cirrhosis should continue antibiotics for up to seven days regardless of the bleeding source
- Variceal bleeding should be treated with vasoactive drugs for up to 5 days
- When used for secondary prevention, aspirin should be continued or reintroduced soon after hemostasis is achieved
- Early reproduction of other antithrombotic drugs is also recommended after hemostasis is achieved to reduce thrombotic events and death

combination with another endoscopic treatment. Thermal coagulation with contact probes achieves hemostasis by coagulating (sealing) the underlying artery in the ulcer bed. Lastly hemoclips can act directly occlude the vessel. Alternative therapies include fibrin sealant or hemostatic powder, but these are less effective. Rebleeding occurs in about 10% of patients; hence, IV PPI therapy should be continued 72 hrs post intervention. PPI have been shown to decrease the risk of rebleeds, but not mortality from UGI bleeds. For hemodynamically stable patients, if rebleeding occurs, options of treatment include repeat EGD or interventional radiology for embolization of GDA. Repeat endoscopic treatment should be attempted first with rebleeds prior to proceeding to another therapy modality even with symptomatic patients. Acute care surgeons would do well to be comfortable with endoscopic methods of hemorrhage control.

Embolization has shown to lower mortality compared to emergent surgery and is successful 90–95%. The goal of embolization is to decrease the blood flow to the bleeding site enough to achieve hemostasis, while collaterals prevent ischemia to adjacent tissues. Failed endoscopic treatment is an indication for embolization by interventional radiology as well as massive GI bleeding that requires over four units of blood or hemorrhagic shock. Embolization can be done with a temporary agent or permanent device. Micro-coils are the preferred agent used for GI bleeds. An angiogram is first done to identify the bleeding site, and then agent is then delivered via a vascular catheter into the selected artery. A completion angiogram is repeated to confirm hemostasis.

Variceal bleeding accounts for about 10% of UGI bleeds and can be treated with combination therapy including medical management (vasopressin and beta blockade) and endoscopic variceal band ligation. Sclerotherapy is also an option, but it is less effective than banding. Variceal ligation is like hemorrhoidal banding, with placement of small elastic bands in the distal esophagus. Rebleeding may require additional therapies designed at decreasing portal hypertension.

Operative intervention for an UGI bleed is required in about 5% of patients and carries a mortality upward of 25–30%. Emergent operative intervention should only be considered in patients who have failed repeat attempts at endoscopic approaches and embolization. In hemodynamically stable and symptomatic patients, endoscopic and radiologic options can be exhausted and repeated before surgical management is considered.

By the time surgery is considered, these patients are usually unstable, and therefore the use of the laparoscopic approach is not typically utilized. Unstable patients may not be able to tolerate the pneumoperitoneum. For the open approach, a midline laparotomy is performed. Bleeding gastric ulcers should be treated with resection if technically feasible due to the risk of malignancy. Intraoperative endoscopy can be useful in identification and localization of the bleeding ulcer. If the location of the ulcer is not amenable for resection, a gastrotomy is most often performed followed by biopsy to rule out malignancy. Here, oversewing of the ulcer for hemostasis is performed. Biopsies should be taken from all four quadrants of the ulcer edge for maximum diagnostic yield. If the ulcer is present along the lesser curvature at the incisura and the ulcer requires resection, an antrectomy with a gastroduodenostomy (Bilroth I) or gastrojejunostomy (Bilroth II) reconstruction should be considered.

For duodenal ulcers, persistent bleeding is typically caused by an ulcer in the posterior wall which has eroded into the gastroduodenal artery. Ligation of the GDA is most effective for hemostasis. The duodenum is mobilized by performing a Kocher maneuver, and a duodenotomy made with a longitudinal incision along the anterior wall of the stomach, starting approximately 2 cm proximal to the pylorus, extending through the pylorus and onto the anterior wall of the duodenum for approximately 3–4 cm in length. The gastroduodenal artery is then ligated by placing three sutures in a figure of eight fashions at the site of the bleeding vessel within the ulcer, in the superior, inferior, and medial positions. This three-point ligation (visualizing the face of a clock: 12, 3, and 6) with permanent suture is imperative

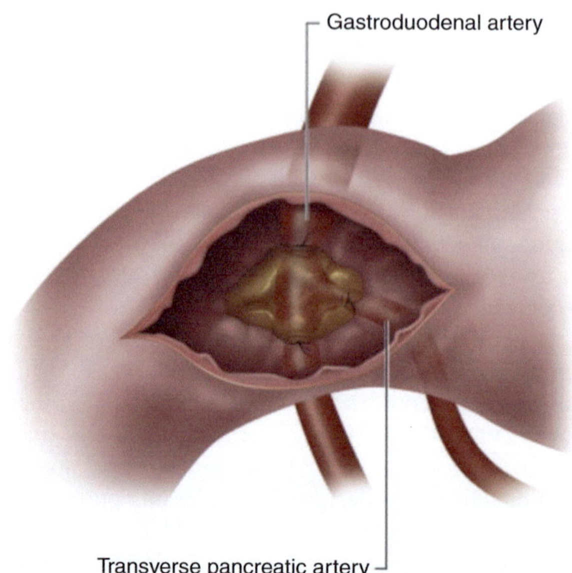

Fig. 1 Three-point ligation of gastroduodenal artery. In Asensio, Cioffi (Eds.) Atlas of Trauma/Emergency Surgical Techniques. Philadelphia, PA: Elsevier/Saunders

given the collateral blood supply from the transverse pancreatic arteries (see Fig. 1). When performing the three-point ligation, it is important to be cognizant of the location of the ampulla of Vater. A probe or small catheter may be used in the ampulla to help identify its location and prevent injury to the common bile duct. After hemorrhage control is obtained, the longitudinal duodenotomy is then closed in a transverse fashion, thereby constructing a Heineke-Mikulicz pyloroplasty.

2 Lower GI Bleed

A patient with lower GI bleed presents with hematochezia, rarely with melena even if the bleed is originating in the right colon. Patients with a lower GI bleed usually have normocytic RBCs, while iron deficiency anemia suggests a chronic bleed. Unlike an UGI bleed, patients usually have normal BUN-creatinine ratio. Any patient presenting with a lower GI bleed should have an upper GI bleed ruled out.

After initial assessment of a patient's hemodynamic stability, a colonoscopy is the next step in diagnosis and treatment. The most common causes of acute severe LGIB include diverticulosis, angioectasia, post-polypectomy bleeding, and ischemic colitis.

A colonoscopy allows for identification of the bleed about 50% of the time. However, an unprepped bowel can decrease the rate of cecal intubation preventing the identification of bleeding sites. It is imperative to carefully inspect the colonic mucosa both on insertion and withdrawal since culprit lesions often bleed intermittently and may be missed when not actively bleeding. The endoscopist should intubate the terminal ileum to rule out proximal blood suggestive of a small bowel lesion or rarely an upper source. An adult or pediatric colonoscope with a large working channel (at least 3.3 mm) should be used because the larger working channel facilitates suctioning of blood, clots, and residual stool and allows for the passage of large diameter (e.g., 10 Fr) endoscopic hemostasis tools. Endoscopic therapy options for acute LGIB include injection (most commonly dilute epinephrine), contact thermal therapies (bipolar/multipolar electrocoagulation, heat probe), noncontact thermal therapy (argon plasma coagulation), through-the-scope clipping devices, and band ligation. Endoscopic clips are an attractive treatment modality for diverticular bleeding. Compared to contact thermal therapies, clips avoid the theoretical risk of transmural injury and perforation in the thin-walled colon. Control of diverticular bleeding using clips can be accomplished either by targeted clip placement directly on the bleeding stigma or by closure of the diverticular orifice in a "zipper-like" fashion resulting in bleeding tamponade (see Fig. 2).

If a colonoscopy is unsuccessful in identification of the source of the bleed, then imaging studies can be helpful in localizing the source (see Fig. 3). Classically, a nuclear scintigraphy (tagged RBC study) was the next line for investigation, as it is highly sensitive for bleeding and can identify bleeding rates of less than 0.5 cc/min. More recently, CT angiography has been used to identify bleeding sources, either to guide future embolization or to guide surgical intervention in an actively bleeding patient who transiently responds to resuscitation. A mesenteric angiogram can allow

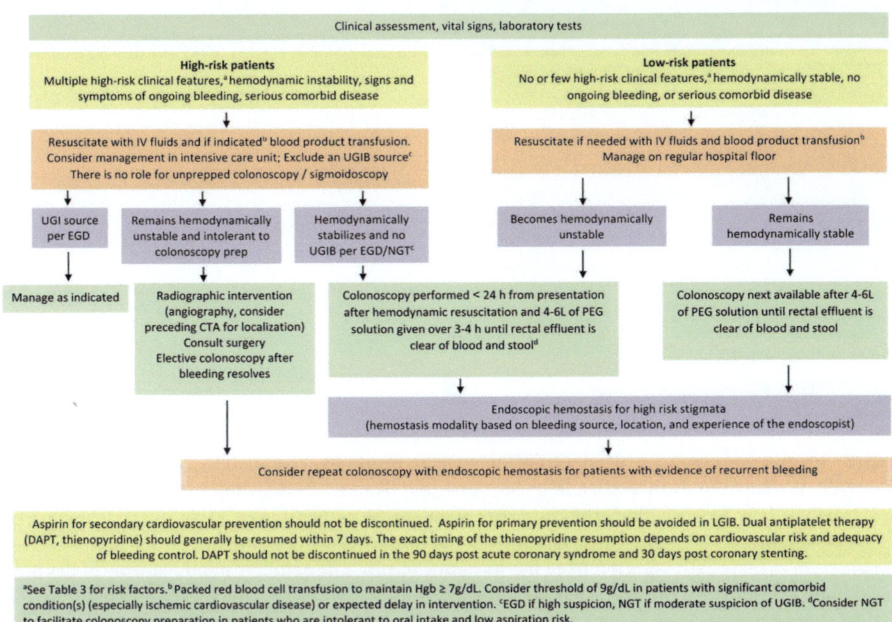

Fig. 2 Algorithm for the management of patients presenting with acute LGIB stratified by bleeding severity. From LL, Gralnek IM. ACG Clinical Guideline: Management of Patients With Acute Lower Gastrointestinal Bleeding [published correction appears in Am J Gastroenterol. 2016 May;111(5):755]. *Am J Gastroenterol.* 2016;111(4):459–474, with permission

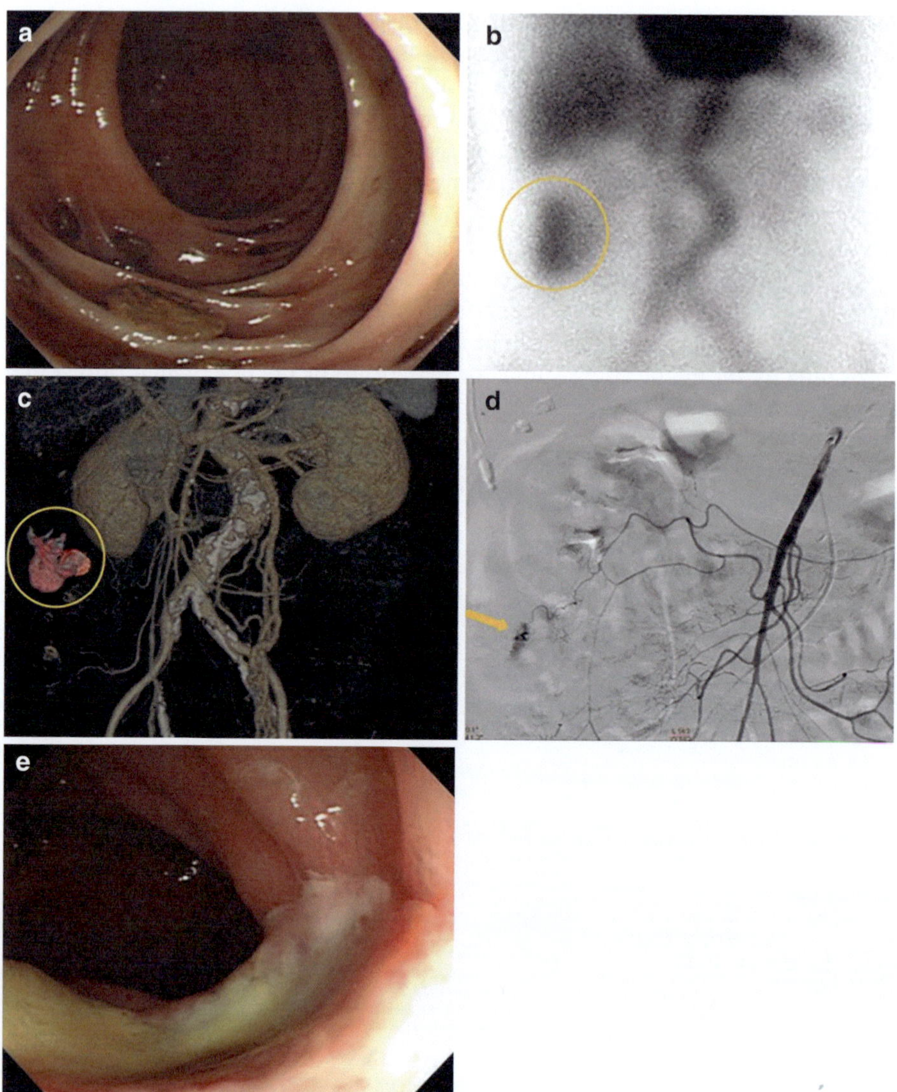

Fig. 3 Identification of LGI bleed. From Takeuchi N, Emori M, Yoshitani M, Soneda J, Takada M, Nomura Y. Gastrointestinal Bleeding Successfully Treated Using Interventional Radiology. *Gastroenterology Res.*, with permission. (**a**) Endoscopy with massive clots over stomach. (**b**) Contrast enhanced CT with extravasation from the posterior walls of the lower stomach body. (**c**) Angiogram reveals extravasation from the posterior gastric artery. (**d**) A microcatheter in the posterior gastric artery. (**e**) The artery has been successfully occluded. (**f**) Endoscopy reveals Bormann 3 type cancer at the posterior walls of the lower gastric body

for treatment as well as diagnosis, although higher rates of bleeding are required for identification (1–2 cc/min). All three of these radiographic modalities will be successful if the patient is actively bleeding at the time of the study. Embolization during angiography can be done as well if an active bleed is identified at that time. As described in UGI bleed, embolization can be done using a temporary or permanent agent. However, there is more concern for ischemia in the colon after embolization because there are fewer collateral vessels in the colon. Patients who undergo embolization for colonic hemorrhage should be closely monitored for ischemia and/or perforation in the post-procedural time frame.

Surgery for continuing massive hemorrhage is reserved for hemodynamic instability, massive transfusion requirements, and persistent hemorrhage despite other interventions. If the bleeding is localized and other interventions continue to fail, a segmental colectomy can be done; however, this is associated with a rebleed rate of up to 15%. On the other hand, the subtotal colectomy has a high morbidity and mortality rate.

A subtotal colectomy is preferred for the hemodynamically unstable patient with an unknown source of bleeding. A large midline incision would be made allowing adequate exposure. The resection would be from terminal ileum to proximal rectum. After resection, if the patient continued to be hemodynamically unstable, a damage control approach should be taken. A temporary abdominal closure would be done, and the patient is left in discontinuity. This allows for further resuscitation in the ICU, and the patient would be brought back when she or he is stable. At the second look laparotomy, a decision can be made if for an ileorectal anastomosis versus an ileostomy.

If the patient is hemodynamically stable, a laparoscopic approach to a segmental colectomy can be attempted. In both, right and left laparoscopic colectomies, the patient will be positioned in a lithotomy position. For a right colectomy, the ports would be placed in similar fashion to a laparoscopic appendectomy. A 12 mm periumbilical port and additional 5 mm ports in the left lower quadrant and suprapubic region are placed, with an additional port in the left upper quadrant. The cecum and the hepatic flexure would be mobilized, taking care not to injure the duodenum which lies below. The 12 mm supraumbilical port can be upsized to allow for extraction of the colon. A laparoscopic left colectomy can be done in a similar fashion with the working ports on the right side of the abdomen. If the patient is adequately resuscitated at the time of surgery, reanastomosis is feasible and should be favored over stoma formation.

3   Small Bowel Bleeding

Massive small bowel bleeding is rare, accounting for 0.4% of all intestinal bleeds; thus, no effective method has been established for diagnosis. If upper and lower endoscopy are negative in the face of continued bleeding, the small bowel needs to be evaluated. A CT angiogram, arteriography, and nuclear scintigraphy can again help with localization of these bleeds. Wireless capsule endoscopy, double balloon enteroscopy, and a radionuclide Meckel's scan can also be used to localize bleeding sites in the small intestine. In patients who are unstable and require exploration, on-table push enteroscopy can be helpful in identifying the bleeding site, as intestinal peristalsis may cause blood to accumulate distal to the site of hemorrhage

Case reports and small studies however have evaluated the usefulness of laparoscopic approach to diagnosis and treatment in resuscitated patients with normal vital signs. A laparoscopic evaluation of the small bowel can help to identify the source of small bowel bleeding if the portion of bowel is filled with blood. The intestinal wall should be explored for local prominence, pitting, overlapping, and abnormal mesentery. The suspected bleeding segment should be palpated carefully with clamps to feel its hardness, flexibility, and activity. If a Meckel's diverticulum is identified while laparoscopically evaluating the bowel, a small bowel resection can be done. The resected bowel should include a few centimeters of small bowel distal to the Meckel's diverticulum, because the bleeding site would likely be distal to the diverticulum.

In conclusion, nonsurgical management, including medical therapy, resuscitation, and correction of coagulopathy, remains the primary management for GI bleeding. The minimally invasive techniques in these diseases focus on endoscopy. Again the acute care surgeon should be familiar with doing therapeutic endoscopy. Endoscopy and interventional radiology treatments decrease mortality in these patients and have high rates of success. Surgery is a last line of treatment as it carries a high morbidity and mortality. The laparoscopic approach can be utilized in selective patients, but as the indication for surgery is most likely to be continued instability, the open approach is most often utilized.

References

1. Lee KKC, You JHS, Wong ICK, Kwong SKS, Lau JYW, Chan TYK, Lau JTF, Leung WYS, Sung JJY, Chung SSC. Cost-effectiveness analysis of high-dose omeprazole infusion as adjuvant therapy to endoscopic treatment of bleeding peptic ulcer. Gastrointest Endosc. 2003;57(2):160. https://doi.org/10.1067/mge.2003.74.
2. Kumar NL, Claggett BL, Cohen AJ, Nayor J, Saltzman JR. Association between an increase in blood urea nitrogen at 24 hours and worse outcomes in acute nonvariceal upper GI bleeding. Gastrointest Endosc. 2017;86(6):1022–1027.e1. https://doi.org/10.1016/j.gie.2017.03.1533. Epub 2017 Apr 2.
3. Colucci G, Stutz M, Rochat S, et al. The effect of desmopressin on platelet function: a selective enhancement of procoagulant COAT platelets in patients with primary platelet function defects. Blood. 2014;123(12):1905–16.
4. Gralnek IM, Dumonceau JM, Kuipers EJ, et al. Diagnosis and management of nonvariceal upper gastrointestinal hemorrhage: European Society of Gastrointestinal Endoscopy (ESGE) guideline. Endoscopy. 2015;47(10):a1–46.

Further Reading

Ahad S, Figueredo EJ. Laparoscopic colectomy. Med Gen Med. 2007;9(2):37.
Ba MC, Qing SH, Huang XC, Wen Y, Li GX, Yu J. Application of laparoscopy in diagnosis and treatment of massive small intestinal bleeding: report of 22 cases. World J Gastroenterol. 2006;12(43):7051–4. https://doi.org/10.3748/wjg.v12.i43.7051.
Blatchford O, Murray WR, Blatchford M. A risk score to predict need for treatment for upper-gastrointestinal haemorrhage. Lancet. 2000;356(9238):1318–21.

Casas A, Gadacz T. Laparoscopic management of peptic ulcer disease. Surg Clin N Am. 1996;76(3):512–22.

Garcia-Tsao G, Abraldes JG, Berzigotti A, Bosch J. Portal hypertensive bleeding in cirrhosis: risk stratification, diagnosis, and management: 2016 practice guidance by the American Association for the study of liver diseases. Hepatology. 2017;65(1):310–35. https://doi.org/10.1002/hep.28906. Epub 2016 Dec 1. Erratum in: Hepatology. 2017 Jul;66(1):304.

Greco L, Koller S, Philp M, Ross H. Surgical management of lower gastrointestinal hemorrhage: an analysis of the ACS NSQIP database. Journal Of Current Surgery. 2017;7(1–2):4–6.

Jordan PH Jr. Surgery for peptic ulcer disease. Curr Probl Surg. 1991;28(4):265–330.

Lau JY, Sung JJ, Lee KK, Yung MY, Wong SK, Wu JC, Chan FK, Ng EK, You JH, Lee CW, Chan AC, Chung SC. Effect of intravenous omeprazole on recurrent bleeding after endoscopic treatment of bleeding peptic ulcers. N Engl J Med. 2000;343(5):310–6. https://doi.org/10.1056/NEJM200008033430501.

Lee CW, Sarosi GA Jr. Emergency ulcer surgery. Surg Clin North Am. 2011;91(5):1001–13. https://doi.org/10.1016/j.suc.2011.06.008.

Leontiadis GI, Sharma VK, Howden CW. Systematic review and meta-analysis of proton pump inhibitor therapy in peptic ulcer bleeding. BMJ. 2005;330(7491):568. https://www.proquest.com/scholarly-journals/systematic-review-meta-analysis-proton-pump/docview/1777629388/se-2?accountid=15172.

Zang L, Wei-Guo H, Yan X-W, Zhang T, Ma J-J, Ye Q, Feng B, Wang M-L, Ai-Guo L, Li J-W. Jie Zhong, and min-Hua Zheng. Journal of Laparoendoscopic & advanced surgical. Techniques. 2010:521–5.

McDonald MP, Broughan TA, Hermann RE, Philip RS, Hoerr SO. Operations for gastric ulcer: a long-term study. Am Surg. 1996;62(8):673–7.

Raphaeli T, Menon R. Current treatment of lower gastrointestinal hemorrhage. Clin Colon Rectal Surg. 2012;25(4):219–27.

Shada AL, Dunst CM, Pescarus R, et al. Laparoscopic pyloroplasty is a safe and effective first-line surgical therapy for refractory gastroparesis. Surg Endosc. 2016;30:1326–32.

Stanley AJ, Laine L. Management of acute upper gastrointestinal bleeding. BMJ. 2019;364:l536. https://doi.org/10.1136/bmj.l536.

Strate LL, Gralnek IM. ACG clinical guideline: management of patients with acute lower gastrointestinal bleeding [published correction appears in Am J Gastroenterol. 2016 May;111(5):755]. Am J Gastroenterol. 2016;111(4):459–74.

Takeuchi N, Emori M, Yoshitani M, Soneda J, Takada M, Nomura Y. Gastrointestinal bleeding successfully treated using interventional radiology. Gastroenterology Res. 2017;10(4):259–67.

Villanueva C, Colomo A, Bosch A, Concepción M, Hernandez-Gea V, Aracil C, Graupera I, Poca M, Alvarez-Urturi C, Gordillo J, Guarner-Argente C, Santaló M, Muñiz E, Guarner C. Transfusion strategies for acute upper gastrointestinal bleeding. N Engl J Med. 2013;368(1):11–21. Erratum in: N Engl J Med 2013 Jun 13;368(24):2341.

Lin HJ, Lo WC, Lee FY, Perng CL, Tseng GY. A prospective randomized comparative trial showing that omeprazole prevents rebleeding in patients with bleeding peptic ulcer after successful endoscopic therapy. Arch Intern Med. 1998;158(1):54–8.

Samakar K, Tschen J, Astudillo A, Wallen J, Garberoglio C. Laparoscopic treatment of bleeding duodenal ulcer. Loma Linda University Medical Center, SAGES; 2012.

Sung JJY, Chan FLK, Chen M, et al. Asia-Pacific working group consensus on nonvariceal upper gastrointestinal bleeding. Gut. 2011;60(9):1170–7.

Bowel Ischemia

Francesco Pata, Antonio Pata, Gianluca Pellino,
Gaetano Gallo, and Giancarlo D'Ambrosio

The term "bowel ischemia" encompasses a wide range of diseases, ranging from self-limiting conditions, usually responding to conservative treatment, to surgical emergencies, associated with high mortality rates. In acute setting, according to anatomy, different pathogenesis, and clinical evolution, we can classify them in two main categories: **acute mesenteric ischemia (AMI)** and **colon ischemia (CI)**, also named ischemic colitis (IC). Bowel ischemia may also be secondary to other pathologies, such as strangulated hernia and intestinal occlusion, but, in these cases, it should be regarded as a complication of the related disease and falls outside the scope of the present chapter.

While *AMI is a surgical emergency with high mortality, CI may be treated conservatively in most cases*, and surgery is indicated in case of gangrene, perforation, or unresponsive disease (Table 1). In this chapter, we provide an overview of the

F. Pata (✉)
Department of Surgery, Nicola Giannettasio Hospital, Corigliano-Rossano, Italy

Department of Pharmacy, Health and Nutritional Sciences, University of Calabria, Rende, Italy

A. Pata
Cardiology Unit, Azienda Ospedaliera Pugliese-Ciaccio, Catanzaro, Italy

G. Pellino
Department of Advanced Medical and Surgical Science, Università degli Studi della Campania "Luigi Vanvitelli", Naples, Italy

Colorectal Surgery, Vall d'Hebron University Hospital, Barcelona, Spain

G. Gallo
Department of Surgery, Sapienza University of Rome, Rome, Italy

G. D'Ambrosio
Department of General Surgery, Surgical Specialties and Organ Transplantation, Sapienza University, Rome, Italy

F. Coccolini et al. (eds.), *Mini-invasive Approach in Acute Care Surgery*,
Hot Topics in Acute Care Surgery and Trauma,
https://doi.org/10.1007/978-3-031-39001-2_18

Table 1 Differences between acute mesenteric ischemia (AMI) and colon ischemia (CI)

	Acute mesenteric ischemia (AMI)	Colon ischemia (CI)
Incidence	1:1000 hospital admission	15–17 cases/100,000 person-years
Site	Small bowel	Large Bowel
Mechanism	Usually occlusive (90%): embolism, arterial trombosis, venous trombosis	Usually not occlusive: transient ipoperfusion +/− colonic wall more prone to ischemia (drugs, medical/surgical conditions)
Clinical features	Acute onset abdominal pain out of proportion in comparison to findings of clinical examination	Abdominal pain, urgency for defecation, rectal bleeding (or bloody diarrhea)
Main Diagnostic tool	CTA (Computed tomography angiography)	Colonoscopy (a CT scan with intravenous contrast is often required before endoscopy to exclude perforation, gangrene or other disease)
Treatment	Usually surgical: resection of ischemic bowel +/− revascularization in occlusive pathology if early recognized	Medical (conservative). Surgery in case of gangrene/fuliminat IC or unresponsive disease for 2–3 weeks
Prognosis	Poor	Favorable
Mortality	50–90% according to lenght of the intestinal segmented affected and the delay of surgery	10% (85% spontaneous resolution in 2–3 weeks)
Special subtype	**Venous Acute Mesenteric Ischaemia (VAMI)**: Mild symptoms, younger patients, usually medical therapy (unfractioned o low-weight heparin) if no gangrene. Better prognosis. Usually associated with hypercoagulable conditions	**Isolated Right Colon Ischemia (IRCI)**: more frequently occlusive mechanism. Less frequently associated with diarrhea/rectal bleeding. Worse prognosis. Fivefold need for surgery and a higher mortality (twofold). Usually associated with atrial fibrillation, coronary artery disease and severe chronic kidney disease

epidemiology, pathogenesis, diagnosis, and clinical management of bowel ischemia, highlighting the role of mini-invasive surgery in this setting.

1 Acute Mesenteric Ischemia

1.1 Introduction

Acute mesenteric ischemia (AMI) is a relatively rare condition, accounting 1 per 1000 acute admissions in Europe and in the USA [1, 2]. The median age is 70 years [3], but any age can be affected. As the incidence increases with the age, many patients present several comorbidities and the clinical features are misleading, the diagnosis is often late, and the high mortality is ranging from 60 to 80% [4]. *"The diagnosis is impossible, the prognosis hopeless, and the treatment useless"*, a frequently cited quote by Cokkinis in 1930 [5], describes the challenge represented by AMI in the current practice.

The common pathogenetic mechanism is represented by an **inadequate perfusion or insufficient venous drainage of a territory tributary of the superior**

mesenteric artery (SMA) sufficient (for amount and time) to injure the small bowel wall, leading, if untreated, to ischemia, gangrene, and perforation. The extension of bowel loop ischemia, the timing of surgery, and preexisting patient diseases are the main determinants of mortality.

1.2   Etiopathogenesis

Four types of AMI can be identified according to the characteristic mechanisms of flow disruption [3, 6–8]:

1. Embolic acute mesenteric ischemia (EAMI) (45%)
2. Thrombotic acute mesenteric ischemia (TAMI) (25%)
3. Nonocclusive mesenteric ischemia (NOMI) (20%)
4. Venous acute mesenteric ischemia (VAMI) (10%)

The etiology may justify some differences in the past medical history, clinical picture, and prognosis. **TAMI** occurs as a complication of an atherosclerotic plaque usually at the origin of the superior mesenteric artery, so patients may have an history of postprandial abdominal pain, weight loss, and "food fear" (*angina abdominis*) and frequently present an history of other atherosclerotic disease and associated factors, as myocardial infarction, stroke, arterial hypertension, and diabetes [9]. As usually involves the origin of SMA, TAMI may result in a global ischemia of the small bowel and right colon, and the prognosis is poor. Emboli usually lodge 3–10 cm distal to the origin of SMA, distally to the origin of pancreatic-duodenal artery and middle colic artery, so **EAMI** spares the first jejunal loops and the transverse colon [10]. Atrial fibrillation and a recent episode of arterial embolism are, respectively, detected in one-half and one-third of patients, and the onset of symptom is dramatic [11]. **NOMI** usually occurs in critically ill, shocked patients for an episode of low cardiac output, with mesenteric hypoperfusion, often exacerbated by vasoactive drugs. As patients are often mechanically ventilated, unconscious ICU patients, the diagnosis is very challenging and clinical presentation misleading.

VAMI is usually a consequence of a slow process, symptoms tend to be milder, with a more insidious outset, and the patients presents lately, some days after the onset of symptoms with a gradually worsening abdominal pain evolving over 3–10 days, but with further delayed presentations in some patients [12]. As the arterial perfusion is preserved and an irreversible ischemia happens lately, a prompt anticoagulant therapy resolves the disease in the majority of cases without surgery. Patients are younger than other groups and hypercoagulable states are the main causative factor.

1.3   Clinical Presentation and Diagnosis

AMI usually presents with acute abdominal pain disproportionated to findings of clinical examination. Nausea, vomiting, and diarrhea may be present [13].

Peritonism, hypotension, fever, and paralytic ileus denote irreversible ischemia and a late stage of the disease. However, clinical presentation is not specific, the diagnosis is challenging, and a proportion of death related to AMI remain undiagnosed. A population-based autopsy-based study in Sweden showed an incidence of AMI of 12.9 per 100,000 person-years [14], more than 20 times higher incidence reported by other population-based studies [15].

No laboratory pathognomonic pattern exists. Leukocytosis, metabolic acidosis with high lactate level, increased serum amylase, lactate dehydrogenase and aspartate aminotransferase are the common laboratory markers.

Plain abdominal X-rays may reveal signs as thumbprinting, thickened bowel wall, pneumatosis intestinalis, portal vein gas, and pneumoperitoneum, especially in the late stages of the disease, but they are not always present, and their absence cannot exclude the diagnosis of AMI [16].

Computed tomography angiography (CTA) represents the gold standard with a sensitivity and a specificity, respectively, of 93.3 and 95.9% [17] and positive and negative predictive values of 97% [18]. It can identify thrombus/embolus in the mesenteric vessels and reveal the effects on bowel wall: thickening, abnormal enhancement, pneumatosis. Renal impairment should not discourage intravenous contrast [19, 20], while oral contrast is not necessary. CTA in NOMI may be misleading: common nonspecific findings are diffuse small bowel hyperenhancement and thickening, luminal dilatation, flat IVC, and ascites ("shock bowel") similar to inflammatory and even infectious diseases [21]. In the early stages, when pneumatosis or perforation is absent, a percutaneous angiography may add further clues to the diagnosis.

As an early diagnosis is the main determinant of prognosis in AMI, a high index of suspicion is required, especially in severe acute abdominal pain with nonspecific findings on abdominal examination occurring in elderly patients with several comorbidities, especially atrial fibrillation, previous MI, recent embolic episodes, diabetes, and hypertension.

1.4 Treatment

The ideal treatment of AMI should be based on the **four Rs**: *resuscitation, rapid diagnosis, revascularization*, and *resection* if an irreversible bowel ischemia has already happened. All these actions should be interpreted nearly simultaneous rather than sequential. Fluid replacement by crystalloids, supplementary oxygen, and wide-spectrum antibiotics (e.g. third-generation cephalosporin and metronidazole) to contrast bacterial translocation are the cornerstone of the medical treatment [22, 23]. In case of diagnosis at an early stage, endovascular treatments, as percutaneous embolectomy in EAMI and percutaneous transluminal angioplasty (PTA) and stenting in TAMI, should be attempted with a close monitoring to detect early findings of ischemia [24]. As the diagnosis usually occurs lately, when ischemia has already occurred, explorative laparotomy with resection of the ischemic bowel and conventional vascular procedures, open embolectomy in EAMI, and bypass in TAMI (antegrade bypass from the supraceliac aorta to the superior mesenteric trunk or renal-mesenteric bypass) must be considered [25]. However, the time frame within any vascular treatment can positively influence the patient outcomes is not defined. It has been estimated that an irreversible ischemia occurs 6 hours after a complete vascular occlusion and within 12 hours after a reduction of 75% of blood flow [26, 27]. The high rate of mortality is often associated with a delayed diagnosis in elderly and compromised patients.

In the real word, diagnosis of AMI usually is performed when some bowel infarction has already occurred and in places when a vascular expertise is not available. In these cases, a prompt explorative laparotomy with resection of all ischemic bowel is necessary. If the patient is unstable or there are doubts about the viability of the remaining bowel, a damage control surgery (DCS) strategy (with resection of all ischemic bowel, laparostomy, and a second-look surgery at 24–48 h to evaluate the need of further resection versus stoma/anastomosis creation) may improve the survival and reduce the risk of unnecessary extensive bowel resection and stoma [28]. Intraoperative Doppler scan can help in differentiating viable from not viable bowel [29]. In case of ischemia of (nearly) all small bowel in elderly and compromised patients, avoiding any resection and proceed to palliative care is a reasonable option [30].

Patients with VAMI present the most favorable outcomes: an *early anticoagulant treatment* by unfractionated heparin (UFH) or low-weight heparins *may avoid surgery* and *reduce the progression of ischemia even after a resection is necessary* due to a late diagnosis [31]. In case of significant bowel involvement, a second look by laparotomy or laparoscopy is suggested to reduce the amount of resected bowel. NOMI requires medical therapy at first, based on fluid resuscitation, removal of any precipitating case, optimization of cardiac input, and elimination of vasopressor drugs. Infusion of vasodilatory agents, as papaverine or prostaglandin E1 (PGE1), has been reported as beneficial in small case series [32, 33]. Laparotomy and resection should be performed when intestinal ischemia occurs [34].

1.5   Role of Laparoscopy

There are not enough evidence to recommend the routinary use of laparoscopy in the management of AMI [35], as the mini-invasive approach is described in case reports and in small case series. No randomized trials have been performed to date. However, laparoscopy seems a reasonable approach in two circumstances [36–38]:

1. As **bedside laparoscopy** in ICU patients: this avoids unnecessary and potentially deleterious explorative laparotomies.
2. For **second-look operations**: to minimize the impact of open surgery in already critical patients when there is a doubt about intestinal viability at the first operation or when the postoperative course suggests a progression of the ischemia in another segment of the small bowel.

Indocyanine green fluorescence may increase the effectiveness of laparoscopy in assessing intestinal perfusion and viability, adding further information to macroscopic evaluation, thus guarantying a tailored surgery and reducing the need of second-look operation or unnecessary extended resections [39]. In a retrospective study of 52 patients with IMA, indocyanine green fluorescence led to a different surgical decision in 18 patients (34.6%) with a clinical benefit in six of those (11.5%) [40]. In other reports, indocyanine green fluorescence led to a resection of ischemic, but macroscopically still not necrotic bowel [41, 42].

2 Colonic Ischemia

2.1 Introduction

Colon ischemia (CI) is the most common ischemic disease of the gastrointestinal tract [43] with an estimated annual incidence rate of 15/17 cases/100,000 in the USA [44]. It is more common in women and in elderly, although cases have been reported also in young patients, usually associated with hypercoagulable states. However, because the manifestations are not specific and self-limiting in several cases, CI is likely underreported [45].

The mortality rate ranges from 4 to 12%, with poor prognosis frequently seen in case of isolate right-side or pancolic involvement and in the fulminant onset of the disease.

CI in intensive care unit (ICU) and isolated right-colon ischemia (IRCI) represent challenging conditions worth of a tailored strategy [46].

2.2 Etiopathogenesis

Colonic ischemia results from a **transient and inadequate perfusion of a colonic tract** sufficient (for ammount and duration) to create an injury of the colonic wall [47]. Unlike AMI, the mechanism is often not occlusive and due to a transient reduction of the blood flow in the colon wall, so that the trigger event is not recognized in many cases [48]. The degree of injury ranges from partial-thickness (self-limiting) to full-thickness (gangrenous) colitis according to the duration and the entity of the trigger event.

The effect of ischemia is exacerbated by the reperfusion that promote [49, 50]:

- Neutrophil chemiotaxis, release of inflammatory mediators and toxic reactive oxygen species
- Increased capillary permeability, with interstitial edema and fluid loss in the third space
- Loss of integrity of the vascular epithelium, favoring bacterial translocation

The colon is particularly susceptible to ischemia because of lower vascularization, in comparison with other intestinal tracts, and less developed and more prone to vasospasm arteriolar vessels (the "vasa recta") [51]. In some individuals, the absence of connections between contiguous vascular areas at the level of the splenic flexure and rectosigmoid junction may further increase the risk, explaining the most frequent localization of CI in splenic flexure and left colon accounting for 75% of cases [52].

Several risk factors have been associated with CI. Among medical conditions, **atrial fibrillation, arterial hypertension, diabetes mellitus, coronary artery disease (CAD)**, and **chronic obstructive pulmonary disease (COPD)** are frequently associated with CI, probably for their effect on atherosclerosis and endothelial disfunction. The latter has been advocated to explain the increased risk of CI in patients with autoimmune diseases.

Particularly, atrial fibrillation, coronary artery disease, and **severe chronic kidney disease** are more common in the IRCI that recognizes more frequently an occlusive mechanism and is associated with a worse prognosis in comparison with other localizations [53] with a fivefold need for surgery and a twofold mortality [54].

Also, constipation and irritable bowel syndrome have been reported as predisposing factors. **Constipation** and fecal impaction may increase intraluminal pressure and reduce blood flow in the colon, lowering the threshold of susceptibility to ischemic events. These mechanisms could explain the anecdotical reports of CI after colonoscopy [55]. **Irritable bowel syndrome** may be associated with constipation and with sympathetic hyperactivity that may impair vasodilatation of colonic microvascular bed as a compensative response to ischemia and is the most likely explanation of the rare episodes of CI after long-distance running in young and otherwise healthy patients [56].

Hypercoagulability states are well-recognized risk factors and the most important ones in younger patients. The more frequent conditions include deficit of protein S, protein C, Leiden mutation of factor V, and antiphospholipid syndrome [56]. Minor thrombophilic abnormalities have been detected in some series although their exact etiological role is uncertain.

Drugs (especially *illicit drugs, immunosuppressants*, and *constipation-inducing* ones) [57] and **surgical operations implying the ligation of the inferior mesenteric artery (IMA)**, such as abdominal aortic aneurysm (AAA) repair or left colonic resections, have been reported as potential predisposing factors [58] although in a small percentage of patients. Previous AAA repair is reported in only a 1–2% of patients with CI [59].

2.3 Clinical Presentation and Diagnosis

The classic triad of symptoms of CI - **abdominal pain, urgency for defecation,** and **rectal bleeding (or bloody diarrhea)** - is present in nearly one-half of patients. Nausea, vomiting, non-bloody diarrhea, and dizziness may be also present [60].

Abdominal pain is usually sudden, cramping, and referred in the left quadrant in the left colonic localizations and in the central abdomen in the right side. It usually anticipates 12–24 hours the rectal bleeding, bright red in the left CI and dark red mixed with feces in IRCI, although rectal bleeding or diarrhea may be absent in the right CI [61].

Symptoms/clinical signs like syncope, peritonism, shock or hypotension should rise the suspicion of acute complications or irreversible disease, such as IRCI and gangrenous or fulminant IC, requiring a prompt surgery.

In the majority of cases, symptoms are self-limiting and resolve in 72 hours. Symptoms not disappearing after 1 or 2 weeks identify no-responder forms tributary of surgery [62].

Physical examination reveals mild or moderate tenderness in the affected abdominal region, with peritonism and guarding when a transmural ischemia occurs.

Blood tests are not pathognomonic. Leukocytosis and increased level of lactates, lactate dehydrogenase, and creatinine kinase are the most frequent although not specific pattern [63].

As the most part of cases do not require urgent surgery, other infective or inflammatory diseases must be excluded to obtain a definitive diagnosis. Stool cultures and detection of *Clostridium difficile* toxins, if diarrhea, should be performed [64].

Imaging is helpful in the differential diagnosis and in the management of severe forms requiring surgery. As mainly nonocclusive in mechanism, no cause is usually detected. Abdominal X-rays have low accuracy. Abdominal Doppler scan, abdominal ultrasound, and MRI although suggestive are not available everywhere, difficult to perform in emergency and operator-dependent.

CT scan with intravenous contrast can exclude other pathologies and identify the colonic segment involved and signs suggestive, although not pathognomonic, of CI [18], such as bowel wall thickening, pericolic fat stranding, surrounding edema, or the "target sign" or "double halo sign." Pneumatosis, free air, and free fluid are suspected for complicated forms and should require a prompt surgical review.

Endoscopy (colonoscopy) represents the most important diagnostic tool in the diagnosis of CI, when fulminant or gangrene forms (requiring urgent surgery) are excluded. It should be performed within 48 h from the diagnosis [65], with minimal insufflation, stopping at the distal-most extent of the disease to avoid unnecessary risks [66]. Carbon dioxide, instead of room air, increases the safety of the procedure, reduces colonic distension, and improves patient comfort [67].

Common endoscopic findings of CI are *erythema and mucosal edema, scattered erosions, longitudinal ulcerations, hemorrhagic spots, purple hemorrhagic nodules*, and the so-called *"colon single-strip sign" (CSSS)*, a longitudinal erythematous band of the mucosa, with erosions or ulcerations, longer more than 5 cm [68]. Biopsies should be performed, unless findings suggestive of gangrene are detected. Biopsies may support the diagnosis but are not pathognomonic, so that an overall review of the patient data is necessary.

Usually, the CI lesions recover in 1–2 weeks, so that, some months after the index admission, a follow-up colonoscopy showing the resolution of the endoscopic findings may indirectly confirm an inconclusive diagnosis at the index admission.

## 2.4	Treatment

The uncomplicated IC is a self-limiting pathology and may require medical therapy. Mild cases resolve by themselves without any therapy in outpatient setting.

Patients with mild to moderate symptoms requiring hospitalization need a conservative therapy based on bowel rest (usually achieved by fasting for 2–3 days, with nasogastric tube placement only in case of paralytic ileus) intravenous fluids, antibiotics, supplemental oxygen, and a low-molecular-weight heparin. Any potential causative or risk factors must be identified and corrected. Antibiotic therapy should be continued for at least 7 days: the American College of Gastroenterology (ACG) suggests a combined therapy of an anti-anaerobic agent (e.g., metronidazole) with an aminoglycoside or a fluoroquinolone or a third-generation cephalosporin [49].

Surgery is reserved for fulminant or gangrene colitis or those with ongoing symptoms for more than 2–3 weeks. Recurrent sepsis in a patient otherwise asymptomatic after an episode of CI may be another indication due to an unhealed bowel allowing bacterial translocation. **IRCI and pancolic involvement are more at risk of complications** and should be evaluated carefully.

Postoperative mortality ranges from 10 to 65% [69] with delayed surgery as important avoidable determinant. Reisefelder et al. [70], in a retrospective study on 177 patients, identified five risk factors associated with high postoperative mortality:

- Subtotal or total colectomy
- Lactate>2.5 mmol/L
- Acute kidney injury
- Low output heart failure (cardiac ejection fraction <20%)
- Pre-and intraoperative catecholamine support

The mortality was 10.5% in absence of the above factors and increased progressively for each factor present. The presence of all five factors was predictive of a 100% mortality. The **ischemic colitis mortality risk (ICMR) score** (Table 2) is an important tool to predict surgical mortality in CI patients.

Surgery consists in the resection of ischemic colonic segment with stoma or anastomosis in line with the operative findings and the patient performance status. Shock or signs of multiple organ disfunction are a contraindication to perform anastomosis [49]. An evaluation of external viability of the unresected bowel may be

Table 2 Ischemic colitis mortality risk (ICMR) score from 49, with permission

Ischemic mortality risk score (ICMR)	Point given
Subtotal or total colectomy	1
Acute kidney injury	1
Lactate >2.5 mmol/L	1
Low output heart failure (cardiac ejection fraction <20%)	1
Pre and intraoperative catecholamine support	1
ICMR points	**Mortality (%)**
0	10.5
1	28.9
2	37.1
3	50.0
4	76.7
5	100

misleading as ischemia may be located only in the inner layers: a macroscopic evaluation of the margins of the resected specimen is then mandatory to ensure a resection with unaffected margins [71].

In high-risk patients, at risk of progression of ischemia or with uncertain surgical margins, a tailored approach based on resection of affected colonic segment without anastomosis or stoma (damage control surgery) and a second-look laparotomy 24–48 hours postoperatively is reasonable. This last advice is not evidence-based and translated by data on the treatment of acute mesenteric ischemia, supported by small case series and retrospective studies.

2.5 Role of Laparoscopy

There is a lack of robust data to support the use of laparoscopy in the management of CI [72]. Laparoscopy may dismiss cases without serosal involvement and theoretically may increase the pressure on the colonic wall, increasing the injury in the affected segment, so that a low-pressure pneumoperitoneum has been suggested [73].

Currently, two potential indications for laparoscopy exist. **Second-look laparoscopy** may be used as a safe alternative to second-look laparotomy to minimize the impact of surgery.

Bedside laparoscopy is another promising tool in the diagnosis of CI in ICU patients. ICU patients are difficult to diagnose, the CT finding may be inconclusive, and a negative laparotomy may negatively impact on an already critical and unstable status. Laparoscopy performed at bedside may reduce the rate of negative laparotomies in ICU patients, as shown in different series [74]. The technique requires a minimum armamentarium and improves management and cost of care of these patients.

2.6 Conclusions

AMI and CI still represent a challenge for acute care surgeons. Despite the advancement in the diagnosis and management of both diseases, the mortality rate is still high, and a delayed diagnosis is an avoidable source of mortality in a quote of patients. Despite other fields, the role of mini-invasive surgery is not supported by robust data, but **bedside** and **second-look laparoscopies are reasonable options**. Probably, the increasing use of indocyanine green fluorescence will guarantee a further spread of laparoscopy in the diagnosis and treatment of ischemic bowel. A high index of suspicion is necessary to promptly recognize the disease, reducing the time frame necessary for patients to undergo surgery.

References

1. Stoney RJ, Cunningham CG. Acute mesenteric ischemia. Surgery. 1993;114(3):489–90.
2. Clair DG, Beach JM. Mesenteric ischemia. N Engl J Med. 2016;374(10):959–68. https://doi.org/10.1056/NEJMra1503884.

3. Tilsed JV, Casamassima A, Kurihara H, Mariani D, Martinez I, Pereira J, Ponchietti L, Shamiyeh A, Al-Ayoubi F, Barco LA, Ceolin M, D'Almeida AJ, Hilario S, Olavarria AL, Ozmen MM, Pinheiro LF, Poeze M, Triantos G, Fuentes FT, Sierra SU, Soreide K, Yanar H. ESTES guidelines: acute mesenteric ischaemia. Eur J Trauma Emerg Surg. 2016;42(2):253–70. https://doi.org/10.1007/s00068-016-0634-0.

4. Oldenburg WA, Lau LL, Rodenberg TJ, Edmonds HJ, Burger CD. Acute mesenteric ischemia: a clinical review. Arch Intern Med. 2004;164(10):1054–62. https://doi.org/10.1001/archinte.164.10.1054.

5. Cokkinis AJ. Observations on the mesenteric circulation. J Anat. 1930;64(Pt 2):200–5.

6. Kärkkäinen JM. Acute mesenteric ischemia: a challenge for the acute care surgeon. Scand J Surg. 2021;110(2):150–8. https://doi.org/10.1177/14574969211007590. Epub 2021 Apr 19.

7. Yasuhara H. Acute mesenteric ischemia: the challenge of gastroenterology. Surg Today. 2005;35(3):185–95. https://doi.org/10.1007/s00595-004-2924-0.

8. Florim S, Almeida A, Rocha D, Portugal P. Acute mesenteric ischaemia: a pictorial review. Insights Imaging. 2018;9(5):673–82. https://doi.org/10.1007/s13244-018-0641-2. Epub 2018 Aug 17.

9. Acosta S. Mesenteric ischemia. Curr Opin Crit Care. 2015;21(2):171–8. https://doi.org/10.1097/MCC.0000000000000189.

10. Liao G, Chen S, Cao H, Wang W, Gao Q. Review: acute superior mesenteric artery embolism: a vascular emergency cannot be ignored by physicians. Medicine (Baltimore). 2019;98(6):e14446. https://doi.org/10.1097/MD.0000000000014446.

11. Wyers MC. Acute mesenteric ischemia: diagnostic approach and surgical treatment. Semin Vasc Surg. 2010;23(1):9–20. https://doi.org/10.1053/j.semvascsurg.2009.12.002.

12. Hmoud B, Singal AK, Kamath PS. Mesenteric venous thrombosis. J Clin Exp Hepatol. 2014;4(3):257–63. https://doi.org/10.1016/j.jceh.2014.03.052. Epub 2014 Apr 13.

13. Bala M, Kashuk J, Moore EE, Kluger Y, Biffl W, Gomes CA, Ben-Ishay O, Rubinstein C, Balogh ZJ, Civil I, Coccolini F, Leppaniemi A, Peitzman A, Ansaloni L, Sugrue M, Sartelli M, Di Saverio S, Fraga GP, Catena F. Acute mesenteric ischemia: guidelines of the World Society of Emergency Surgery. World J Emerg Surg. 2017;12:38. https://doi.org/10.1186/s13017-017-0150-5.

14. Acosta S. Epidemiology of mesenteric vascular disease: clinical implications. Sem Vasc Surg. 2010;23:4–8.

15. Huerta C, Rivero E, Montoro MA, Garcia Rodriguez LA. Risk factors for intestinal ischaemia among patients registered in a UK primary care database: a nested case control study. Aliment Pharmacol Ther. 2011;33:969–78.

16. Dhatt HS, Behr SC, Miracle A, Wang ZJ, Yeh BM. Radiological evaluation of bowel ischemia. Radiol Clin N Am. 2015;53(6):1241–54. https://doi.org/10.1016/j.rcl.2015.06.009.

17. Yikilmaz A, Karahan OI, Senol S, et al. Value of multislice computed tomography in the diagnosis of acute mesenteric ischemia. Eur J Radiol. 2011;80:297–302.

18. Olson MC, Fletcher JG, Nagpal P, Froemming AT, Khandelwal A. Mesenteric ischemia: what the radiologist needs to know. Cardiovasc Diagn Ther. 2019;9(Suppl 1):S74–87. https://doi.org/10.21037/cdt.2018.09.06.

19. Mcdonald JS, Mcdonald RJ, Comin J. Frequency of acute kidney injury following intravenous contrast medium administration: a systematic review and meta-analysis. Radiology. 2013;267:119–28.

20. Garzelli L, Nuzzo A, Copin P, Calame P, Corcos O, Vilgrain V, Ronot M. Contrast-enhanced CT for the diagnosis of acute mesenteric ischemia. AJR Am J Roentgenol. 2020;215(1):29–38. https://doi.org/10.2214/AJR.19.22625. Epub 2020 May 6.

21. Mirvis SE, Shanmuganathan K, Erb R. Diffuse small-bowel ischemia in hypotensive adults after blunt trauma (shock bowel): CT findings and clinical significance. AJR Am J Roentgenol. 1994;163(6):1375–9. https://doi.org/10.2214/ajr.163.6.7992732.

22. Klar E, Rahmanian PB, Bücker A, Hauenstein K, Jauch KW, Luther B. Acute mesenteric ischemia: a vascular emergency. Dtsch Arztebl Int. 2012;109(14):249–56. https://doi.org/10.3238/arztebl.2012.0249. Epub 2012 Apr 6.

23. Wong PF, Gilliam AD, Kumar S, Shenfine J, O'Dair GN, Leaper DJ. Antibiotic regimens for secondary peritonitis of gastrointestinal origin in adults. Cochrane Database Syst Rev. 2005;(2):CD004539. https://doi.org/10.1002/14651858.CD004539.pub2.
24. Acosta S, Björck M. Modern treatment of acute mesenteric ischaemia. Br J Surg. 2014;101(1):e100–8. https://doi.org/10.1002/bjs.9330. Epub 2013 Nov 20.
25. Bobadilla JL. Mesenteric ischemia. Surg Clin North Am. 2013;93(4):925–40, ix. https://doi.org/10.1016/j.suc.2013.04.002. Epub 2013 May 16.
26. Robinson JWL, Mirkovitch V, Winistorfer B, Saegesser F. Response of the intestinal mucosa to ischaemia. Gut. 1981;22:512–27. https://doi.org/10.1136/gut.22.6.512.
27. Boley SJ, Brandt LJ, Veith FJ. Ischemic disorders of the intestine. Curr Probl Surg. 1978;15(4):1–85. https://doi.org/10.1016/S0011-3840(78)80018-5.
28. Ordoñez CA, Parra M, García A, Rodríguez F, Caicedo Y, Serna JJ, Salcedo A, Franco J, Toro LE, Ordoñez J, Pino LF, Guzmán M, Orlas C, Herrera JP, Aristizábal G, Pata F, Di Saverio S. Damage control surgery may be a safe option for severe non-trauma peritonitis management: proposal of a new decision-making algorithm. World J Surg. 2021;45(4):1043–52. https://doi.org/10.1007/s00268-020-05854-y. Epub 2020 Nov 5.
29. Sartini S, Calosi G, Granai C, Harris T, Bruni F, Pastorelli M. Duplex ultrasound in the early diagnosis of acute mesenteric ischemia: a longitudinal cohort multicentric study. Eur J Emerg Med. 2017;24(6):e21–6. https://doi.org/10.1097/MEJ.0000000000000378.
30. Parys S, Daneshmand A, Sieunarine K, Watanabe Y. The effect of comorbidity on early clinical decision making in acute mesenteric ischemia. Acta Chir Belg. 2021;122:341. https://doi.org/10.1080/00015458.2021.1916281.
31. Acosta S, Salim S. Management of acute mesenteric venous thrombosis: a systematic review of contemporary studies. Scand J Surg. 2021;110(2):123–9. https://doi.org/10.1177/1457496920969084. Epub 2020 Oct 29.
32. Mitsuyoshi A, Obama K, Shinkura N, Ito T, Zaima M. Survival in nonocclusive mesenteric ischemia: early diagnosis by multidetector row computed tomography and early treatment with continuous intravenous high-dose prostaglandin E(1). Ann Surg. 2007;246(2):229–35. https://doi.org/10.1097/01.sla.0000263157.59422.76.
33. Björck M, Koelemay M, Acosta S, Bastos Goncalves F, Kölbel T, Kolkman JJ, Lees T, Lefevre JH, Menyhei G, Oderich G, et al. Editor's choice—management of the diseases of mesenteric arteries and veins: clinical practice guidelines of the European Society of Vascular Surgery (ESVS). Eur J Vasc Endovasc Surg. 2017;53(4):460–510. https://doi.org/10.1016/j.ejvs.2017.01.010.
34. Alvi AR, Khan S, Niazi SK, Ghulam M, Bibi S. Acute mesenteric venous thrombosis: improved outcome with early diagnosis and prompt anticoagulation therapy. Int J Surg. 2009;7(3):210–3. https://doi.org/10.1016/j.ijsu.2009.03.002. Epub 2009 Mar 28.
35. Cocorullo G, Falco N, Fontana T, Tutino R, Salamone G, Gulotta G. Update in laparoscopic approach to acute mesenteric ischemia. In: Agresta CF, editor. Emergency laparoscopy. Springer International Publishing; 2016. p. 179–84. https://doi.org/10.1007/978-3-319-29620-3_13.
36. Bergamini C, Alemanno G, Giordano A, et al. The role of bed-side laparoscopy in the management of acute mesenteric ischemia of recent onset in post-cardiac surgery patients admitted to ICU. Eur J Trauma Emerg Surg. 2020;48(1):87–96. https://doi.org/10.1007/s00068-020-01500.
37. Yanar H, Taviloglu K, Ertekin C, Ozcinar B, Yanar F, Guloglu R, Kurtoglu M. Planned second-look laparoscopy in the management of acute mesenteric ischemia. World J Gastroenterol. 2007;33(24):3350–3. https://doi.org/10.3748/wjg.v13.i24.3350.
38. Cocorullo G, Mirabella A, Gulotta G, Mandalà V. Laparoscopy in acute mesenteric ischemia. In: Mandalà V, editor. The role of laparoscopy in emergency abdominal surgery. Updates in surgery. Milano: Springer; 2012. https://doi.org/10.1007/978-88-470-2327-7_9.
39. Boni L, David G, Mangano A, Dionigi G, Rausei S, Spampatti S, Cassinotti E, Fingerhut A. Clinical applications of indocyanine green (ICG) enhanced fluorescence in laparoscopic surgery. Surg Endosc. 2015;39(7):2046–55. https://doi.org/10.1007/s00464-014-3895-x. Epub 2014 Oct 11.

40. Mehdorn M, Ebel S, Köhler H, Gockel I, Jansen-Winkeln B. Hyperspectral imaging and indocyanine green fluorescence angiography in acute mesenteric ischemia: a case report on how to visualize intestinal perfusion. Int J Surg Case Rep. 2021;82:105853. https://doi.org/10.1016/j.ijscr.2021.105853. Epub 2021 Apr 1.
41. Karampinis I, Keese M, Jakob J, et al. Indocyanine Green tissue angiography can reduce extended bowel resections in acute mesenteric ischemia. J Gastrointest Surg. 2018;22:2117–24. https://doi.org/10.1007/s11605-018-3855-1.
42. Nakagawa Y, Kobayashi K, Kuwabara S, Shibuya H, Nishimaki T. Use of indocyanine green fluorescence imaging to determine the area of bowel resection in non-occlusive mesenteric ischemia: a case report. Int J Surg Case Rep. 2018;51:352–7. https://doi.org/10.1016/j.ijscr.2018.09.024.
43. Alemanno G, Somigli R, Prosperi P, Bergamini C, Maltinti G, Giordano A, Valeri A. Combination of diagnostic laparoscopy and intraoperative indocyanine green fluorescence angiography for the early detection of intestinal ischemia not detectable at CT scan. Int J Surg Case Rep. 2016;26:77–80. https://doi.org/10.1016/j.ijscr.2016.07.016. Epub 2016 Jul 19.
44. Suh DC, Kahler KH, Choi IS, Shin H, Kralstein J, Shetzline M. Patients with irritable bowel syndrome or constipation have an increased risk for ischaemic colitis. Aliment Pharmacol Ther. 2007;25(6):681–92. https://doi.org/10.1111/j.1365-2036.2007.03250.x.
45. Stamatakos M, Douzinas E, Stefanaki C, Petropoulou C, Arampatzi H, Safioleas C, Giannopoulos G, Chatziconstantinou C, Xiromeritis C, Safioleas M. Ischemic colitis: surging waves of update. Tohoku J Exp Med. 2009;218(2):83–92. https://doi.org/10.1620/tjem.218.83.
46. Longo WE, Ballantyne GH, Gusberg RJ. Ischemic colitis: patterns and prognosis. Dis Colon Rectum. 1992;35:726–30.
47. Green BT, Tendler DA. Ischemic colitis: a clinical review. South Med J. 2005;98(2):217–22. https://doi.org/10.1097/01.SMJ.0000145399.35851.10.
48. Washington C, Carmichael JC. Management of ischemic colitis. Clin Colon Rectal Surg. 2012;25(4):228–35. https://doi.org/10.1055/s-0032-1329534.
49. Brandt LJ, Feuerstadt P, Longstreth GF, Boley SJ; American College of Gastroenterology. ACG clinical guideline: epidemiology, risk factors, patterns of presentation, diagnosis, and management of colon ischemia (CI). Am J Gastroenterol. 2015;110(1):18–44; quiz 45. https://doi.org/10.1038/ajg.2014.395. Epub 2014 Dec 23.
50. Hung A, Calderbank T, Samaan MA, Plumb AA, Webster G. Ischaemic colitis: practical challenges and evidence-based recommendations for management. Front Gastroenterol. 2019;12(1):44–52. https://doi.org/10.1136/flgastro-2019-101204.
51. Misiakos EP, Tsapralis D, Karatzas T, Lidoriki I, Schizas D, Sfyroeras GS, Moulakakis KG, Konstantos C, Machairas A. Advents in the diagnosis and management of ischemic colitis. Front Surg. 2017;4:47. https://doi.org/10.3389/fsurg.2017.00047.
52. Elder K, Lashner BA, Al Solaiman F. Clinical approach to colonic ischemia. Cleve Clin J Med. 2009;76(7):401–9. https://doi.org/10.3949/ccjm.76a.08089.
53. Flobert C, Cellier C, Berger A, Ngo A, Cuillerier E, Landi B, Marteau P, Cugnenc PH, Barbier JP. Right colonic involvement is associated with severe forms of ischemic colitis and occurs frequently in patients with chronic renal failure requiring hemodialysis. Am J Gastroenterol. 2000;95(1):195–8. https://doi.org/10.1111/j.1572-0241.2000.01644.x.
54. Sotiriadis J, Brandt LJ, Behin DS, Southern WN. Ischemic colitis has a worse prognosis when isolated to the right side of the colon. Am J Gastroenterol. 2007;102(10):2247–52. https://doi.org/10.1111/j.1572-0241.2007.01341.x.
55. Lee SO, Kim SH, Jung SH, Park CW, Lee MJ, Lee JA, Koo HC, Kim A, Han HY, Kang DW. Colonoscopy-induced ischemic colitis in patients without risk factors. World J Gastroenterol. 2014;20(13):3698–702. https://doi.org/10.3748/wjg.v20.i13.3698.
56. Cohen DC, Winstanley A, Engledow A, Windsor AC, Skipworth JR. Marathon-induced ischemic colitis: why running is not always good for you. Am J Emerg Med. 2009;27(2):255.e5–7. https://doi.org/10.1016/j.ajem.2008.06.033.

57. Longstreth GF, Yao JF. Diseases and drugs that increase risk of acute large bowel ischemia. Clin Gastroenterol Hepatol. 2010;8(1):49–54. https://doi.org/10.1016/j.cgh.2009.09.006. Epub 2009 Sep 16.
58. Gurakar M, Locham S, Alshaikh HN, Malas MB. Risk factors and outcomes for bowel ischemia after open and endovascular abdominal aortic aneurysm repair. J Vasc Surg. 2019;70(3):869–81. https://doi.org/10.1016/j.jvs.2018.11.047. Epub 2019 Mar 6.
59. Ultee KH, Zettervall SL, Soden PA, Darling J, Bertges DJ, Verhagen HJ, Schermerhorn ML, Vascular Study Group of New England. Incidence of and risk factors for bowel ischemia after abdominal aortic aneurysm repair. J Vasc Surg. 2016;64(5):1384–91. https://doi.org/10.1016/j.jvs.2016.05.045. Epub 2016 Jul 27.
60. Flynn AD, Valentine JF. Update on the diagnosis and management of colon ischemia. Curr Treat Options Gastroenterol. 2016;14(1):128–39. https://doi.org/10.1007/s11938-016-0074-2.
61. Sun D, Wang C, Yang L, Liu M, Chen F. The predictors of the severity of ischaemic colitis: a systematic review of 2823 patients from 22 studies. Color Dis. 2016;18:949–58. https://doi.org/10.1111/codi.13389.
62. Brandt LJ, Boley SJ. AGA technical review on intestinal ischemia. Am Gastrointest Assoc Gastroenterol. 2000;118(5):954–68. https://doi.org/10.1016/s0016-5085(00)70183-1.
63. Theodoropoulou A, Koutroubakis IE. Ischemic colitis: clinical practice in diagnosis and treatment. World J Gastroenterol. 2008;14(48):7302–8. https://doi.org/10.3748/wjg.14.7302.
64. Dignan CR, Greenson JK. Can ischemic colitis be differentiated from C difficile colitis in biopsy specimens? Am J Surg Pathol. 1997;21(6):706–10. https://doi.org/10.1097/00000478-199706000-00011.
65. Screenarasimhaiah J. Diagnosis and managemente of ischemic colitis. Curr Gastroenterol Rep. 2005;7(5):421–6.
66. Montoro MA, Brandt LJ, Santolaria S, et al. Clinical patterns and outcomes of ischaemic colitis: results of the working Group for the Study of Ischaemic Colitis in Spain (CIE study). Scand J Gastroenterol. 2011;46:236–46.
67. Brandt LJ, Boley SJ, Sammartano R. Carbon dioxide and room air insufflation of the colon. Effects on colonic blood flow and intraluminal pressure in the dog. Gastrointest Endosc. 1986;32:324–9.
68. Zuckerman GR, Prakash C, Merriman RB, Sawhney MS, DeSchryver-Kecskemeti K, Clouse RE. The colon single-stripe sign and its relationship to ischemic colitis. Am J Gastroenterol. 2003;98(9):2018–22. https://doi.org/10.1111/j.1572-0241.2003.07633.x.
69. Rania H, Mériam S, Rym E, Hyafa R, Amine A, Najet BH, Lassad G, Mohamed TK. Ischemic colitis in five points: an update 2013. Tunis Med. 2014;92(5):299–303.
70. Reissfelder C, Sweiti H, Antolovic D, et al. Ischemic colitis: who will survive? Surgery. 2011;149:585–92.
71. Urbanavičius L, Pattyn P, de Putte DV, Venskutonis D. How to assess intestinal viability during surgery: a review of techniques. World J Gastrointest Surg. 2011;3(5):59–69. https://doi.org/10.4240/wjgs.v3.i5.59.
72. Amore Bonapasta S, Lazzaro S, Passafiume F, Santoni S, Grassi GB, Longo G. Laparoscopic management of acute, severe colon ischaemia: demanding emergency extended left hemicolectomy with completely intracorporeal anastomosis—a video vignette. Color Dis. 2019;21(12):1454–5. https://doi.org/10.1111/codi.14812. Epub 2019 Aug 21.
73. Peris A, Matano S, Manca G, Zagli G, Bonizzoli M, Cianchi G, Pasquini A, Batacchi S, Di Filippo A, Anichini V, Nicoletti P, Benemei S, Geppetti P. Bedside diagnostic laparoscopy to diagnose intraabdominal pathology in the intensive care unit. Crit Care. 2009;13(1):R25. https://doi.org/10.1186/cc7730. Epub 2009 Feb 25.
74. Alemanno G, Prosperi P, Di Bella A, Socci F, Batacchi S, Peris A, Pieri M, Olivo G, Quilghini P, Fontanari P, Stefàno P, Giordano A, Iacopini V, Bergamini C, Valeri A. Bedside diagnostic laparoscopy for critically ill patients in the intensive care unit: retrospective study and review of literature. J Minim Access Surg. 2019;15(1):56–62. https://doi.org/10.4103/jmas.JMAS_232_17.

General Surgery Emergencies in Pregnancy

Goran Augustin

1 General Considerations

The pregnant patient should be placed in a left lateral position to relieve pressure on the inferior vena cava. This is more important in pregnancy when CO2 pneumoperitoneum puts additional pressure on the inferior vena cava. Pregnancy is a hypercoagulable state. To avoid thromboembolic events, sequential compression stockings are routinely employed. Some also administer a prophylactically low dose of heparin or LMWH. However, evidence regarding the optimal perioperative prevention strategy of thromboembolic events during pregnancy is scarce. No incidents of DVT or PE were documented [1]. Fetal monitoring during laparoscopy in pregnancy is not necessary. Preoperative and postoperative fetal monitoring is adequate. During operation, fetal well-being is indirectly estimated through maternal CO2 and O2 levels.

2 Acute Appendicitis

2.1 Indications

Conservative management of acute appendicitis (AA) is more commonly employed in pregnancy and ranges from 5.8 to 19% of cases [2–4]. Nonoperative therapy is based on broad-spectrum antibiotics [5]. An abdominal MRI should be performed before the commencement of conservative treatment [6–10]. There is no consensus on the route, type, and duration of antibiotic therapy, typically lasting 3–10 days [7, 9, 11]. The most significant shortcoming of conservative treatment is a 25% failure rate even with uncomplicated AA in the first and second trimesters [5].

G. Augustin (⊠)
School of Medicine University of Zagreb, University Hospital Centre Zagreb, Croatian Academy of Medical Sciences, Zagreb, Croatia

© The Author(s), under exclusive license to Springer Nature Switzerland AG 2023
F. Coccolini et al. (eds.), *Mini-invasive Approach in Acute Care Surgery*,
Hot Topics in Acute Care Surgery and Trauma,
https://doi.org/10.1007/978-3-031-39001-2_19

2.2   Treatment

Appendectomy is the most common non-obstetric surgical procedure performed in pregnancy [12]. However, several uncertainties regarding the optimal abdominal wall approach for suspected AA in pregnancy exist [13]. There is no consensus regarding the specific abdominal wall approach used for suspected AA in pregnancy. Four systematic reviews (SRs) comparing open appendectomy (OA) versus laparoscopic appendectomy (LA) for suspected AA reported inconsistent findings [14–17]. There were significant differences in included studies, analyzed outcomes, and reported magnitude and direction of effect sizes from meta-analyses (MAs). All SRs included observational studies and had critically low methodological quality [18]. OA and LA are equally safe and effective with similar obstetric outcomes. LA is preferred due to less uterine manipulation, faster recovery, less pain, and better cosmesis. Single-port laparoscopy is also used. The method is feasible, but with (1) a high (33%) rate of conversion to standard or reduced-port laparoscopic appendectomy and (2) an increased rate of wound complications (8%) [19].

2.3   Prognosis

Fetal loss is arguably the most important obstetric outcome considering the effect of different approaches to appendectomy in pregnancy. All four SRs [14–17] reported a significantly higher fetal loss rate after LA than OA, although all included a different number of studies. The study by McGory et al. [20] predominantly affected the result because it included more than half of the total number of participants in all studies within analyzed SRs. Only McGory et al. [20] have shown that LA is significantly worse than OA for fetal loss. There are many limitations of that study, and their findings should be interpreted cautiously [18]. The remaining studies reported no significant difference in fetal loss between LA and OA.

3   Acute Cholecystitis

3.1   Indications

Recurrence rates after conservative treatment are 31–92%, decreasing as pregnancy advances [21–25]. Also, the disease is often more severe at the time of relapse [26]. Compared with patients managed surgically, nonoperative management is associated with a significantly higher rate of labor induction and preterm delivery requiring neonatal intensive care [26], fetal death [24], and a spontaneous abortion rate of 12% in the first trimester [27]. Therefore, conservative treatment of acute cholecystitis during pregnancy is not recommended, except until the late third trimester. There are difficulties in performing laparoscopic cholecystectomy (LC) after 35 weeks of gestation. After conservative therapy, as bridge therapy, LC is performed postpartum.

3.2   Treatment

There have been no published randomized controlled trials (RCTs) comparing open (OC) and laparoscopic cholecystectomy (LC) in pregnancy. LC carries a decreased risk of spontaneous abortion in the first trimester and premature contractions [28, 29] or preterm delivery [29, 30] in the third trimester. Previously, LC was mainly performed in the puerperium, while OC during pregnancy [31].

The only significant differences between LC and OC were that patients underwent LC on average 5 weeks of gestation earlier than those with OC. The serum alkaline phosphatase was significantly higher with the OC. No PTDs occurred after first-trimester LC in many studies [30, 32, 33]. 10.7% of pregnant patients with acute cholecystitis underwent OC in the USA between 1999 and 2006 [34]. The conversion rate to OC in pregnancy in Australia was 13% [35], while meta-analysis found only 3.8% [36]. LC is the treatment of choice in pregnant patients with gallbladder disease, regardless of the trimester [37].

3.3   Prognosis

LC is associated with decreased risks for fetal, maternal, and surgical complications. The average length of hospital stay is 3.2 days after LC and 6.0 days after OC [36].

4   Acute Pancreatitis

4.1   Indications

In pregnancy, as in the general population, initial management is mainly medical. Surgical treatment of acute pancreatitis (AP) has two aspects—operative intervention for the AP itself and management of local (biliary tract disease, pancreatic tumor) or distant (primary hyperparathyroidism, hypertriglyceridemia, etc.) cause of the AP.

Surgery for necrotizing AP in pregnancy should be delayed as long as possible [38]. Resolution is achieved in most patients (78.9%) with conservative treatment. Therefore, the indications for surgery and antibiotics are [38–42] (a) pancreatic necrosis and infection (3–4 weeks after the onset of symptoms), (b) extensive intra-abdominal exudates, and (c) clinical deterioration. In pregnancy, there are no published series relating to the laparoscopic management of necrotizing pancreatitis.

4.2   Treatment

Percutaneous drainage, endoscopic drainage, or minimally invasive surgical techniques are gaining wider acceptance. Decompression and percutaneous drainage avoid or delay surgery in most patients with severe AP [38, 41]. For patients with pancreatic abscess, drainage is recommended [40]. Necrosectomy is deferred as late as possible, and it can be performed during the CS through midline laparotomy.

The only indication for laparoscopy in the general population is biliary AP. Patients with common bile duct stones should undergo LC within 24–48 h after ERCP to shorten the hospitalization, avoid readmission, and reduce the possibility of recurrent biliary events in the interval between ERCP and LC [43, 44]. ERCP for treating CBD stones and acute cholangitis in pregnancy is preferred to the surgical approach [45–52]. For biliary AP, the principles are the same as in the nonpregnant population. With mild AP, LC is recommended during the same hospitalization and with severe AP when the inflammation subsides.

4.3 Prognosis

Due to the lack of performance of laparoscopy for AP in pregnancy, no studies compare maternal and obstetric/fetal outcomes between methods. LC for indications other than AP during pregnancy shows better outcomes for both the mother and fetus. Maternal and fetal outcomes depend primarily on the severity and cause of AP.

5 Visceral Perforation

5.1 Perforated Peptic Ulcer

5.1.1 Treatment

A perforated peptic ulcer is extremely rare during pregnancy, with less than 100 cases published. Diffuse peritonitis from perforated peptic ulcers commonly results in preterm labor or spontaneous abortion even before treatment. All reported cases were treated with midline laparotomy, despite many cases in the general population now being treated by laparoscopy.

5.1.2 Prognosis

There are two important predictors of fetal outcome from perforated peptic ulcers during pregnancy. The first predictor is related to long-standing peptic ulcer disease with its treatment during pregnancy. The second predictor is the presence of peritonitis. The diagnosis is often made late in pregnancy resulting in peritonitis with severe obstetric consequences.

5.2 Bowel Perforation

5.2.1 Treatment

There are different causes of bowel perforation, including ischemia, colon cancer, and intestinal endometriosis. The appropriate management of these patients may be challenging, and for good outcomes, a multidisciplinary approach is mandatory.

The best approach is en bloc resection of endometriosis and associated segment of a perforated bowel. For small bowel perforation, resection with anastomosis or ileostomy when prolonged peritonitis is present is recommended. With sigmoid colon perforation, Hartmann's operation is the procedure of choice [53]. For obstructive colon cancer, treatment is surgical. The resection of the diseased segment with proximal colostomy and closure of the rectal stump or mucous fistula are the procedures with the lowest reported mortality rates [54–56].

Surgical management of perforated intra-abdominal viscus is usually complex due to diffuse peritonitis and enlarged gravid uterus. Therefore, when encountered, a midline laparotomy is often required. Due to the high incidence of preterm labor, this is also the incision of choice to deliver a viable fetus.

5.2.2 Prognosis

Endometriosis as a cause of bowel perforation should always be confirmed histologically; decidualized endometriosis involving the entire intestinal wall was found in 88% of cases. Fetal survival is 100%, with a mean gestational age near term [57, 58] in patients with intestinal perforation. Maternal survival is also 100%.

Of four pregnant patients with obstructed colon carcinoma [54–56, 59], one died (maternal mortality of 25%). Perinatal mortality is 50%, probably due to prolonged peritonitis.

6 Symptomatic Abdominal Wall Hernia

6.1 Treatment

During pregnancy, even symptomatic hernias are not operatively repaired. There are no reported cases of incarceration during pregnancy or delivery caused by a groin hernia with a first symptomatic manifestation during pregnancy [60].

Many authors claim that mesh hernioplasties should not be performed in women who plan future pregnancies. The rationale is that the abdominal wall becomes more rigid, with less compliance which is essential for the normal abdominal wall distension to accommodate the growing uterus. Moreover, the prerequisite for laparoscopic hernia repair, in most cases, is mesh. Therefore, laparoscopic mesh hernioplasty can be safely performed only after the last pregnancy. Another advantage of open umbilical or inguinal hernia repair is the simultaneous operation when CS is indicated. Through the (extended) skin incision for CS, both umbilical (vertical midline skin incision) and inguinal (Pfannenstiel incision) hernias can be repaired.

6.2 Prognosis

Results have shown an increased risk of recurrence if abdominal wall hernias are operatively repaired during pregnancy. The risk is twofold higher if the patient becomes pregnant after surgical repair. Therefore, the recommendation is to perform hernioplasty after the last pregnancy.

7 Symptomatic Diaphragmatic Hernia

7.1 Indications

There is no strict consensus about indications for the operative treatment of diaphragmatic hernia (DH) during pregnancy. For asymptomatic patients, some recommend CS after fetal lung maturity with simultaneous hernia repair always before the onset of labor. The recommendation is based upon maternal and fetal morbidity being 55% and 27%, respectively, when vaginal delivery was attempted before the DH repair [61]. Others [62] recommend vaginal delivery with (1) planned induction of labor (to avoid precipitous labor at a remote site), (2) regional anesthesia to help prevent the urge to bear down, and (3) the use of instrumentation to shorten the second stage of labor.

7.2 Treatment

7.2.1 Open Approach

The open approach may be transabdominal, thoracoabdominal, or transthoracic.

The *transthoracic approach* is indicated for previously operated DH by the transabdominal approach due to dense intra-abdominal adhesions [63–65]. Under normal circumstances, the best surgical approach is *lateral thoracotomy* at the level of the seventh or eighth rib [66] because it provides a better view of the diaphragm while it requires one-lung ventilation. If strangulation has occurred, the incision should be planned as a *thoracoabdominal approach* for adequate exposure and easier access to the bowel, particularly if the colon is involved. Also, a separate laparotomy is an option. Some prefer the transthoracic approach due to the limited intra-abdominal space from the gravid uterus [67].

The *transabdominal approach* enables good access to (1) herniated parenchymal organs such as the liver and spleen [68] when mobile cecum is present or (2) anterior (Morgagni) DH. The transabdominal approach is preferred because it is less invasive [69]. However, some prefer the transthoracic approach in longer-lasting hernias to treat pleuroperitoneal adhesions. On the other hand, the transabdominal approach is better in pregnancy if CS is indicated or other intra-abdominal pathologic findings are removed, such as gallbladder stones. Most cases are explored through midline laparotomy, although a subcostal incision can be performed [70]. Midline laparotomy is better if abdominal organ resection is anticipated.

7.2.2 Laparoscopic Approach

Recently, the laparoscopic approach has gained popularity [71–78]. The advantages are avoiding laparotomy, which increases the rate of abdominal wall disruption during and after delivery and postoperative hernia. The disadvantage is that CS requires a separate incision. Simultaneous Pfannenstiel incision for CS, when the laparoscopic procedure is completed, results in excellent cosmetic results. Also, the laparoscopic operation can be undertaken after vaginal delivery [77, 78] or CS [79] as a secondary procedure.

With a *lateral approach*, the patient is positioned in frank right lateral decubitus with double-lumen endotracheal intubation. An electronic fetal monitoring device is placed on the right lower part of the abdomen. The lateral position has many advantages over the more traditional *supine position*. First, it permits a complete view of the diaphragm, the subdiaphragmatic space, and the thorax. In this position, gravity helps retract the spleen, the stomach, and the uterus without manipulation. This reduces the risk of iatrogenic injury, especially to the gravid uterus. Also, if needed, a thoracoscopy could be easily accomplished without any repositioning. A more pronounced right lateral decubitus reduces the risk of inferior vena cava compression by a posterolateral displacement of the uterus. This position could be tried preoperatively with fetal and maternal monitoring (for 1 h) to ensure maternal hemodynamic stability and fetal well-being [71].

8 Intestinal Obstruction

8.1 Treatment

8.1.1 Intussusception

Most patients are explored by laparotomy, but laparoscopy is more frequently used to minimize abdominal wall trauma and shorten postoperative hospital stay [80, 81]. After exploration, the further procedure depends on the viability of the intestine and the presence of the lead point. The manual reduction can be attempted in small bowel intussusception if the segment involved is viable and if malignancy is not suspected (palpated or checked with intraoperative enteroscopy) [80]. The manual reduction should be performed to push the intussuscipiens rather than pulling the bowel due to a lower risk of bowel wall tearing. Resection of the bowel segment is indicated in the presence of [82] (1) gangrenous bowel, (2) recurrent intussusceptions, and (3) the leading point is present. The leading point should be resected, and additional procedures depend on the histopathological diagnosis.

Maternal prognosis, both after resection for ischemic bowel or without bowel resection, is excellent [80–84]. Higher rates of spontaneous abortion and preterm labor are present [83], particularly if perforation with peritonitis occurs. If intussusception presents during the puerperium, it is easier to indicate diagnostic imaging modalities with radiation; therefore, the diagnosis could be made earlier. The problem is that intussusception is sometimes mistaken for postdelivery ileus delaying the diagnostic workup.

8.1.2 Small Bowel Volvulus

All cases of small bowel volvulus were treated by laparotomy. Laparoscopy could be used in the early stages because detorsion leads to restitution, without additional more complex laparoscopic procedures such as intestinal resection.

Early diagnosis and management are essential to avoid infarction of the bowel. The rate of bowel resection is still high, around 68%, over the last 20 years [85]. Maternal and fetal mortality decreased from 6–20% and 22–50% [86] to 3–15% and 22%, respectively (another 14% of newborns with proven asphyxia) [85, 87].

8.1.3 Sigmoid Volvulus

In the absence of peritonitis and during the second trimester of gestation, early studies recommend detorsion by mini-laparotomy to shorten the operating time. In contrast, sigmoid resection with anastomosis may be performed after puerperium [88, 89]. Sigmoid resection is recommended due to the high incidence of recurrence [90, 91]. Such management could be performed by laparoscopy. Others recommend anastomosis after sigmoidectomy during the first and second trimesters [92]. Hartmann's procedure is safer, eliminating the risk of anastomotic dehiscence with its deleterious consequences on the mother and fetus. The growing uterus could compress the anastomosis, causing ischemia, or compress the colon distal to the anastomosis, increasing the risk of anastomotic dehiscence. In the third trimester, if sufficient intestinal exposure cannot be obtained due to the enlarged uterus, a CS is required [93]. After detorsion, the deflated loop could be on the left side of the abdomen and should be replaced. This can be done by slipping the loop of the bowel over the fundus of the uterus. Compression by the uterus may be a contributing factor in obstruction when the volvulus is partial. The entire bowel should be examined for other areas of obstruction. Intestinal viability should be assessed cautiously. If viable, the bowel can be derotated and left in situ [94, 95], but recurrent sigmoid volvulus in the general population is around 50%; therefore, resection during the index operation with or without anastomosis is recommended [93].

9 Acute Crohn's Disease

9.1 Indications

The indications for surgery in pregnant women with Crohn's disease (CD) are not different from the general population and include intestinal obstruction or perforation, bleeding, or abscess. Only 2–2.7% of CD pregnant patients require surgery [96, 97]. The approach should be multidisciplinary, and surgery should be performed at a tertiary center with neonatal, pediatric, and obstetric departments.

9.2 Treatment

The most common location for surgical intervention is terminal ileum, including free or contained small bowel perforation [98] or terminal ileitis with abscesses and fistula or stenosis [99]. Half of the patients present in the second trimester, with a similar incidence in the first and less than 10% in the third [98, 99]. Ileocecal resection is the most common procedure performed (66.7%), followed by small bowel resection (20%), subtotal colectomy (6.7%), and restoration of bowel continuity (6.7%) [99]. A laparoscopic approach is preferred but completed in only 20% of patients [98, 99]. Only several cases of image-guided percutaneous drainage of an intra-abdominal abscess are published [98].

9.2.1 Terminal Ileitis/Acute Appendicitis

If acute appendicitis is suspected, laparoscopic exploration is recommended. If an indication for bowel resection exists (abscess adjacent to active ileocecal disease, bowel perforation, bowel obstruction), ileocolic resection can be completed by laparoscopy or conversion to midline laparotomy. There is an issue with bowel resection when the active ileocecal CD is present without perforation, obstruction, or adjacent abscess [100]. During exploration, when the active disease is found, resection is preferable to prevent exacerbation later in pregnancy. The severity of the CD, not the operation itself, is the leading cause of the poor fetal outcome.

9.3 Prognosis

Intra-abdominal surgery performed during the first trimester is associated with an increased risk of miscarriage; for planned procedures in the second trimester, the risk is lower. In the third trimester, a laparotomy may be complicated by premature delivery and technical difficulties. However, the severity of the CD, not the operation, determines the maternal and fetal risk.

9.3.1 Maternal Outcome

Increased maternal morbidity is due to the consequences of acute abdominal conditions requiring emergency surgery and the underlying chronic inflammatory condition itself and all comorbid conditions related to it. There is a threefold increase in the incidence of gestational diabetes in patients with IBD compared to healthy controls, regardless of gestational corticosteroid use [101]. There is a significantly higher rate of gestational diabetes among UC patients using ART than CD patients (29.4% vs. 6.1%) [102]. Higher maternal thromboembolic complications and malnutrition/poor weight gain in pregnant IBD patients are confirmed [103, 104]. Perioperative complications depend mainly on the severity of CD. There are no comparisons between open or laparoscopic procedures.

9.3.2 Fetal Outcome

Active disease at conception is associated with a higher rate of fetal loss, preterm birth (twofold), LBW (threefold), and small for gestational age infants [105–115]. Women with CD have 1.9 times the risk of fetal abdominal wall defects [116]. The association between CD and abdominal wall defects was found and is declining. It is unlikely that the introduction of biologics increased the risk of wall defects and that folic acid food fortification could have been beneficial [116]. Preterm delivery is further associated with disease flares during pregnancy [108, 117]. The overall preterm delivery rate among surgically treated patients is 79% [98].

A meta-analysis including more than 700 patients with CD reported a normal pregnancy in 83% (71–93% in individual studies). Fetal malformations were observed in 1% of all pregnancies, and the frequency of spontaneous abortions and stillbirths was similar to that observed in the general population [118]. Studies with all CD subgroups during pregnancy did not find significantly different perinatal outcomes (105–142 g less than children born to mothers without CD and a higher risk of LBW and preterm birth) compared to the general population even before the era of biologics.

A typical resection segment is terminal ileum, and loss of the terminal ileum's capacity for nutrient and vitamin absorption could predispose to smaller birth weight. Secondly, the fact that resection had previously occurred may serve as a marker of greater disease severity. The rate of previous surgery for CD is similar between pregnant women and nonpregnant women with CD [105]. There is a correlation between length of bowel resection or active disease at the time of conception and an increased risk of spontaneous abortion compared to a reference population and women with UC [119]. Operated patients during pregnancy after 1983 had a premature delivery rate of 40% [98].

The difference in the distribution of the CD lesions may be a significant factor for different perinatal outcomes. Surgical intervention for large bowel CD has a worse perinatal outcome compared to ileal CD [120, 121]. With the resection of terminal ileitis, fetal mortality is 0% [121]. One explanation for the worse perinatal outcome with colonic CD is the higher rate of postoperative complications [120, 121].

Up to 1962, all women with the first episode of surgically treated terminal ileitis delivered prematurely, and perinatal mortality was 43% [122]. After 1983, perinatal mortality in operated CD patients during pregnancy is 5%, but premature birth is 79% [98].

There are no comparisons between open or laparoscopic procedures.

10 Splenic Rupture

10.1 Treatment

There are no criteria or guidelines for the nonoperative management of pregnant patients. However, to be eligible for nonoperative management, patients should meet several criteria based on data on the general population [123]: (1) hemodynamic stability, (2) the absence of peritoneal signs, and (3) the absence of other abdominal injuries requiring surgery. In many instances, bleeding from the spleen of any cause can be successfully treated by radiologic interventional techniques.

10.1.1 Traumatic Splenic Rupture

Surgical treatment for traumatic splenic rupture includes a midline incision to facilitate access, and visualization for both exploration and potential CS is recommended. CS in patients with intraperitoneal bleeding due to splenic rupture has two goals: (1) adequate surgery for the ruptured spleen cannot be undertaken because a term-sized uterus prevents adequate exposure of the splenic fossa and (2) CS is necessary to prevent intrauterine death due to maternal hypoxia or hypotension. Generally, methods used for a ruptured spleen include splenectomy, partial splenectomy, or spleen-preserving methods. The bleeding should be stopped because further bleeding can lead to fetal loss. For splenic artery aneurysm rupture, percutaneous embolization is one option, especially in symptomatic patients without rupture or contained rupture. Another option is resection of the aneurysm, if not intraparenchymal. When rupture occurs, splenectomy is the only definitive treatment option.

The laparoscopic approach is rarely used. There are several cases of blunt trauma causing a splenic rupture [75, 124]. Laparoscopic procedures are indicated in early presentations because, in delayed presentation, blood clots obscure the operative field, and there is difficulty in visualization. Also, in hemodynamically unstable patients, definitive treatment must be swift; therefore, laparotomy is recommended [125]. Another indication for laparoscopic approach is early splenic pregnancy in symptomatic or hemodynamically stable patients [126]. The third indication is stable patients with asymptomatic or symptomatic patients with splenic artery aneurysms but without rupture.

10.1.2 Splenic Pregnancy

The laparoscopic approach is increasingly used for suspected splenic pregnancy as both a diagnostic and therapeutic tool. For early splenic pregnancy, even with hemoperitoneum, but in hemodynamically stable patients, laparoscopic treatment is optimal [127, 128].

There are no recommendations for the type of procedure. Partial splenectomy or wedge resection, including ectopic pregnancy, can be made. Essential steps are atraumatic mobilization of the spleen, temporary splenic artery occlusion avoiding injury to pancreatic parenchyma, the use of topical hemostatic agents, and the use of absorbable mesh [125].

10.2 Prognosis

10.2.1 Spontaneous Splenic Rupture

Due to the rarity of the condition, the maternal and fetal outcome for every etiology is difficult to estimate. Therefore, the outcomes are mainly presented for the whole group of splenic ruptures. In the conservatively treated group, the maternal mortality was 100% [129]. Up to 2008, the maternal mortality rate in a spontaneous splenic rupture in pregnancy was 14.3% [130]. The fetal mortality rate in a spontaneous splenic rupture in pregnancy is also declining [130].

10.2.2 Splenic Pregnancy

Despite being a life-threatening condition, no mortality has been reported for splenic pregnancy [125]. This may be related to misdiagnosis as a spontaneous splenic rupture and publication bias in not reporting fatal outcomes.

References

1. Nasioudis D, Tsilimigras D, Economopoulos KP. Laparoscopic cholecystectomy during pregnancy: a systematic review of 590 patients. Int J Surg. 2016;27:165–75.
2. Cheng HT, Wang Y-C, Lo HC, et al. Laparoscopic appendectomy versus open appendectomy in pregnancy: a population-based analysis of maternal outcome. Surg Endosc. 2015;29:1394–9.
3. Abbasi N, Patenaude V, Abenhaim HA. Management and outcomes of acute appendicitis in pregnancy—population-based study of over 7000 cases. BJOG. 2014;121:1509–14.
4. Cai Y-L, Yang S-S, Peng D-Z, Jia Q-B, Li F-Y, Ye H, et al. Laparoscopic appendectomy is safe and feasible in pregnant women during second trimester. Medicine (Baltimore). 2020;99:–e21801.
5. Joo JI, Park HC, Kim MJ, Lee BH. Outcomes of antibiotic therapy for uncomplicated appendicitis in pregnancy. Am J Med. 2017;130:1467–9.
6. Amitai MM, Katorza E, Guranda L, Apter S, Portnoy O, Inbar Y, et al. Role of emergency magnetic resonance imaging in the workup of suspected appendicitis in pregnant women. Isr Med Assoc J. 2016;18:600–4.
7. Augustin G, di Saverio S. MRI is mandatory for the assignment into antibiotic treatment or appendectomy group of patients during pregnancy. Am J Med. 2020;133:e208.
8. Young BC, Hamar BD, Levine D, Roque H. Medical management of ruptured appendicitis in pregnancy. Obstet Gynecol. 2009;114:453–6.
9. Ajjarapu A, Moreira N. Successful non-surgical management of acute, uncomplicated appendicitis in pregnancy: a case report. Proc Obs Gynecol. 2020;9:8.
10. Chung J, Berryman RP. An atypical case of a common pregnancy issue: appendicitis-like hyperemesis gravidarum. Case Rep Med. 2020;2020:6959605.
11. Liu J, Ahmad M, Wu J, Tong XJ, Zeng HZ, Chan FS-Y, et al. Antibiotic is a safe and feasible option for uncomplicated appendicitis in pregnancy—a retrospective cohort study. Asian J Endosc Surg. 2020;14:207.
12. Rasmussen AS, Christiansen CF, Ulrichsen SP, Uldbjerg N, Nørgaard M. Non-obstetric abdominal surgery during pregnancy and birth outcomes: a Danish registry-based cohort study. Acta Obstet Gynecol Scand. 2020;99(4):469–76. https://pubmed.ncbi.nlm.nih.gov/31774546/.
13. Di Saverio S, Podda M, De Simone B, Ceresoli M, Augustin G, Gori A, et al. Diagnosis and treatment of acute appendicitis: 2020 update of the WSES Jerusalem guidelines. World J Emerg Surg. 2020;15:27.
14. Frountzas M, Nikolaou C, Stergios K, Kontzoglou K, Toutouzas K, Pergialiotis V. Is the laparoscopic approach a safe choice for the management of acute appendicitis in pregnant women? A meta-analysis of observational studies. Ann R Coll Surg Engl. 2019;101:235–48.
15. Chakraborty J, Kong JC, Su WK, Gourlas P, Gillespie C, Slack T, et al. Safety of laparoscopic appendicectomy during pregnancy: a systematic review and meta-analysis. ANZ J Surg. 2019;89:1373.
16. Lee SH, Lee JY, Choi YY, Lee JG. Laparoscopic appendectomy versus open appendectomy for suspected appendicitis during pregnancy: a systematic review and updated meta-analysis. BMC Surg. 2019;19(1):41.
17. Prodromidou A, Machairas N, Kostakis ID, Molmenti E, Spartalis E, Kakkos A, et al. Outcomes after open and laparoscopic appendectomy during pregnancy: a meta-analysis. Eur J Obstetr Gynecol Reprod Biol. 2018;225:40–50.
18. Augustin G, Boric M, Barcot O, Puljak L. Discordant outcomes of laparoscopic versus open appendectomy for suspected appendicitis during pregnancy in published meta-analyses: an overview of systematic reviews. Surg Endosc. 2020;34:4245–56.
19. Cho IS, Bae SU, Jeong WK, Baek SK. Single-port laparoscopic appendectomy for acute appendicitis during pregnancy. J Minim Access Surg. 2021;17(1):37–42. https://pubmed.ncbi.nlm.nih.gov/31929222/.

20. McGory ML, Zingmond DS, Tillou A, et al. Negative appendectomy in pregnant women is associated with a substantial risk of fetal loss. J Am Coll Surg. 2007;205:534–40.
21. Swisher SG, Schmit PJ, Hunt KK, et al. Biliary disease during pregnancy. Am J Surg. 1994;168:576–81.
22. Dixon NP, Faddis DM, Silberman H. Aggressive management of cholecystitis during pregnancy. Am J Surg. 1987;154(3):292–4.
23. Glasgow RE, Visser BC, Harris HW, Patti MG, Kilpatrick SJ, Mulvihill SJ. Changing management of gallstone disease during pregnancy. Surg Endosc. 1998;12(3):241–6. http://www.ncbi.nlm.nih.gov/pubmed/9502704.
24. Jelin EB, Smink DS, Vernon AH, Brooks DC. Management of biliary tract disease during pregnancy: a decision analysis. Surg Endosc. 2008;22(1):54–60. http://www.ncbi.nlm.nih.gov/pubmed/17713817.
25. Jackson H, Granger S, Price S, et al. Diagnosis and laparoscopic treatment of surgical disease during pregnancy: an evidence-based review. Surg Endosc. 2008;22:1917–27.
26. Lu EJ, Curet MJ, El-Sayed YY, Kirkwood KS. Medical versus surgical management of biliary tract disease in pregnancy. Am J Surg. 2004;188(6):755–9. http://www.ncbi.nlm.nih.gov/pubmed/15619495.
27. McKellar DP, Anderson CT, Boynton CJ, et al. Cholecystectomy during pregnancy without fetal loss. Surg Gynecol Obs. 1992;174:465–8.
28. Barone JE, Bears S, Chen S, et al. Outcome study of cholecystectomy during pregnancy. Am J Surg. 1999;177:232–6.
29. Curet MJ, Allen D, Josloff RK, Pitcher DE, Curet LB, Miscall BG, et al. Laparoscopy during pregnancy. Arch Surg. 1996;131(5):546–50.
30. Graham G, Baxi L, Tharakan T. Laparoscopic cholecystectomy during pregnancy: a case series and review of the literature. Obs Gynecol Surv. 1998;53:566–74.
31. Álvarez-Villaseñor AS, Mascareño-Franco HL, Agundez-Meza JJ, Cardoza-Macías F, Fuentes-Orozco C, Rendón-Félix J, et al. Cholelithiasis during pregnancy and postpartum: prevalence, presentation and consequences in a referral hospital in Baja California Sur. Gac Med Mex. 2017;153:146–52.
32. Affleck DG, Handrahan DL, Egger M, Price R. The laparoscopic management of appendicitis and cholelithiasis during pregnancy. Am J Surg. 1999;178:523–9.
33. Rollins MD, Chan KJ, Price R. Laparoscopy for appendicitis and cholelithiasis during pregnancy: a new standard of care. Surg Endosc. 2004;18:237–41.
34. Kuy S, Roman SA, Desai R, Sosa JA. Outcomes following cholecystectomy in pregnant and nonpregnant women. Surgery. 2009;146:358–66.
35. Paramanathan A, Walsh SZ, Zhou J, Chan S. Laparoscopic cholecystectomy in pregnancy: an Australian retrospective cohort study. Int J Surg. 2015;18:220–3.
36. Sedaghat N, Cao AM, Eslick GD, Cox MR. Laparoscopic versus open cholecystectomy in pregnancy: a systematic review and meta-analysis. Surg Endosc. 2017;31(2):673–9.
37. https://www.sages.org/publications/guidelines/guidelines-for-diagnosis-treatment-and-use-of-laparoscopy-for-surgical-problems-during-pregnancy/.
38. Hernandez A, Petrov MS, Brooks DC, et al. Acute pancreatitis in pregnancy: a 10-year single center experience. J Gastrointest Surg. 2007;11:1623–7.
39. Pezzilli R, Zerbi A, Di Carlo V, et al. Practical guidelines for acute pancreatitis. Pancreatology. 2010;10:523–35.
40. Wada K, Takada T, Hirata K, et al. Treatment strategy for acute pancreatitis. J Hepatobiliary Pancreat Sci. 2010;17:79–86.
41. Hasibeder WR, Hasibeder C, Rieger M, et al. Critical care of the patient with acute pancreatitis. Anaesth Intensive Care. 2009;37:190–206.
42. Nathens AB, Curtis RJ, Beale RJ, et al. Management of the critically ill patient with severe acute pancreatitis. Crit Care Med. 2004;32:2524–36.
43. Chandler CF, Lane JS, Ferguson P, Thonpson JE, et al. Prospective evaluation of early versus delayed laparoscopic cholecystectomy for the treatment of acute cholecystitis. Am Surg. 2000;66:896–900.

44. de Vries A, Donkervoort SC, van Geloven AA, Pierik EGJM. Conversion rate of laparoscopic cholecystectomy after endoscopic retrograde cholangiography in the treatment of choledocholithiasis: does the time interval matter? Surg Endosc. 2005;19:996–1001.
45. Sungler P, Heinerman PM, Steiner H, et al. Laparoscopic cholecystectomy and interventional endoscopy for gallstone complications during pregnancy. Surg Endosc. 2000;14:267–71.
46. Al-Akeely MH. Management of complicated gallstone disease during pregnancy. Saudi J Gastroenterol. 2003;9(3):135–8. http://www.ncbi.nlm.nih.gov/pubmed/19861817.
47. Baillie J, Cairns SR, Putman WS, Cotton PB. Endoscopic management of choledocholithiasis during pregnancy. Surg Gynecol Obs. 1990;171:1–4.
48. Tham TC, Vandervoort J, Wong RC, et al. Safety of ERCP during pregnancy. Am J Gastroenterol. 2003;98:308–11.
49. Barthel JS, Chowdhury T, Miedema BW. Endoscopic sphincterotomy for the treatment of gallstone pancreatitis during pregnancy. Surg Endosc. 1998;12:394–9.
50. Gupta R, Tandan M, Lakhtakia S, et al. Safety of therapeutic ERCP in pregnancy-an Indian experience. Indian J Gastroenterol. 2005;24:161–3.
51. Jamidar PA, Beck GJ, Hoffman BJ, et al. Endoscopic retrograde cholangiopancreatography in pregnancy. Am J Gastroenterol. 1995;90:1263–7.
52. Tang SJ, Mayo MJ, Rodriguez-Frias E, et al. Safety and utility of ERCP during pregnancy. Gastrointest Endosc. 2009;69:453–61.
53. Costa A, Sartini A, Garibaldi S, Cencini M. Deep endometriosis induced spontaneous colon rectal perforation in pregnancy: laparoscopy is advanced tool to confirm diagnosis. Case Rep Obs Gynecol. 2014;2014:907150.
54. Sung JF, Salvay HB, Hansman MF, Taslimi MM. Stercoral perforation of the colon with favorable pregnancy outcome. Obstet Gynecol. 2009;113(2 Pt 2):491–2. http://www.ncbi.nlm.nih.gov/entrez/query.fcgi?cmd=Retrieve&db=PubMed&dopt=Citation&list_uids=19155931.
55. Matsushita T, Yomoto Y, Fukushima K, et al. Stercoral perforation of the colon during pregnancy. J Obs Gynaecol Res. 2011;37:1685–8.
56. Costales AB, Agarwal AK, Chauhan SP, Refuerzo JS, Taub EA. Stercoral perforation of the colon during pregnancy: a case report and review of the literature. Am J Perinatol Reports. 2015;5:e25–9.
57. Maggiore ULR, Ferrero S, Mangili G, Bergamini A, Inversetti A, Giorgione V, et al. A systematic review on endometriosis during pregnancy: diagnosis, misdiagnosis, complications and outcomes. Hum Reprod Update. 2016;22:70–103.
58. Wollenschlaeger M, Carlan SJ, McWhorter J, Kuffskie M, Madruga M. Spontaneous sigmoid colon rupture secondary to endometriosis in the third trimester of pregnancy. J Gynecol Surg. 2018;34:40–2.
59. Russell W. Stercoraceous ulcer. Am Surg. 1976;42:416–20.
60. Lechner M, Fortelny R, Öfner D, Mayer F. Suspected inguinal hernias in pregnancy—handle with care! Hernia. 2014;18:375–9.
61. Kurzel RB, Naunheim KS, Schwartz RA. Repair of symptomatic diaphragmatic hernia during pregnancy. Obstet Gynecol. 1988;71:869–71. http://ovidsp.ovid.com/ovidweb.cgi?T=JS&PAGE=reference&D=med3&NEWS=N&AN=3285266.
62. Genc MR, Clancy TE, Ferzoco SJ, Norwitz E. Maternal congenital diaphragmatic hernia complicating pregnancy. Obstet Gynecol. 2003;102(5 Pt 2):1194–6.
63. Stephenson B, Stamatakis J. Late recurrence of a congenital diaphragmatic hernia. Case report. BJOG An Int J Obstet Gynaecol. 1991;98:110–1.
64. Craddock D, Hall J. Strangulated diaphragmatic hernia complicating pregnancy. Br J Surg. 1968;55:559–60.
65. Fardy H. Vomiting in late pregnancy due to diaphragmatic hernia. Case report. BJOG An Int J Obstet Gynaecol. 1984;91:390–2.
66. Hamaji M, Burt BM, Ali SO, Cohen DM. Spontaneous diaphragm rupture associated with vaginal delivery. Gen Thorac Cardiovasc Surg. 2013;61:473–5.
67. Suhardja TS, Vaska A, Foley D, Gribbin J. Adult Bochdalek hernia in a pregnant woman. ANZ J Surg. 2019;89:E162.

68. Myers BF, McCabe CJ. Traumatic diaphragmatic hernia: occult marker of serious injury. Ann Surg. 1993;218:783–90.
69. Aydin Y, Altuntas B, Ulas AB, et al. Morgagni hernia: transabdominal or transthoracic approach? Acta Chir Belg. 2014;114:131–5.
70. Hernández-Aragon M, Rodriguez-Lazaro L, Crespo-Esteras R, et al. MR-L. Bochdalek diaphragmatic hernia complicating pregnancy in the third trimester: case report. Obs Gynecol Cases Rev. 2015;2(5):057. https://clinmedjournals.org/articles/ogcr/clinmed-international-library-ogcr-2-057.pdf.
71. Julien F, Drolet S, Lévesque I, Bouchard A. The right lateral position for laparoscopic diaphragmatic hernia repair in pregnancy: technique and review of the literature. J Laparoendosc Adv Surg Tech A. 2011;21:67–70.
72. Brusciano L, Izzo G, Maffettone V, et al. Laparoscopic treatment of Bochdalek hernia without the use of a mesh. Surg Endosc. 2003;17:1497–8.
73. Wieman E, Pollock G, Moore BT, Serrone R. Symptomatic right-sided diaphragmatic hernia in the third trimester of pregnancy. JSLS. 2013;17:358–60.
74. Debergh I, Fierens K. Laparoscopic repair of a Bochdalek hernia with incarcerated bowel during pregnancy: report of a case. Surg Today. 2014;44:753–6.
75. Rolton DJ, Lovegrove RE, Dehn TC. Laparoscopic splenectomy and diaphragmatic rupture repair in a 27-week pregnant trauma patient. Surg Laparosc Endosc Percutan Tech. 2009;19(4):e159–60. http://www.ncbi.nlm.nih.gov/pubmed/19692872.
76. Palanivelu C, Rangarajan M, Maheshkumaar GS, Parthasarathi R. Laparoscopic mesh repair of a Bochdalek diaphragmatic hernia with acute gastric volvulus in a pregnant patient. Singap Med J. 2008;49:e26–8.
77. Šenkyrik M, Lata J, Husová L, Díte P, Husa P, Horálek F, et al. Unusual Bochdalek hernia in puerperium. Hepato-Gastroenterology. 2003;50(53):1449–51.
78. Watkin DS, Hughas S, Thompson MH. Herniation of colon through the right diaphragm complicating the puerperium. J Laparoendosc Surg. 1993;3:583–6.
79. Olaru AI, Uzochukwu I, Sheehan K, Greene R. Bochdalek diaphragmatic hernia rupture in pregnancy: a case report. Ann Clin Cas Rep. 2017;2:1275.
80. Harma MI, Harma M, Karadeniz G, et al. Idiopathic ileoileal invagination two days after cesarean section. J Obs Gynaecol Res. 2011;37:160–2.
81. Steinberg LS, Nisenbaum HL, Horii SS, et al. Post-cesarean section pain secondary to intus-suscepting colonic adenocarcinoma. Ultrasound Obs Gynecol. 1997;10:362–5.
82. Kocakoc E, Bozgeyik Z, Koc M, Balaban M. Idiopathic postpartum intussusception: a rare cause of acute abdominal pain. Med Princ Pr. 2010;19(2):163–5. http://www.ncbi.nlm.nih.gov/pubmed/20134182.
83. Bosman W-MPF, Bosman HT, Hedeman Joosten PP, Ritchie ED. Ileocaecal intussusception due to submucosal lipoma in a pregnant woman. BMJ Case Rep. 2014;2014:bcr2013203110.
84. Tutar O, Kocak B, Velidedeoglu M, et al. Small bowel intussusception in a pregnant woman with Peutz–Jeghers syndrome. Scott Med J. 2014;59:e9–13. https://www.ncbi.nlm.nih.gov/pubmed/?term=Small+bowel+intussusception+in+a+pregnant+woman+with+Peutz–Jeghers+Syndrome.
85. Cong Q, Li X, Ye X, et al. Small bowel volvulus in mid and late pregnancy: can early diagnosis be established to avoid catastrophic outcomes? Int. Int J Clin Exp Med. 2014;7:4538–43.
86. Dilbaz S, Gelisen O, Caliskan E, et al. Small bowel volvulus in pregnancy. Eur J Obs Gynecol Reprod Biol. 2003;111:204–6.
87. Gaikwad A, Ghongade D, Kittad P. Fatal midgut volvulus: a rare cause of gestational intestinal obstruction. Abdom Imaging. 2010;35:288–90.
88. De U, De KK. Sigmoid volvulus complicating pregnancy: case report. Indian J Med Sci. 2005;59:317–9.
89. James D. Intestinal obstruction during late pregnancy caused by volvulus of sigmoid colon. BMJ. 1950;2:24.
90. Bandler M, Friedman S, Roberts M. Recurrent volvulus of the sigmoid colon during pregnancy complicated by toxemia of pregnancy. Am J Gastroenterol. 1964;42:447–53.

91. Alshawi J. Recurrent sigmoid volvulus in pregnancy: report of a case and review of the literature. Dis Colon Rectum. 2005;48:1811–3.
92. Twité N, Jacquet C, Hollemaert S, et al. Intestinal obstruction in pregnancy. Rev Med Brux. 2006;27:104–9.
93. Allen JR, Helling TS, Langenfeld M. Intraabdominal surgery during pregnancy. Am J Surg. 1989;158(6):567–9.
94. Serafeimidis C, Waqainabete I, Creaton A, et al. Sigmoid volvulus in pregnancy: case report and review of literature. Clin Cas Rep. 2016;30:759–61. https://www.ncbi.nlm.nih.gov/pubmed/27525078.
95. Palmucci S, Lanza ML, Gulino F, Scilletta B, Ettorre GC. Diagnosis of a sigmoid volvulus in pregnancy: ultrasonography and magnetic resonance imaging findings. J Radiol Case Rep. 2014;8(2). http://www.radiologycases.com/index.php/radiologycases/article/view/1766.
96. Mogadam M, Korelitz BI, Ahmed SW, Dobbins WO, Baiocco PJ. The course of inflammatory bowel disease during pregnancy and postpartum. Am J Gastroenterol. 1981;75(4):265–9. http://europepmc.org/abstract/med/7258171.
97. Goettler CE, Stellato TA. Initial presentation of Crohn's disease in pregnancy. Dis Colon Rectum. 2003;46:406–10.
98. Killeen S, Gunn J, Hartley J. Surgical management of complicated and medically refractory inflammatory bowel disease during pregnancy. Color Dis. 2017;19:123–38.
99. Germain A, Chateau T, Beyer-Berjot L, Zerbib P, Lakkis Z, Amiot A, et al. Surgery for Crohn's disease during pregnancy: a nationwide survey. United Eur Gastroenterol J. 2020;8:736–40.
100. Boreham PF, Soltau DH. Pregnancy and Crohn's disease. BMJ. 1970;2:541.
101. Leung YPY, Kaplan GG, Coward S, Tanyingoh D, Kaplan BJ, Johnston DW, et al. Intrapartum corticosteroid use significantly increases the risk of gestational diabetes in women with inflammatory bowel disease. J Crohns Colitis. 2015;9:223–30.
102. Lavie I, Lavie M, Doyev R, Fouks Y, Azem F, Yogev Y. Pregnancy outcomes in women with inflammatory bowel disease who successfully conceived via assisted reproduction technique. Arch Gynecol Obs. 2020;302(3):611–8.
103. Nguyen GC, Boudreau H, Harris ML, Maxwell CVGB. Outcomes of obstetric hospitalizations among women with inflammatory bowel disease in the United States. Clin Gastroenterol Hepatol. 2009;7:329–34.
104. Moser MA, Okun NB, Mayes DC, Bailey RJ. Crohn's disease, pregnancy, and birth weight. Am J Gastroenterol. 2000;95(4):1021–6. http://www.nature.com/ajg/journal/v95/n4/pdf/ajg2000260a.pdf.
105. Triantafillidis G, Gikas A, et al. Pregnancy and inflammatory bowel disease in Greece: a prospective study of seven cases in a single hospital setting. Ann Gastroenterol. 2007;20:29–34.
106. Cornish J, Tan E, Teare J, et al. A meta-analysis on the influence of inflammatory bowel disease on pregnancy. Gut. 2007;56:830–7.
107. Fedorkow DM, Persaud D, Nimrod CA. Inflammatory bowel disease: a controlled study of late pregnancy outcome. Am J Obstet Gynecol. 1989;160:998–1001.
108. Morales M, Berney T, Jenny A, Morel P, Extermann P. Crohn's disease as a risk factor for the outcome of pregnancy. Hepato Gastroenterol. 2000;47(36):1595–8.
109. Fonager K, Sørensen HT, Olsen J, Dahlerup JF, Rasmussen SN. Pregnancy outcome for women with Crohn' s disease: a follow-up study based on linkage between national registries. Am J Gastroenterol. 1998;93(12):2426–30.
110. Hanan IM, Kirsner JB. Inflammatory bowel disease in the pregnant woman. Clin Perinatol. 1985;12(3):669–82. http://www.ncbi.nlm.nih.gov/entrez/query.fcgi?cmd=Retrieve&db=PubMed&dopt=Citation&list_uids=2865025.
111. Nielsen OH, Andreasson B, Bondesen S, Jarnum S. Pregnancy in ulcerative colitis. Scand J Gastroenterol. 1983;18(6):735–42. http://www.ncbi.nlm.nih.gov/pubmed/6669937.
112. Kornfeld D, Cnattingius S, Ekbom A. Pregnancy outcomes in women with inflammatory bowel disease—a population-based cohort study. Am J Obs Gynecol. 1997;177(4):942–6. http://www.ncbi.nlm.nih.gov/entrez/query.fcgi?cmd=Retrieve&db=PubMed&dopt=Citation&list_uids=9369849.

113. Nørgård B, Fonager K, Sørensen HT, Olsen J. Birth outcomes of women with ulcerative colitis: a nationwide danish cohort study. Am J Gastroenterol. 2000;95(11):3165–70.
114. Dominitz JA, Young JCC, Boyko EJ. Outcomes of infants born to mothers with inflammatory bowel disease: a population-based cohort study. Am J Gastroenterol. 2002;97(3):641–8.
115. Bush MC, Patel S, Lapinski RH, Stone JL. Perinatal outcomes in inflammatory bowel disease. J Matern Fetal Neonatal Med. 2004;15(4):237–41. http://www.ncbi.nlm.nih.gov/entrez/query.fcgi?cmd=Retrieve&db=PubMed&dopt=Citation&list_uids=15280131.
116. Auger N, Côté-Daigneault J, Bilodeau-Bertrand M, Arbour L. Inflammatory bowel disease and risk of birth defects in offspring. J Crohns Colitis. 2020;14(5):588–94.
117. Reddy SI, Wolf JL. Management issues in women with inflammatory bowel disease. J Am Osteopat Assoc. 2001;101:S17–23.
118. Miller J. Inflammatory bowel disease in pregnancy: a review. J R Soc Med. 1986;79:221–5.
119. Nielsen OH, Andreasson B, Bondesen S, Jacobsen O, Jarnum S. Pregnancy in Crohn's disease. Scand J Gastroenterol. 1984;19(6):724–32.
120. Schofield PF, Turnbull RB, Hawk WA. Crohn's disease and pregnancy. BMJ. 1970;2:364.
121. Hill J, Clark A, Scott NA. Surgical treatment of acute manifestations of Crohn's disease during pregnancy. J R Soc Med. 1997;90(2):64–6.
122. Blair JS, Allen N. Crohn's disease presenting acutely during pregnancy. J Obs Gynaecol Br Commonw. 1962;69:648–51.
123. Ochsner MG. Factors of failure for nonoperative management of blunt liver and splenic injuries. World J Surg. 2001;25(11):1393–6. http://www.ncbi.nlm.nih.gov/pubmed/11760740.
124. Latic F, Delibegovic S, Latic A, et al. Urgent laparoscopic splenectomy after traumatic splenic rupture in pregnancy. Acta Inf Med. 2009;17:231–2.
125. Antequera A, Babar Z, Balachandar C, Johal K, Sapundjieski M, Qandil N. Managing ruptured splenic ectopic pregnancy without splenectomy: case report and literature review. Reprod Sci. 2021;28(8):2323–30. https://pubmed.ncbi.nlm.nih.gov/33638134/.
126. Wu L, Jiang X, Ni J. Successful diagnosis and treatment of early splenic ectopic pregnancy: a case report. Med (United States). 2018;97(17):e0466. https://pubmed.ncbi.nlm.nih.gov/29703001/.
127. Biolchini F, Giunta A, Bigi L, Bertellini C, Pedrazzoli C. Emergency laparoscopic splenectomy for haemoperitoneum because of ruptured primary splenic pregnancy: a case report and review of literature. ANZ J Surg. 2010;80:55–7.
128. Yagil Y, Beck-Razi N, Amit A, et al. Splenic pregnancy: the role of abdominal imaging. J Ultrasound Med. 2007;26:1629–32.
129. Denehy T, McGrath EW, Breen JL. Splenic torsion and rupture in pregnancy. Obs Gynecol Surv. 1988;43:123–31.
130. Wang C, Tu X, Li S, et al. Spontaneous rupture of the spleen: a rare but serious case of acute abdominal pain in pregnancy. J Emerg Med. 2011;41:503–6.

Nonspecific Abdominal Pain

Gaetano Gallo ⓘ, Monica Ortenzi, Mario Guerrieri,
Francesco Virdis, Marta Goglia, and Salomone Di Saverio

1   Epidemiology

There is no consensus regarding the definition of acute nonspecific abdominal pain (NSAP). However, it can be considered as abdominal pain with no other obvious clinical presentations, with no strictly defined time duration, not accompanied by signs of peritonitis, hemodynamic instability, or other obvious clinical presentations requiring an emergency surgical operation, and which does not consist primarily of a urogenital complaint [1–3].

Although it remains a "diagnosis of exclusion" [4], it is considered responsible for a great number of emergency surgical admissions; specifically, 5–10% of all admissions to the emergency department (ED) are caused by acute abdominal pain. Interestingly, 40% or more of those patients will be discharged without a formal diagnosis, up to 35% will be admitted, and roughly 56% will be misdiagnosed

G. Gallo (✉)
Department of Medical and Surgical Sciences, University of Catanzaro, Catanzaro, Italy
e-mail: gallog@unicz.it

M. Ortenzi · M. Guerrieri
Department of General and Emergency Surgery, Polytechnic University of Marche,
Ancona, Italy

F. Virdis
Trauma and Acute Care Surgery Unit, Niguarda Ca Granda Hospital, Milan, Italy

M. Goglia
Department of General Surgery, "La Sapienza" University of Rome—Sant'Andrea University
Hospital, Rome, Italy

S. Di Saverio
Department of General Surgery, University of Insubria, University Hospital of Varese, ASST
Sette Laghi, Regione Lombardia, Italy

    271
F. Coccolini et al. (eds.), *Mini-invasive Approach in Acute Care Surgery*,
Hot Topics in Acute Care Surgery and Trauma,
https://doi.org/10.1007/978-3-031-39001-2_20

[5–9]. In a survey published by the World Organisation of Gastroenterology Research Committee (OMGE) which analyzed 10,320 patients with acute abdominal pain, 3507 of them (34%) were complaining of NSAP [10].

Many of these patients refer persistent symptoms and are difficult to be discharged; they often undergo multiple, expensive investigations and have repeated admissions to the ED [1].

Furthermore, the increased morbidity and associated healthcare costs resulting from delayed diagnosis or misdiagnosis deserve a renewed search for a more accurate approach to its evaluation. Although attempts have been made, no evidence-based clinical guideline nor diagnostic algorithms for the exclusion of NSAP requiring urgent intervention have been developed or validated to date [6, 9, 11, 12].

The underlying conditions of NSAP comprise a spectrum of undiagnosed conditions, both somatic and functional; [4] for example, in children, NSAP may predict organic and functional disease in the adulthood in about 10% of patients [13]. Previous studies indicated that NSAP may predict higher mortality respect to the general population and increased risk for various alimentary tract diseases during the 20-year follow-up [14]. Consequently, it can be argued that not all cases of NSAP are self-limited, short-lived, and harmless [15]. Among young women, for anatomic, physiologic, and pregnancy motivations, NSAP may be caused by a great variety of causes, including pelvic inflammatory disease (PID), appendicitis, ectopic pregnancy, torsion of the adnexa, etc. [14, 16] Moreover, 1–2% of those patients diagnosed with NSAP will receive a malignancy diagnosis within a year [17]. In general, NSAP can be classified as a symptomatology that requires urgent treatment or a nonurgent condition [18]; therefore, an early and accurate diagnosis plays a pivotal role for an accurate management of this condition, resulting in better outcomes and greater diagnostic and therapeutic solutions [18]. Its correct and standardized both diagnostic and therapeutic management still represent a challenge [6].

Nevertheless, the most important part of the evaluation remains a thorough history and a careful physical examination given the wide variety of disorders which may cause abdominal pain.

The physician is called to establish a differential diagnosis, plan appropriate imaging studies, and determine whether surgery is necessary.

The management of acute NSAP could be divided into three stages (Fig. 1): the first one includes patient's medical history, physical examination, baseline investigations, and formulation of differential diagnosis. The second stage involves the use of radiological techniques, when needed. The third stage should be represented by diagnostic laparoscopy [13, 14].

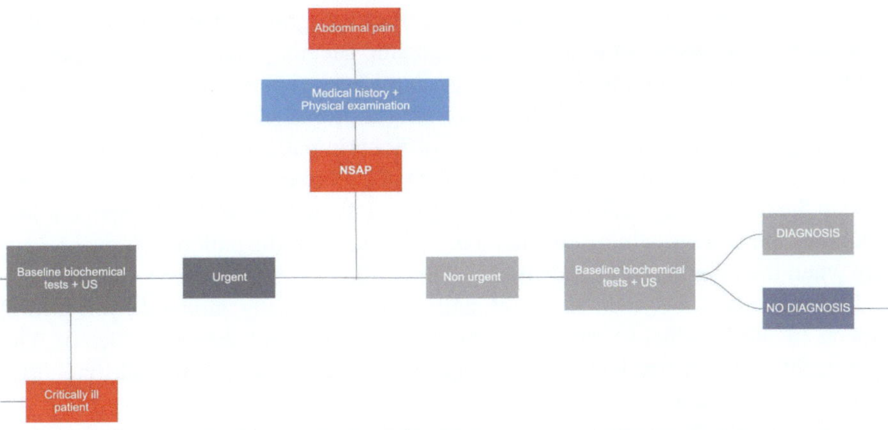

Fig. 1 Flowchart for nonspecific acute abdominal pain

2 First Stage: Baseline Investigations

A thorough physical examination is recommended as the first step in the diagnostic assessment of acute abdominal pain. Traditionally, based on medical history, physical examination, and laboratory parameters, a physician would decide whether additional investigations are necessary or not. However, it has been demonstrated that clinical evaluation may not be highly accurate and specific in the diagnosis of NSAP. Likewise, diagnostic adjuncts such as laboratory studies seem to not significantly increase the diagnostic accuracy. The literature demonstrates how the diagnosis based on medical history and physical examination is correct in no more than 43–59% of patients with abdominal pain [18–20]), while the rate of correct diagnosis with the adjunct of laboratory parameters ranges between 46 and 48% [18, 21, 22]). The diagnostic accuracy increased when urgent and nonurgent conditions were differentiated as primary outcome. A correct anamnesis, physical examination, and laboratory values showed high sensibility for urgent and nonurgent differentiation while low specificity for a specific diagnosis [21].

The diagnosis of acute NSAP has been highly discussed throughout the years, and many suggestions have been formulated. In 1990, Lavelle and Kanagaratnam introduced usefulness index test for the assessment of usefulness of clinical observations [23, 24]. DeDombal et al. have suggested that the proportion of correct diagnoses can be greatly increased by the use of structured questionnaires and diagnostic programs on computer [25]. However, although computer-aided diagnosis can improve diagnostic rates by at least 20%, these programs are unpopular. In addition, no scoring systems that increase diagnostic accuracy were found for patients with acute abdominal pain. Several factors have been reported to possibly contribute to a low accuracy. First of all, performing a proper physical examination and collecting sufficient information could be difficult in patients belonging to extreme age groups (pediatric and elderly population). Furthermore, an interobserver difference in the diagnostic accuracy has been reported. In daily practice, the resident first examines the patient, while staff members will examine the patient afterward, usually when the imaging has been already done [18].

The agreement between residents and staff is generally moderate for several aspects of medical history and physical examination ($\kappa = 0.29$–0.74) [9, 10]. The agreement between residents and emergency physicians for additional diagnostic imaging is sufficient ($\kappa = 0.6$) [26].

Generally, residents and tutors are moderately in agreement regarding the anamnestic assessment of the patients as well as regarding the physical examination, while the agreement on additional diagnostic imaging is considered to be sufficient.

Research of differences in diagnostic accuracy between residents and specialist physicians is hampered by a methodological difficulty. The presentation can change over time, and so it can differ between the time of examination. This variability could influence the reliability of the comparison. For these reasons, some authors have suggested the opportunity to have preliminary examinations carried out by two different observers, ideally under the same circumstances. Outpatient reevaluation of those ones suspected of nonurgent conditions led to a change in diagnosis in 35% of patients after clinical reevaluation, a change in management in 19% of cases, and a change from conservative to surgical treatment in 4.5% of patients [18, 27]. Moreover, outpatient reevaluation of patients suspected of nonurgent conditions after clinical evaluation and the performance of ultrasound led to a change in diagnosis in 18% of cases, change in management in 13%, and a change from conservative to surgical treatment in 3% of patients [18, 27].

3 Second Stage: Imaging Studies

Since the first step of examination is often insufficient to reach a diagnosis, additional imaging modalities could be used to increase diagnostic certainty. Several imaging modalities such as conventional (plain) radiography, ultrasound, CT scan, and magnetic resonance imaging (MRI) have been increasingly used over the years [4, 18]. Plain abdominal radiographs have played fundamental, even though controversial, roles in the assessment of NSAP. Some institutions still propose the use of a combination of plain chest radiography and the upright and supine plain abdominal radiographs as known as the acute abdominal series (AAS), as the first radiological screening in all patients with abdominal pain [4, 18]. The purpose of GAPEDES phase 1 study was to determine whether it was possible to derive a sensitive, easy to run, and reproducible clinical guideline for the evaluation of

NSAP using history, physical examination, commonly available laboratory studies, AAS, and NHCT as potential inputs [6]. However, this guideline demonstrated low sensitivity and accuracy, not higher than 56% [18, 21, 28]. Indeed, it could be misleading in the workup of acute abdominal pain [29, 30]. Concerning the ultrasound (US) examination, the rate of correct diagnosis ranges from 53 to 83% of cases, according to the literature [21, 31–33]. Not surprisingly, when compared with computed tomography, the sensitivity and specificity of ultrasound are definitely lower. However, ultrasound is widely available, cheap, and easy to run; also, during on-call hours, it carries no risk of ionizing radiation exposure or contrast-induced nephropathy, despite having a major drawback in the possibility of interobserver variability.

Previous studies have demonstrated how an early use of CT in the diagnostic workup of acute abdominal pain has led to a correct diagnosis in 96.8% of cases [4, 34], when combined with the previous investigations. Ideally, except for few patients, such as children or pregnant women, in which US or MRI should be considered the method of choice, CT should be considered the gold standard to guide treatment and avoid harmful delays [21, 30].

It is important to remember that computed tomography has major downsides such as the risk of contrast-induced nephropathy and exposure to ionizing radiation. The steering group advises the use of intravenous contrast in preference to other methods of contrast administration. Oral contrast administration delays computed tomography for hours, and other methods of contrast administration provide little additional information. However, the use of intravenous contrast media could lead to contrast-induced nephropathy (CIN) even if this evidence is based on studies with intra-arterial contrast administration. More recent studies have demonstrated that the risk of CIN is minimal when the eGFR (glomerular filtration rate) is above 45 mL/min/1.73 m^2 [35–37]. Preventive measures such as prehydration can decrease the risk of CIN. In daily practice, this might not be possible for every patient. In urgent situations, correctly diagnosing the underlying pathology (and subsequently earlier start of treatment) is more important than the possible risk of CIN. Therefore, computed tomography can be performed without preventive measures and without prior ultrasound in critically ill patients [18].

Due to the downsides of CT, an ultrasound is still preferred as the first imaging modality. Only in critically ill patients, a computed tomography should be performed without a prior ultrasound; in other cases, a CT scan is recommended only when the ultrasound is negative or inconclusive [18, 21].

No trials have been performed analyzing the diagnostic value of MRI in patients with acute abdominal pain. Nowadays, some studies have demonstrated that MRI is sufficiently accurate to diagnose appendicitis and diverticulitis [18, 38, 39]. The advantage of MRI over computed tomography is that no administration of contrast media is necessary and that there is no ionizing radiation exposure. The downside is that MRI scanners are not yet widely available and that the assessment of MRI images needs specific training [40]. For pregnant women with a suspicion of an urgent cause, an MRI should be contemplated, because of the serious consequences of a missed diagnosis [18, 38, 39].

It has to be noted that, although the advanced utilization of modern imaging did not decrease the rate of NSAP, the rate of emergency surgery in NSAP was greatly decreased from 4% to 0.5% [15].

4 Wait and See Policy

Hospitalization followed by active clinical observation, traditionally defined as "wait and see," has been the most widely used method in the clinical management of patients with nontypical clinical signs. The predictive value of clinical diagnosis reached with this method, which varies with the underlying cause, has been estimated between 68 and 92% [14].

Previous studies demonstrated how approximately half of the patients admitted for observation is likely to undergo a surgical procedure during the first admission.

However, on the one hand, this method entails risks for the patients because of possible complications such as peritonitis, hemorrhage, or infertility; on the other hand, laparotomy might be unnecessarily performed [16, 41].

A recent RCT (randomized controlled trial) demonstrated how patients who underwent delayed laparoscopy had a mean operative time equal to the mean operative time in early laparoscopy group, and there was no higher morbidity nor mortality. Therefore, the authors concluded that delaying surgery in NSAP patients does not increase operative risks or jeopardize clinical results.

Furthermore, this kind of approach could help avoiding unnecessary surgical procedures under general anesthesia [14, 45], and although patients treated by early laparoscopy had a shorter hospital stay (3.7 vs. 4.7 days) and more accurate diagnosis (83% vs. 45%), the greater accuracy did not show clear clinical benefits (recurrent pain at 12 months: 16% vs. 25%, not significant) [42].

In other words, delaying the decision to submit patients with persistent symptoms and without a definite diagnosis to a laparoscopy of 24–72 h from admissions could reduce the number of unnecessary surgical operations.

5 Third Stage: Diagnostic Laparoscopy

So far, if the diagnosis remains uncertain or CT is not accessible, the next step in the management of NSAP should be represented by diagnostic laparoscopy (DL).

The available studies on the value of diagnostic laparoscopy in case of NSAP have enrolled patient samples not representative for the current clinical practice. These studies have not included preoperative imaging in the diagnostic assessment.

Few RCTs compared the role of early laparoscopy with the traditional "wait and see" approach in the management of NSAP [13, 14, 43].

Two of these studies presented at least one major limitation, such as the limited number of patients, [13] insufficient preoperative evaluation, [43] and enrolling both males and females. Furthermore, in these studies, the diagnostic laparoscopy itself is used as reference diagnosis.

Another RCT focused on acute right iliac fossa pain in young women and concluded that, on the one hand, early laparoscopy results in a higher number of definite diagnosis and in a shorter hospital stay when compared with active observation. On the other hand, morbidity, mortality, and costs are similar [14]. In addition, in patients submitted to laparoscopy, the policy to remove the appendix, if no other clear causes of pain were found, was adopted in accordance with the data showing that the external inspection of the appendix at laparoscopy is an unreliable finding for the presence of appendicitis [14, 44]. Greason et al. [44] showed that routine appendectomy during diagnostic laparoscopy does not increase morbidity and does not prolong hospital stay. However, the study clearly showed that removing a "normal looking" appendix has a limited clinical role when the follow-up is adequate.

The actual literature has demonstrated that, in selected patient populations where no prior diagnostic imaging has been performed, a diagnostic laparoscopy can accurately diagnose the cause of the abdominal pain in 80–94% of patients [14, 18, 41, 43]. Postoperative complications have been reported in 3.5–25% of patients after diagnostic laparoscopy [18, 41, 42, 44, 45].

Contraindications for DL do not differ from the ones for exploratory laparotomy, except for patients unable to tolerate pneumoperitoneum and those with a tense and distended abdomen (i.e., clinically suspected abdominal compartment syndrome) [14, 46].

In the past few years, imaging modalities have significantly improved in diagnostic accuracy. Treatment of the causes of acute abdominal pain has been modified thought the years and it does not always involve a surgical approach. Compared with imaging modalities, diagnostic laparoscopy has a higher risk of complications.

Reported complications range from severe complications such as septic shock and enterocutaneous fistula to wound infections.

Therefore, based on the current literature, no conclusions can be drawn on the added value of a laparoscopy in the diagnostic pathway of patients with acute abdominal pain. However, laparoscopy should not be used in the diagnostic pathway of patients when no sufficient prior imaging has been performed. Only in patients with a high suspicion of an underlying life-threatening cause, with inconclusive imaging, a DL could be contemplated.

6   Conclusions

Although attempts have been made toward developing consensus guidelines and diagnostic algorithms, no prospective evidence-based clinical guidelines for the exclusion of NSAP have been developed or validated to date [4, 14, 18]. The necessity to achieve a correct diagnosis and a systematic approach to NSAP should be useful in order to reduce the admission rate for NSAP because of the costs and morbidity associated with this condition in terms of excessive hospital stay, multiple investigations, and unnecessary surgical explorations [4, 14, 18]. In other words, what Poulin et al. wrote still remains actual: "management of acute NSAP needs to be periodically adjusted to get the best outcomes at the lowest costs and with the least invasive and most appropriate diagnostic tools" [46].

Conflict of Interest All authors declare no personal conflict of interest.

Ethical Approval Not required.

References

1. Sheridan WG, White AT, Havard T, Crosby DL. Non-specific abdominal pain: the resource implications. Ann R Coll Surg Engl. 1992;74(3):181–5.
2. Lewis FR, Holcroft JW, Boey J, Dunphy JE. Appendicitis: a critical review of diagnosis and treatment in 1000 cases. Arch Surg. 1975;110:677–84.
3. Alvarado A. A practical score for the early diagnosis of acute appendicitis. Ann Emerg Med. 1986;15:557–64.
4. Carlucci M, et al. Nonspecific abdominal pain. In: Emergency laparoscopy. Cham: Springer; 2016. p. 73–8.
5. Cervellin G, Mora R, Ticinesi A, Meschi T, Comelli I, Catena F, Lippi G. Epidemiology and outcomes of acute abdominal pain in a large urban emergency department: retrospective analysis of 5,340 cases. Ann Transl Med. 2016;4(19):362. https://doi.org/10.21037/atm.2016.09.10.
6. Gerhardt RT, Nelson BK, Keenan S, Kernan L, MacKersie A, Lane MS. Derivation of a clinical guideline for the assessment of nonspecific abdominal pain: the guideline for abdominal pain in the ED setting (GAPEDS) phase 1 study. Am J Emerg Med. 2005;23(6):709–17. https://doi.org/10.1016/j.ajem.2005.01.010.
7. Irvin TT. Abdominal pain: a surgical audit of 1190 emergency admissions. Br J Surg. 1989;76(11):1121–5.
8. Brewer RJ, Golden GT, Hitch DC, et al. Abdominal pain—an analysis of 1000 consecutive cases in a university hospital emergency room. Am J Surg. 1976;131:219–23.
9. Adams ID, Chan M, Clifford PC, et al. Computer aided diagnosis of acute abdominal pain: a multicentre study. BMJ. 1986;293:800–4.
10. De Dombal FT. The OMGE acute abdominal pain survey. Progress report, 1986. Scand J Gastroenterol. 1988;23:35–42.
11. American College of Emergency Physicians. Clinical policy for the initial approach to patients presenting with a chief complaint of nontraumatic acute abdominal pain. Ann Emerg Med. 1994;23(4):906–22.
12. American College of Emergency Physicians. Clinical policy: critical issues for the initial evaluation and management of patients presenting with a chief complaint of nontraumatic acute abdominal pain. Ann Emerg Med. 2000;36:406–15.
13. Decadt B, Sussman L, Lewis MP, et al. Randomized clinical trial of early laparoscopy in the management of acute non-specific abdominal pain. Br J Surg. 1999;86:1383–6.
14. Morino M, Pellegrino L, Castagna E, Farinella E, Mao P. Acute nonspecific abdominal pain: a randomized, controlled trial comparing early laparoscopy versus clinical observation. Ann Surg. 2006;244(6):881–6; discussion 886–8. https://doi.org/10.1097/01.sla.0000246886.80424.ad.
15. Fagerström A, Paajanen P, Saarelainen H, Ahonen-Siirtola M, Ukkonen M, Miettinen P, Paajanen H. Non-specific abdominal pain remains as the most common reason for acute abdomen: 26-year retrospective audit in one emergency unit. Scand J Gastroenterol. 2017;52(10):1072–7. https://doi.org/10.1080/00365521.2017.1342140. Epub 2017 Jun 28.
16. Paterson-Brown S. Emergency laparoscopy surgery. Br J Surg. 1993;80(279–283):3.

17. Ferlander P, Elfström C, Göransson K, von Rosen A, Djärv T. Nonspecific abdominal pain in the Emergency Department: malignancy incidence in a nationwide Swedish cohort study. Eur J Emerg Med. 2018;25(2):105–9. https://doi.org/10.1097/MEJ.0000000000000409.
18. Gans SL, Pols MA, Stoker J, Boermeester MA, Expert Steering Group. Guideline for the diagnostic pathway in patients with acute abdominal pain. Dig Surg. 2015;32(1):23–31. https://doi.org/10.1159/000371583. Epub 2015 Jan 28.
19. Kraemer M, Yang Q, Ohmann C. Acute Abdominal Pain Study Group: classification of subpopulations with a minor and a major diagnostic problem in acute abdominal pain. Theor Surg. 1993;8:6–14.
20. Hancock DM, Heptinstall M, Old JM, Lobo FX. Computer aided diagnosis of acute abdominal pain. The practical impact of a 'theoretical exercise'. Theor Surg. 1987;2:99–105.
21. Lameris W, van Randen A, van Es HW, van Heesewijk JP, van Ramshorst B, Bouma WH, et al. Imaging strategies for detection of urgent conditions in patients with acute abdominal pain: diagnostic accuracy study. BMJ. 2009;338:b2431.
22. Laurell H, Hansson LE, Gunnarsson U. Diagnostic pitfalls and accuracy of diagnosis in acute abdominal pain. Scand J Gastroenterol. 2006;41:1126–31.
23. Eskelinen M, Lipponen P. Usefulness index in nonspecific abdominal pain—an aid in the diagnosis? Scand J Gastroenterol. 2012;47(12):1475–9. https://doi.org/10.3109/00365521.2012.733951. Epub 2012 Oct 24.
24. Lavelle SM, Kanagaratnam B. The information value of clinical data. Int J Biomed Comput. 1990;26:203–9.
25. de Dombal FT, Leaper DJ, Staniland JR, McCann AP, Horrocks JC. Computer-aided diagnosis of acute abdominal pain. Br Med J. 1972;2(5804):9–13. https://doi.org/10.1136/bmj.2.5804.9.
26. Pines J, Uscher Pines L, Hall A, Hunter J, Srinivasan R, Ghaemmaghami C. The interrater variation of ED abdominal examination findings in patients with acute abdominal pain. Am J Emerg Med. 2005;23:483–7.
27. Toorenvliet BR, Bakker RF, Flu HC, Merkus JW, Hamming JF, Breslau PJ. Standard outpatient re-evaluation for patients not admitted to the hospital after emergency department evaluation for acute abdominal pain. World J Surg. 2010;34:480–6.
28. MacKersie AB, Lane MJ, Gerhardt RT, Claypool HA, Keenan S, Katz DS, et al. Nontraumatic acute abdominal pain: unenhanced helical CT compared with three-view acute abdominal series. Radiology. 2005;237:114–22.
29. Heesewijk JP, van Ramshorst B, Bouma WH, et al. Imaging strategies for detection of urgent conditions in patients with acute abdominal pain: diagnostic accuracy study. BMJ. 2009;339:b2431.
30. van Randen A, Lamris W, Luitse JS, Gorzeman M, Hesselink EJ, Dolmans DE, et al. The role of plain radiographs in patients with acute abdominal pain at the ED. Am J Emerg Med. 2011;29:582–589.e2.
31. Lindelius A, Trngren S, Sondn A, Pettersson H, Adami J. Impact of surgeon-performed ultrasound on diagnosis of abdominal pain. Emerg Med J. 2008;25:486–91.
32. Allemann F, Cassina P, Rthlin M, Largiadr F. Ultrasound scans done by surgeons for patients with acute abdominal pain: a prospective study. Eur J Surg. 1999;165:966–70.
33. Nural MS, Ceyhan M, Baydin A, Genc S, Bayrak IK, Elmali M. The role of ultrasonography in the diagnosis and management of non-traumatic acute abdominal pain. Intern Emerg Med. 2008;3:349–54.
34. Wilson DH, Wilson PD, Walmsley RG, et al. Diagnosis of acute abdominal pain in the accident and emergency department. Br J Surg. 1977;64:250–4.
35. Katzberg RW, Newhouse JH. Intravenous contrast medium-induced nephrotoxicity: is the medical risk really as great as we have come to believe? Radiology. 2010;256:21–8.
36. Rudnick M, Feldman H. Contrast-induced nephropathy: what are the true clinical consequences? Clin J Am Soc Nephrol. 2008;3:263–72.
37. Rao QA, Newhouse JH. Risk of nephropathy after intravenous administration of contrast material: a critical literature analysis. Radiology. 2006;239:392–7.

38. Heverhagen JT, Zielke A, Ishaque N, Bohrer T, El-Sheik M, Klose KJ. Acute colonic diverticulitis: visualization in magnetic resonance imaging. Magn Reson Imaging. 2001;19:1275–7.
39. Leeuwenburgh MM, Wiarda BM, Wiezer MJ, Vrouenraets BC, Gratama JW, Spilt A, et al. Comparison of imaging strategies with conditional contrast-enhanced CT and unenhanced MR imaging in patients suspected of having appendicitis: a multicenter diagnostic performance study. Radiology. 2013;268:135–43.
40. Leeuwenburgh MM, Wiarda BM, Bipat S. Acute appendicitis on abdominal MR images: training readers to improve diagnostic accuracy. Radiology. 2012;264:455–63.
41. Gaita'n H, Angel E, Sa'nchez J, et al. Laparoscopic diagnosis of acute lower abdominal pain in women of reproductive age. Int J Gynecol Obstet. 2002;76:149–58.
42. Champault G, Rizk N, Lauroy J, et al. Right iliac fosse in women: conventional diagnostic approach versus primary laparoscopy. A controlled study (65 cases). Ann Chir. 1993;47:316–9.
43. Grunewald B, Keating J. Should the 'normal' appendix be removed at operation for appendicitis? J R Coll Surg Edinb. 1993;38:158–60.
44. Greason KL, Rappold JF, Liberman MA. Incidental laparoscopic appendectomy for acute right lower quadrant abdominal pain. Surg Endosc. 1998;12:223–5.
45. Poulin EC, Schlachta CM, Mamazza J. Early laparoscopy to help diagnose acute non-specific abdominal pain. Lancet. 2000;355:861–3.
46. Olsen JB, Myre'n CJ, Haahr PE. Randomized study of the value of laparoscopy before appendectomy. Br J Surg. 1993;80:922–3.

Management of Bariatric Surgery Early and Delayed Complications

Uri Kaplan

1   Introduction

According to the World Health Organization (WHO), obesity rates have almost tripled in the last four decades [1]. It carries a significant public health concern and is associated with increased risk to develop chronic diseases such hypertension, diabetes mellitus, hyperlipidemia, and obstructive sleep apnea. Obesity negatively influences patient's morbidity and mortality.

Bariatric surgical procedures have been shown to be the best treatment option for achieving sustained weight loss and remission of obesity-related comorbidities [2, 3]. Nowadays, most bariatric cases are performed in centers of excellence by trained bariatric surgeons as part of multidisciplinary teams. These factors improve significantly the outcome of bariatric surgery.

The rapid development of laparoscopic instrumentation in the early 1990s had led to surge in bariatric procedures. Data comparing laparoscopic to open gastric bypass found that laparoscopic approach was associated with less complications, shorter hospital stay, and equivalent loss of excess weight [4]. In the last 20 years, with further advancement of laparoscopic bariatric surgery, this approach has become the standard of care. Nowadays, postoperative admissions are short, and some bariatric procedures are performed in outpatient clinics.

The aim of this chapter is to review both early and late bariatric procedure complications. We'll provide diagnostic tools and treatment option for patients who present to the emergency department.

U. Kaplan (✉)
General Surgery B, Emek Medical Center, Afula, Israel

Rappaport Faculty of Medicine, Technion—Israel Institute of Technology, Haifa, Israel

© The Author(s), under exclusive license to Springer Nature Switzerland AG 2023   281
F. Coccolini et al. (eds.), *Mini-invasive Approach in Acute Care Surgery*,
Hot Topics in Acute Care Surgery and Trauma,
https://doi.org/10.1007/978-3-031-39001-2_21

1.1   General

1.2   Epidemiology

Obesity has become a global epidemic and currently is one of the major public health challenges. According to the WHO, in 2016, 39% of adults (more than 1.9 billion) in the world were overweight (defined as body mass index (BMI) $\geq$25 kg/m^2) and 13% (over 650 million) were obese (defined as BMI $\geq$30 kg/m^2) [1]. In 2014, the global prevalence of morbid obesity (BMI $\geq$40 or BMI $\geq$35 with at least one obesity-related comorbidity) was 0.64% in men and 1.6% in women [5]. There are disparities in the prevalence of obesity across countries. This trend continues within the country among sex, age, ethnic group, and socioeconomic status [6].

Commonly performed bariatric procedures have a morbidity rate between 5 and 10%. In 5% of them, the complications will happen at home [7]. With that being said, the rate of emergency department (ED) visits of bariatric patients is much higher. The rate of ED visits, within 30 days of surgery, is around 11% of patients. The readmission rate is between 4.4 and 5.5%. Around 50% of those visits and readmissions occur in hospitals other than the one where the bariatric procedure was performed [8, 9].

1.3   Types of Bariatric Surgery

Knowledge regarding the gastrointestinal tract anatomical changes post-bariatric surgery is a key factor in the management of patients with post-surgical complications.

Historically, bariatric procedures were classified as either restrictive, reducing the volume of food patients can digest; malabsorptive, reducing the absorption of food at the mucosal level; or both. However, it is reasonable to associate the beneficial influence of surgery on the body adipose system as the key factor for bariatric surgery success [10]. The influence of bariatric surgery on the adipose system is beyond the scope of this chapter.

Clinical practice guidelines for bariatric surgery are well established [11, 12]. The fifth International Federation for the Surgery of Obesity and Metabolic Disorders (IFSO) global registry report contains data from over 60 countries on over 833,000 operations [13]. According to it, in 2019, the four most common operations worldwide were sleeve gastrectomy (SG) (58.6%), Roux-en-Y gastric bypass (RYGB) (31.2%), omega anastomosis gastric bypass/mini gastric bypass (OAGB/MGB) (4.1%), and adjustable gastric band (AGB) (3.7%). Over the last decade, there is a trend toward reduction in gastric banding and RYGB, while there is a rise in SG and OAGB/MGB procedures. Nowadays, almost all bariatric procedures are performed laparoscopically (99.1%) [13]. Currently, there is no evidence regarding which operation suits each patient, and that is the main reason for many operative options.

1.3.1   Sleeve Gastrectomy (SG)

The operation was developed as a first stage for duodenal switch operation however, due to comparable outcomes, became a stand-alone procedure. Most of the stomach (approximately 70–80%) is excised. The procedure starts with denuding the greater curvature from its blood supply starting 4–6 cm proximal to the pylorus up to the angle of His. A bougie, between 34 and 42 French, is inserted along the lesser curvature, and using a linear stapler, the fundus body and antrum of the stomach are excised creating a tubular pouch. The excised part of the stomach is removed (Fig. 1.I). The procedure is safe (mortality rate of 0.1–0.2%) with low complication rate [14, 15].

1.3.2 Roux-En-Y Gastric Bypass (RYGB)

The operation is considered the gold standard of bariatric surgery. The procedure involves the creation of a small proximal gastric pouch of approximately 30 mL. The pouch is separated from the rest of the stomach which is left in situ. The small bowel is divided 50–150 cm distal to the duodenojejunal (DJ) flexure. The distal limb of small bowel is anastomosed to the gastric pouch in an antecolic or retrocolic fashion. This limb is called the Roux limb. The proximal part, termed biliopancreatic limb (BP limb), is anastomosed 50–150 cm distal to the gastrojejunostomy anastomosis (Fig. 1.II). The proximal anastomosis is termed gastrojejunostomy

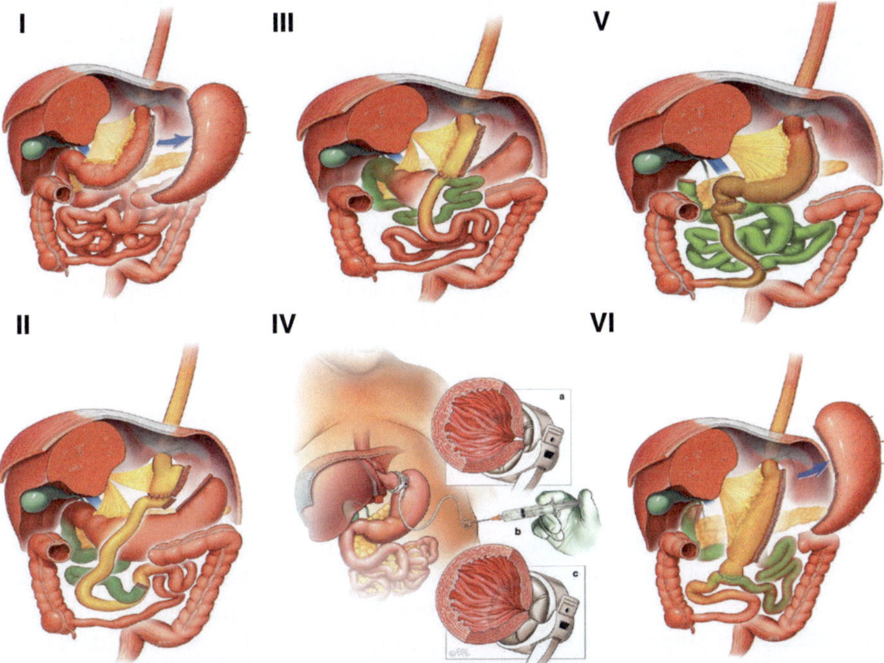

Fig. 1 Common bariatric surgeries: I, sleeve gastrectomy; II, Roux-en-Y gastric bypass; III, omega anastomosis gastric bypass/mini gastric bypass; IV, adjustable gastric banding (a-deflated band, b-subcutaneous port, c-inflated band); V, duodenal switch; VI, single anastomosis duodeno-ileal anastomosis with sleeve gastrectomy (SADI-S). Reprinted from Ramos AC, Carraso HJ, Bastos EL. (2021). Bariatric Procedures: Anatomical and Physiological Changes. Bhaskar AG, Kantharia N, Baig S, Priya P, Lakdawala M, Sancheti MS (Eds). Management of Nutritional and Metabolic Complications of Bariatric Surgery. (pp. 41–50). Springer Nature

(GJ) and the distal anastomosis is called jejuno-jejunostomy (JJ). Any mesenteric defects are closed. The procedure is safe with slightly higher morbidity and mortality compared to SG with no statistical significance [14, 15].

1.3.3 Omega Anastomosis Gastric Bypass/Mini Gastric Bypass (OAGB/MGB)

OAGB/MGB is a recent modification of the RYGB. The procedure is easier to perform. It begins with the creation of a long and narrow proximal gastric pouch which ends at the area of the gastric incisura. The rest of the stomach is left in situ. The small bowel, approximately 200 cm from the DJ flexure, is anastomosed in an antecolic loop fashion to the gastric pouch (Fig. 1.III). The procedure is safe with comparable results to the RYGB [16].

1.3.4 Adjustable Gastric Banding (AGB)

The band is an inflatable silicone ring connected by the tube to a subcutaneous injection port. The band is located around the angle of His creating a small gastric pouch of around 30 mL. The band lies in the 2-to-8 o'clock position and usually secured with gastro-gastric sutures overlying the fundus to the proximal pouch. Insertion or aspiration of fluid from the band, via the subcutaneous port, adjusts the degree of constriction (Fig. 1.IV). The procedure is safe with low complication rate [17].

1.3.5 Other Bariatric Surgeries

Duodenal switch (DS) involves the creation of gastric sleeve followed by division of the duodenum in his first part. The ileum is divided 250 cm proximal to the ileocolic valve and is anastomosed to the duodenum in a Roux-en-Y fashion (Fig. 1.V). Single anastomosis duodeno-ileostomy (SADI) is similar to DS in terms of the gastric sleeve and duodenum division. However, the ileum is anastomosed to the duodenum in a loop fashion 250–300 cm from the ileocolic valve (Fig. 1.VI). Both procedures are mainly malabsorptive with acceptable safety [18].

2 Classification of Bariatric Surgery Complications

Complication post-bariatric surgery can be classified according to the type of surgery, initial presentation, or time from surgery. Almost all bariatric surgeries are performed in minimally invasive technique which enables short hospital stay post-surgery. For that reason, most patients will be evaluated by general surgeons and not bariatric surgeons. We will discuss early complication, which occurs up to 30 days from surgery, and late complication, which occurs more than 30 days from surgery, separately. In each part, we'll discuss the complication according to the initial presentation. In general, the three main complaints to the emergency department will be bleeding, obstruction, and sepsis. The classification is summarized in Table 1.

Table 1 Complication of common bariatric surgeries

Early (less than 30 days' postop)			
	SG	RYGB/OAGB/MGB	AGB
General	Cardiopulmonary complications (including PE, MI)		
Bleeding	Staple line hemorrhage (intraluminal or extraluminal)	Staple line hemorrhage (intraluminal or extraluminal)	Hemorrhage (intraperitoneal)
Obstruction	Sleeve stricture	Anastomosis stenosis (GJ, JJ)	
	Port site hernia		
Sepsis	Staple line leak	Staple line leak	Esophageal/gastric perforation
		Anastomosis leak	
Late (more than 30 days' postop)			
General	Nutritional deficiencies/cholelithiasis		
Bleeding	Esophagitis	Bleeding marginal ulcer	Esophagitis
Obstruction	Sleeve twist	Internal hernia Small bowel adhesion	Band overtight Band erosion Band slippage
	Port site hernia/small bowel adhesion		
Sepsis	Staple line leak	Perforated marginal ulcers	Port/band infection

Postop postoperative; *SG* sleeve gastrectomy; *RYGB* Roux-en-Y gastric bypass; *OAGB* omega anastomosis gastric bypass; *MGB* mini gastric bypass; *AGB* adjustable gastric banding; *PE* pulmonary embolism; *MI* myocardial infarct; *GJ* gastrojejunostomy; *JJ* jejuno-jejunostomy

2.1 Early Complications

Early complications can be classified to nonsurgical, mainly related to general anesthesia and immobilization, and surgical, specific to the procedure itself.

2.1.1 Nonsurgical Complication

The nonsurgical complications are similar to other operative procedures and include cardiorespiratory complication and thromboembolic events.

Cardiorespiratory complications are usually present with chest pain or discomfort, shortness of breath, and tachycardia. Analysis of death within 30 days of surgery found that cardiac causes account for 28% of death and pulmonary embolism for 17% [19]. Bariatric population are predisposed to thromboembolic events due to numerous factors, including obesity itself, immobility, hypoventilation syndrome, and venous stasis disease. The rate of deep vein thrombosis (DVT) or pulmonary embolism (PE), up to 30 days post-bariatric surgery, is 2.2%, with a death rate of 0.03% [20]. Patient with chest pain and shortness of breath should have immediate 12-lead ECG, measurement of myocardial enzymes, and chest X-ray. While massive PE is usually fatal, a low threshold for CT angiogram can contribute to rapid diagnosis.

2.1.2 Surgical Complication

Bleeding
Although massive bleeding post-bariatric surgery is usually diagnosed during the perioperative admission, patient can present with hemorrhagic shock and even exsanguination. The main reasons for bleeding are staple lines, mesenteric or omental vessels, and iatrogenic injuries. In early postoperative period, port site bleeding should be in the differential diagnosis. The incidence of postoperative bleeding ranges from 0.5 to 4% [21]. The rate of reoperation due to bleeding ranges from 0.8 to 2.5% of all postoperative bleeding post-bariatric surgery [22]. Bleeding can be intraperitoneal or intraluminal. The clinical symptoms are tachycardia, oliguria, and decrease in hemoglobin (Hb) level. Gastrointestinal (GI) bleeding can also present with vomiting of blood, hematochezia, or melena. Intraperitoneal bleeding presents as abdominal discomfort or abdominal pain and even as peritonitis.

Staple line is the most common cause for bleeding in patients post-SG. Erosion at the staple line can cause intraperitoneal or intraluminal bleeding. Bleeding will occur in 0–20% of cases; however, only 1.4% will require reoperation due to major bleeding [23]. Early bleeding post-RYGB or OAGB/MGB results mainly due to staple line. The rate of bleeding post-RYGB is 1–4%. Common sites for bleeding post-RYGB are gastric remnant staple line (40%) followed by GJ (30%) and JJ (30%). Major bleeding in OAGB/MGB occurs in 0.2–28.6% of cases with 0.3–0.58% of these cases necessitate intervention including reoperation [23].

Obstruction
The prevalence of early post-bariatric surgery obstruction is low. The most common reason is stricture. The main reason for obstruction post-SG is stricture, usually at the incisura angularis (Fig. 2). The common causes for obstruction in the early phase are food intolerance and tissue edema. In RYGB or OAGB/MGB, the main reason is stricture at the anastomosis sites. Strictures in the GJ anastomosis or JJ anastomosis, in case of RYGB, are the main cause for early obstruction. The causes for GJ or JJ stricture are tension and/or ischemia at the anastomosis. Blood clot at the JJ can obstruct the anastomosis. Unlike the GJ anastomosis, which can present more slowly (up to weeks), JJ anastomosis stenosis has more acute presentation and more difficult to diagnose, due to altered anatomy. They present with epigastric pain or discomfort due to remnant distension and even as peritonitis due to gastric remnant perforation [23]. The rate of GJ stricture in OAGB/MGB is rare and was reported around 0.2% in revision cases [24]. The main causes are uneven traction during pouch creation and narrow anastomosis [23]. AGB is designed to partially cause obstruction in the cardia of the stomach. As such, patient can present with symptoms that resemble obstruction. With that being said, the rate of early obstruction is very low.

Systemic Inflammatory Response Syndrome (SIRS)/Sepsis
Gastrointestinal leak is the most common cause for sepsis post-bariatric surgery. Although early recognition is difficult in morbidly obese patient, prompt diagnosis

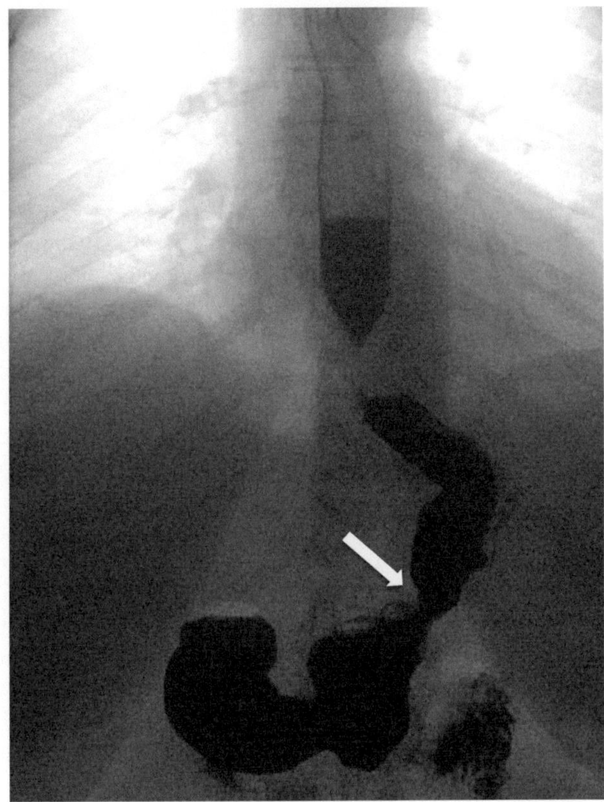

Fig. 2 Upper gastrointestinal contrast swallow test showing narrowing of the sleeve (white arrow)

is crucial and can minimize the risk of developing chronic fistula or progression to septic shock. The etiology of leaks can be divided into technical issues and patient-related issues. The most common presentation is tachycardia, fever, and abdominal pain. The patient will usually be described as ill-appearing.

Staple line leak is the most dreadful complication of SG. The rate of staple line leak is 1–3% in primary cases and more than 10% in revision procedures [25]. The most common site is near the GEJ. The main two reasons are ischemia and distal obstruction due to stenosis, twist or kink at the incisura angularis. Leak should be categorized according to their occurrence time post-surgery: acute, less than 7 days; early, within 1–6 weeks; late, within 6–12 weeks; and chronic, more than 12 weeks [26].

Small bowel leaks post-RYGB and OAGB/MGB are usually diagnosed earlier, within 3 days of surgery. The rate of leak post-RYGB ranged from 0.1 to 5.8% [23]; however, this rate is gradually decreasing and today it is around 0.3% [27]. The most common sites for leaks are at the GJ anastomosis. Other sites include gastric remnant staple line, JJ anastomosis, and along the small bowel due to iatrogenic injuries. The rates of leaks post-OAGB/MGB are 0.8–1.6% in primary cases and 4.08% in revisional procedures [23].

Esophageal or gastric perforation can present to the emergency department 48 h post-AGB surgery. This complication is rare but should be considered.

2.2 Late Complications

2.2.1 Nonsurgical Complication

Nutritional deficiencies are common post-bariatric procedures. The most common are anemia due to iron, B12, or folic acid deficiency, abnormalities in bone metabolism, and other vitamin and mineral deficiency. Thiamine (B1) deficiency can occur within 8–15 weeks post-surgery and is related to inadequate repletion and persistent vomiting. Acute presentation, such as Wernicke's encephalopathy, can present with nutritional polyneuropathy, ophthalmoparesis, ataxia, and confusion. Early initiation of supplement can prevent permanent deficits, and recovery typically occurs within 3–6 month [28]. Vitamins and trace element levels should be assessed frequently in the first 2 years and afterward annually.

Cholelithiasis formation is common post-bariatric surgery due to rapid weight loss. The incidence of gallstone formation ranges from 10 to 38% [29]. During rapid weight loss, cholesterol travels from adipose tissue to bile forming high saturation index. This, in turn, encourages cholesterol crystals that eventually form to stones. The progression of asymptomatic cholelithiasis to symptomatic ones is less than 5%, and the rate of cholecystectomy after RYGB is 6.8% [29]. Choledocholithiasis is infrequent post-RYGB, with rate of 0.2–5.3% of cases with cholelithiasis [27]. As in any patient who present with right upper quadrant abdominal pain, biliary disease could be the cause for the emergency department (ED) visit.

2.2.2 Surgical Complication

Bleeding

The effect of SG on gastroesophageal reflux disease (GERD) is inconclusive [30]. However, patients who suffer from severe GERD can present with upper GI bleeding due to erosive esophagitis. The main cause for late bleeding in patients post-RYGB and OAGB/MGB is bleeding marginal ulcer (MU). MU is an ulcer that develops at the GJ anastomosis, usually at the jejunal side, with multifactorial etiology. The incidence of MU is 0.6–16%, of which 9.27% will require surgical intervention [31]. Symptoms include heartburn, epigastric pain, nausea, and vomiting. Risk factors include nonsteroidal anti-inflammatory medications (NSAIDs) or corticosteroid treatment, nicotine use, and *Helicobacter pylori* infection.

Obstruction

Bariatric surgery patients, like any other general surgery patients, can suffer from post-surgery intra-abdominal adhesions. The rate of intestinal obstruction due to adhesion in bariatric patients is 13.7% [32]. Bariatric patients are prone to develop incisional hernia due to their excess weight and comorbidities. The rate of port site hernia post-bariatric surgery has been reported to be as high as 37% [33]. The rate of symptomatic or incarcerated port site hernia is not well documented, and for that, reason is unknown. Symptoms include nausea, vomiting, and usually focal abdominal pain around one or more of the surgical scars.

Twisting and kinking of the gastric sleeve are the main reasons for obstruction after SG. They account for 1.4% of SG surgeries and the average interval for diagnosis is 37 days [34]. Late obstruction in AGB can be caused by band slippage or overtighten of the band. The rate of slippage is 4.93% [35]. Band slippage can involve prolapse of the posterior pouch, anterior pouch, or concentric. It can deteriorate to ischemia of the gastric wall if left untreated and should be considered if symptoms do not respond to percutaneous decompression. Band erosion means reported rate is 1.46% (0.23–32.65%) [36]. Most cases do not mandate emergency treatment unless the presenting symptom is peritonitis or infection. Most cases will be asymptomatic, however, others can present as loss of restriction, bleeding, port infection, or dysphagia. Proximal migration can cause obstruction of the gastro-esophageal junction (GEJ).

Internal hernia (IH) is the most common and dreadful cause for small bowel obstruction after RYGB or OAGB/MGB. It can occur at any time post-surgery but mainly has a late presentation. The incidence ranges from 1 to 5.8%. If not treated surgically, IH has a mortality rate of over 50% [37]. Post-RYGB reconstruction, the small bowel can pass through the new anatomic space. This passage can cause twisting, obstruction, and even incarceration of the small bowel. Nowadays, most RYGB is performed in an antecolic approach which means there are two anatomic spaces: between the two mesenteries of the small bowel at the area of the JJ anastomosis and between the mesentery of the Roux limb, the meso of the transverse colon, and the retroperitoneum. The latter is referred as Petersen's hernia. In a retrocolic approach, a third space is the defect in the meso-transverse colon (Fig. 3). The most common site for IH is the JJ mesenteric defect. Patients have intermittent obstruction and usually do not vomit. The episodic abdominal pain usually delays the diagnosis and imaging may also be negative. Patients with suspected diagnosis of internal hernia and negative imaging may need to undergo diagnostic laparoscopy. In OAGB/MGB, there is only one anatomic space that can cause IH which resembles Petersen's hernia in RYGB. OAGB/MGB has lower rate of internal hernia compared to the RYGB [16].

SIRS/Sepsis

As mentioned before, the most common cause for sepsis post-bariatric surgery is gastrointestinal leak. Leaks post-SG can be diagnosed 3 months' post-surgery. Perforated marginal ulcer is another cause for bariatric patients to present with sepsis. The rate of perforated marginal ulcer post-RYGB is 0.83% [38].The etiology and outcome of this not well understood.

Abdominal Pain/Discomfort

Abdominal pain is a common complaint for patient post-bariatric procedure. Abdominal pain was presented in 21.6% of the bariatric patients who present to the ED. In 33.4% of these patients, no explanation of the pain was found [39]. The

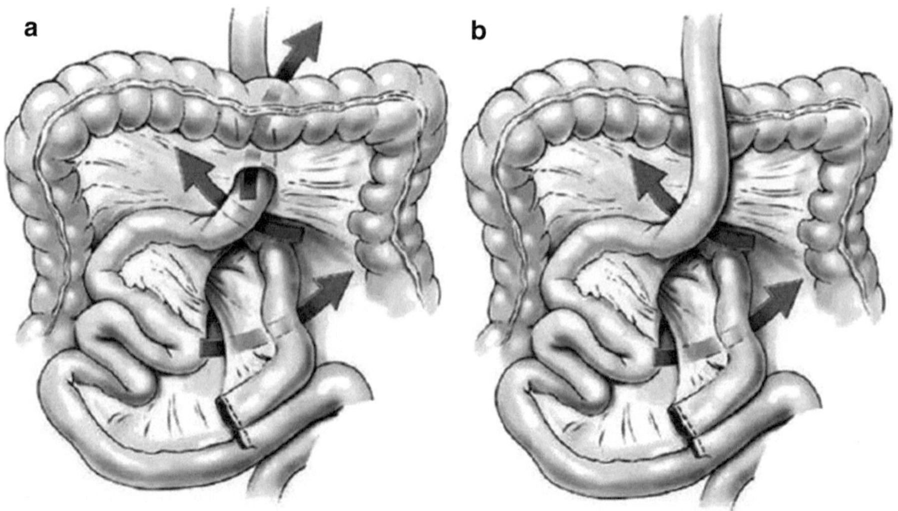

Fig. 3 Mesenteric defects in Roux-en-Y gastric bypass: (**a**) Retrocolic approach creating three defects. (**b**) Antecolic approach creating two defects. Reprinted from Palermo M, Acquafresca PA, Serra E. (2020). Closing the mesentery defects. Ettinger J, Azaro E, Weiner R, Higa KD, Neto MG, Teixeira AF, Jawad M (Eds). Gastric bypass bariatric and metabolic surgery perspectives. (pp. 181–185). Springer Nature

pathologic features that contribute to the pain are divided into surgical, nonsurgical, and psychological or behavioral. These patients usually undergo numerous tests including imaging, endoscopy, and even surgery.

3 Diagnosis

Most bariatric patients will present with complaints of abdominal pain. Emergency department physician needs to complete the diagnosis based on the patients chief complaint and the procedure they have had. Other abdominal pathologies such as pancreatitis, appendicitis, diverticulitis, nephrolithiasis, and hepatitis should be included in the differential diagnosis.

3.1 Clinical Presentation

Any patient who arrives to the emergency department (ED) should initially be assessed and stabilized according to ABCs (airway, breathing, and circulation). Initial treatment warrants a special consideration in the obese patient.

3.1.1 Airway

Patient may present with inadequate oxygenation due to problems with airway. It's essential to be prepared for difficult airway management due to their habitus and difficulties in landmark identification. Preparing an adequate airway management strategy is of paramount importance. Placing the patient in ramped position and adequate preoxygenation are always imperative, and apneic oxygenation, using high flow nasal cannula, should be considered [40].

3.1.2 Breathing

Tachypnea can present as an indicator for pulmonary or cardiac disease; however, it may be an indicator for systemic acidotic process. Obese patients have reduced functional residual capacity and as a result suffer from limited oxygen reserve [40]. Calculation of tidal volume during mechanical ventilation should be based on ideal body weight and not actual weight.

3.1.3 Circulation

Tachycardia in obese patients should be taken seriously as it can serve as a clue for underline pathology [41]. It can indicate hypovolemia due to dehydration or bleeding, and it can also be the presenting symptom of pulmonary embolus or anastomotic leak. Hypotension is usually a sign of hypovolemia, due to bleeding, dehydration, or sepsis. Resuscitation should be initiated with IV crystalloid in case of hypovolemia or packed red blood cell transfusion in case of active GI bleeding.

3.1.4 History

Abdominal pain is the most common principal diagnosis associated with ED visits followed by metabolic disorders and infection [9], whereas abdominal pain nausea/vomiting and dehydration are the main symptoms associated with ED visits. A focused history can help narrow the differential diagnosis. Initial assessment should be in the search for evidence of obstruction, GI bleeding, or infection/sepsis. A meticulous question regarding the nature of the pain can assist the diagnosis. Epigastric pain can indicate GEJ or GJ anastomosis pathology, whereas dull or nonspecific pain could indicate small bowel pathology. Hematemesis, melena, or hematochezia is obvious sign of GI bleeding but can be seen in GI perforation as well. Particular importance should be given to the bariatric procedure itself. Type and time since surgery could give clues regarding the diagnosis. Surgical report is the preferable method; however, surgery that was performed in foreign country or long interval time since surgery could make it difficult to know which procedure the patient had. Medical history including underlying comorbidities, which can alter the initial treatment, as well as current medication and recent medication withhold should be sought.

3.1.5 Physical Examination

Abdominal examination could be misleading in the obese patient. The wide distance between the skin and abdominal wall muscle can make it harder to identify signs of peritonitis. Signs of wound infection or localized pain should be sought. Focal tenderness, guarding, and rebound will be difficult to elicit. A benign abdominal examination should not give a false assumption that abdominal pathology is not present.

3.2 Tests

3.2.1 Laboratory Tests

Initial tests should include complete blood cell count, renal and liver function, lipase, blood gases, and CRP. In case of suspected cardiac ischemia, troponin level should be obtained. Elevated liver enzymes could be seen in gallbladder disease or obstruction of biliopancreatic limb along with elevated lipase. Lactic acidosis can be found in bowel ischemia or sepsis. Blood cultures should be taken in any patients with suspected sepsis or fever. Type and crossed blood products should be prepared in bleeding patients.

3.2.2 Imaging Studies

During the early postoperative period, chest X-ray can help in patients with dyspnea for the diagnosis of atelectasis, effusion, or pneumonia. Free air under the diaphragm, in instable patient with abdominal pain, can be seen. Plain X-ray can determine the position of gastric band. The correct position should be in 1–2 to 7–8 position as seen in Fig. 4. Other positions of the band may indicate slippage of the band. Contrast swallow study assists in the diagnosis of leaks at the area of anastomosis or along the staple line; however, the low sensitivity (22–75%) and the high availability of computed tomography in the ED, resulted that contrast swallow study is rarely performed. The use of ultrasound (US) in bariatric patient is questionable due to their habitus. However, patients with suspected gallbladder disease may benefit from US exam.

CT is the main diagnostic tool in the assessment of bariatric patient at the ED and should be considered in the early assessment of patients with signs of obstruction or sepsis. In clinically stable patients with suspected bariatric surgery complication, CT of the abdomen and pelvis with intravenous and small amount of oral contrast has

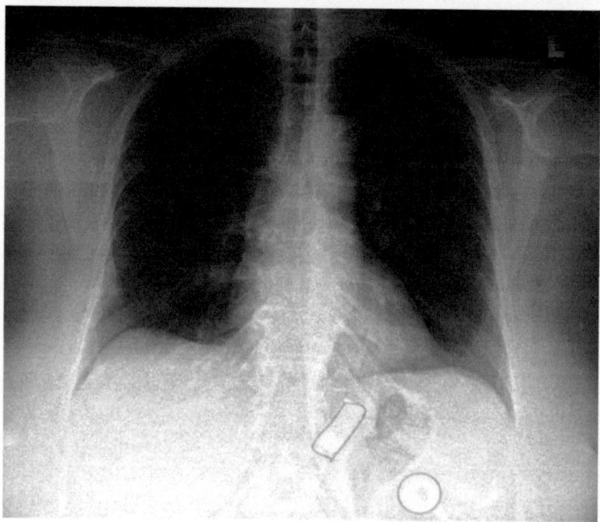

Fig. 4 X-ray study showing a normally positioned gastric band at approximately 45° to the spine. The band and port are outlined in gray line

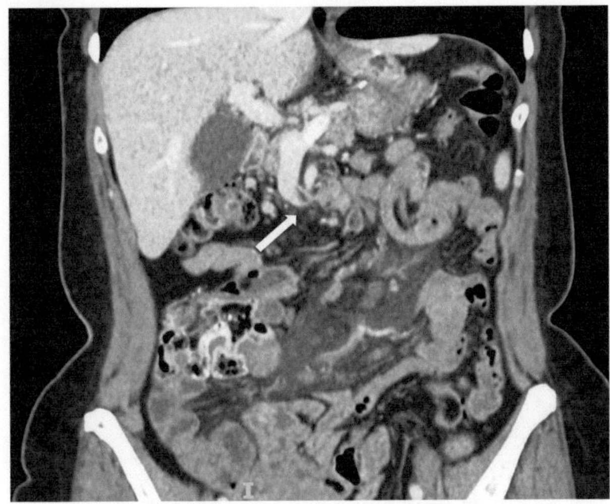

Fig. 5 CT scan image shows superior mesenteric vein beaking sign. Internal hernia was diagnosed in this post-RYGB patient during diagnostic laparoscopy

higher sensitivity and specificity than contrast swallow study in identifying leak along with the ability to identify abscess, internal hernia, and other pathologies [42]. The addition of the chest to the study can help in ruling out PE or other pulmonary complications. CT detects leaks in the GJ anastomosis or in SG in 60–80% of the cases [43].

CT has a major role in the diagnosis of internal hernia (IH) which is one of the most difficult pathologies to identify. There are several signs for internal hernia in CT exam including swirled mesentery, small bowel obstruction (SBO), hurricane eye, and superior mesenteric vein (SMV) beaking (Fig. 5). The overall accuracy and sensitivity for diagnosis of IH were mesenteric swirl and SBO; however, SMV beaking with SBO had the highest specificity [44]. In case of clinical suspicion, negative CT study does not rule out the diagnosis and surgery should be considered.

3.2.3 Endoscopy

Endoscopy is the modality of choice in the diagnosis and treatment of bleeding complication. It can diagnose MU and treat active bleeding. Band erosion is easily diagnosed during endoscopy and, in certain conditions, can be treated by endoscopy. Stricture, leaks, and fistula can also be diagnosed and treated [45]. Most cases of GI bleeding necessitate early endoscopic intervention. Endoscopy is the modality of choice in the diagnosis of band erosion. The decision regarding the use of endoscopy during the diagnosis and treatment of other complication mandates a consultation between the surgeon and the gastroenterologist.

4 Differential Diagnosis

The differential diagnosis should be assessed according to the time since surgery, presenting symptoms, and type of procedure. The differential diagnosis is summarized in Table 1.

5 Treatment

Initial assessment and treatment of bariatric surgery complications is summarized in Algorithm 1.

5.1 Medical Treatment

Initial treatment should start with rapid assessment of hemodynamic stability. Most patients will require IV crystalloid fluids. Antiemetic and PPI medication should be considered. Urgent surgical consult should be ordered in unstable patients post-bariatric surgery. The decision regarding explorative laparotomy vs. laparoscopy will be decided based on surgeon experience and preference.

5.1.1 Bleeding

The treatment of patients, who present with GI bleeding, should include the initiation of IV proton pump inhibitors (PPI) and blood sample for type and cross. Antidote for anticoagulation treatment should be considered based on

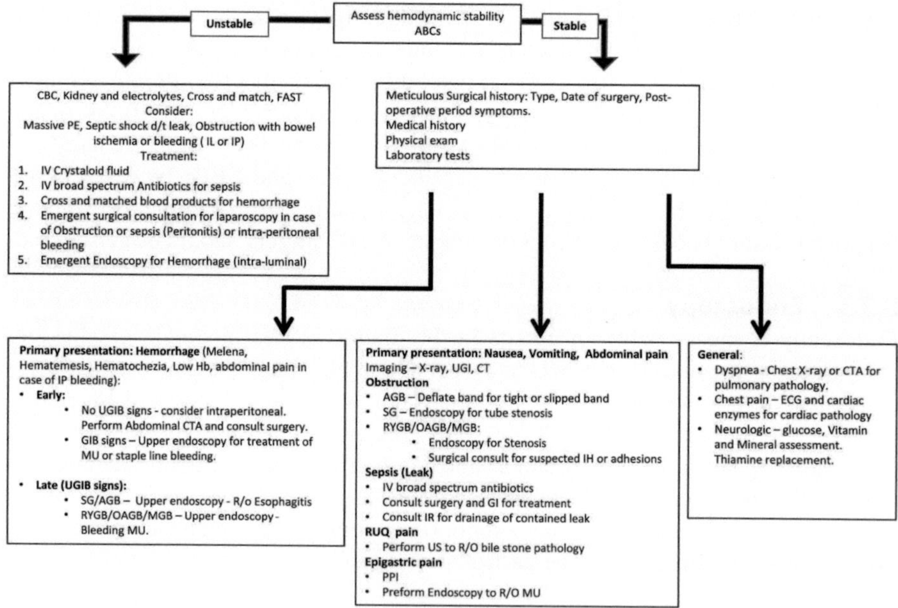

Algorithm 1 Emergency department assessment and treatment for patient with bariatric surgery complications. *ABC* airway, breathing, circulation; *CBC* complete blood count; *FAST* focal assessment sonography for trauma; *IL* intraluminal; *IP* intraperitoneal; *Hb* hemoglobin; *GIB* gastrointestinal bleeding; *CTA* computed tomography angiography; *MU* marginal ulcer; *UGI* upper gastrointestinal contrast study; *US* ultrasound; *PPI* proton pump inhibitors; *ECG* electrocardiogram. *AGB* adjustable gastric banding; *SG* sleeve gastrectomy; *RYGB* Roux-en-Y gastric bypass

hemodynamic status and type of procedure planned. Upper endoscopy for diagnosis and treatment should be ordered in patients with intraluminal bleeding. Esophagitis or gastritis can be treated conservatively. Bleeding MU will usually respond well to nonsurgical treatment. It includes PPI, sucralfate, and treating causative factors. The indication for surgical intervention includes bleeding that does not respond to conservative treatment including endoscopy.

5.1.2 Obstruction

Patients with obstructive symptoms are usually dehydrated. The initial treatment should include IV fluids, electrolyte supplementations, and urinary output assessment. Endoscopy is used for the final diagnosis and treatment in case of stenosis post-SG or at the GJ anastomosis. Dilatation is performed with gradual pneumatic balloon dilatation. Multiple sessions are usually required. IH is treated surgically. Any patient with suspected IH should have immediate surgical consult.

Slipped or overinflated gastric band can be treated by deflation of the band. Band deflation should be performed under strict aseptic condition by any general surgeon. Port site can be difficult to palpate but usually the patient know the exact place. A non-coring needle, Huber needle, is preferably used; however, any needle can be used. The port should be held firmly between the thumb and index finger of the nondominant hand, and the needle should be inserted at the doom of the port until it touches the metallic base of the port. After complete aspiration of the fluid, immediate resolution of symptoms should be made. Patient with complete resolution should be sent to his bariatric surgeon. If symptoms do not resolve, surgical exploration is warrant.

5.1.3 Sepsis

The treatment of staple line leak post-SG is challenging. Initial management and the course of treatment are based on time of occurrence and septic condition of the patient [46]. After blood cultures, a broad-spectrum IV antibiotics, covering gram-negative, anaerobic, and gram-positive, in case of wound complication, should be initiated. Patients who are ill-appearing or hemodynamically unstable should have emergent surgical consult. While "contained cause" (e.g,. abscess, contained leak) can be treated conservatively, patients with signs of peritonitis warrant prompt surgical intervention. Initial treatment of leaks includes no oral intake (NPO), IV fluids, PPI, and parenteral nutrition. Percutaneous drainage of collection should be made by interventional radiology (IR). Surgical consult, as well as contacting the bariatric surgeon, is warrant. Other treatment options include stent, double pigtail drain inserted endoscopically, glue, and surgical washout and drainage. In proximal leaks after SG, conservative treatment should last at least 12 weeks before reoperation is considered [25].

Early leaks post-RYGB or OAGB/MGB can be treated conservatively with NPO and parenteral nutrition. Other treatment options include endoscopic stents and over the scope clips. The success rate of RYGB is higher than OAGB/MGB due to the fact that bile and pancreatic fluids do not pass at the anastomosis site.

Patient with the diagnosis of perforated MU is usually ill-appearing and the treatment is surgical.

5.2   Surgical Treatment

Patients with bariatric surgery complication and signs of peritonitis or unstable patients should have emergent surgical consultation for prompt surgical intervention. The decision on laparoscopic or open intervention is decided based on surgeon experience. If the patient is stable, transfer to bariatric excellence center is recommended due to surgical experience and supporting multidisciplinary team.

Surgical intervention for bleeding MU who failed endoscopic treatment can include suture of the ulcer with absorbable sutures under endoscopy surveillance, longitudinal enterotomy with suture of the ulcer bed followed by transverse closure of the enterotomy, or redo the GJ anastomosis. The recurrence rate of MU after surgical intervention is 24% after 12 months [31]. The treatment for perforated MU is similar to the treatment of anastomosis leak post-RYGB or OAGB/MGB. The surgical treatment includes primary suture or omental Graham patch with or without gastrostomy to the remnant stomach. Redo of the GJ anastomosis is another surgical option.

Acute SG leak can be treated with surgical irrigation and drainage of the staple line. Re-suture is an option; however, it is not recommended in patients of postoperative day 3–4 or friable tissue. Surgical treatment, after failed conservative treatment, can include total gastrectomy with Roux-en-Y esophagojejunostomy or Roux-en-Y fistulo-jejunostomy.

Obstruction at the JJ warrants surgical treatment. CT scan can help in identifying the precise location—at the BP limb, Roux limb, or both. It can also identify whether the cause is blood clot or not. In case of blood clot, enterotomy with clot removal is an option. Stenosis at the JJ anastomosis warrants redo of the stenotic part or resection of the JJ with reconstruction of a new JJ anastomosis.

The treatment for IH is emergent surgical exploration. In most cases, the bowel in Petersen's hernia traverses from left to right and in case of mesenteric hernia at the area of JJ anastomosis from right to left. Running the small bowel from the ileocecal valve to the DJ flexure can help with orientation during surgery. During surgery, after returning the bowel to their anatomic place, mesenteric defects are closed with nonabsorbable sutures.

Acute band slippage that does not respond to percutaneous band deflation is an indication for urgent surgical intervention. Laparoscopic band removal is usually the treatment of choice. After lysis of adhesion, the band is unclipped or cut and removed. Special attention should be made to divide the band capsule in order to relieve the obstruction symptoms. Skin incision above the port site, removal of the port and the connecting tube end the procedure. Band erosion is usually not treated operatively unless the presenting symptoms are peritonitis or infection. Band erosion above 50% of its circumference can be treated endoscopically. Subcutaneous removal of the port before the procedure is mandated. In case of peritonitis or infection, the treatment of choice is laparoscopic removal of the eroded band, repair of gastric wall, and drainage.

5.3   Prognosis

Bariatric procedures are safe. The mortality rate ranges from 0.03 to 0.2% and is constantly decreasing in the last 20 years. The 30 days' serious adverse event rate is less than 6%. The rates of early reoperation and readmission are 0.5–3% and 2.8–4.8% for SG, respectively, and 0.7–5% and 4.7–6.5% for RYGB [46]. Long-term studies found that the rates of reoperations or re-interventions range from 5 to 22.1% [47].

References

1. World Health Organiztion. Obesity and overweight fact sheet. 2020. http://www.who.int/news-room/factsheets/detail/obesity-and-overweight. Accessed 13 Mar 2021.
2. Buchwald H, Avidor Y, Braunwald E, et al. Bariatric surgery: a systematic review and meta-analysis. JAMA. 2004;292(14):1724–37.
3. Colquitt JL, Pickett K, Loveman E, Frampton GK. Surgery for weight loss in adults. Cochrane Database Syst Rev. 2014;2014(8):CD003641.
4. Nguyen NT, Goldman C, et al. Laparoscopic versus open gastric bypass: a randomized study of outcomes, quality of life, and costs. Ann Surg. 2001;234(3):279–91.
5. Meisinger C, Ezzati M, Di Cesare M. Trends in adult body-mass index in 200 countries from 1975 to 2014: a pooled analysis of 1698 population-based measurement studies with 19.2 million participants. 2016.
6. McLaren L. Socioeconomic status and obesity. Epidemiol Rev. 2007;29(1):29–48.
7. Bradley JF III, Ross SW, Christmas AB, et al. Complications of bariatric surgery: the acute care surgeon's experience. Am J Surg. 2015;210(3):456–61.
8. Telem DA, Yang J, Altieri M, et al. Rates and risk factors for unplanned emergency department utilization and hospital readmission following bariatric surgery. Ann Surg. 2016;263(5):956–60.
9. Mora-Pinzon MC, Henkel D, Miller RE, et al. Emergency department visits and readmissions within 1 year of bariatric surgery: a statewide analysis using hospital discharge records. Surgery. 2017;162(5):1155–62.
10. Miras AD, Le Roux CW. Mechanisms underlying weight loss after bariatric surgery. Nat Rev Gastroenterol Hepatol. 2013;10(10):575.
11. Mechanick JI, Youdim A, Jones DB, et al. Clinical practice guidelines for the perioperative nutritional, metabolic, and nonsurgical support of the bariatric surgery patient2013 update: cosponsored by American Association of Clinical Endocrinologists, the Obesity Society, and American Society for Metabolic & Bariatric Surgery. Endocr Pract. 2013;19(2):337–72.
12. Di Lorenzo N, Antoniou SA, Batterham RL, et al. Clinical practice guidelines of the European Association for Endoscopic Surgery (EAES) on bariatric surgery: update 2020 endorsed by IFSO-EC, EASO and ESPCOP. Surg Endosc. 2020;34(6):2332–58.
13. Ramos A, Kow L, Brown W, et al. 5th IFSO Global Registry Report. Int Fed Surg Obes Metab Disord. 2019.
14. Kumar SB, Hamilton BC, Wood SG, Rogers SJ, Carter JT, Lin MY. Is laparoscopic sleeve gastrectomy safer than laparoscopic gastric bypass? A comparison of 30-day complications using the MBSAQIP data registry. Surg Obes Relat Dis. 2018;14(3):264–9.
15. Peterli R, Wölnerhanssen BK, Peters T, et al. Effect of laparoscopic sleeve gastrectomy vs laparoscopic Roux-en-Y gastric bypass on weight loss in patients with morbid obesity: the SM-BOSS randomized clinical trial. JAMA. 2018;319(3):255–65.

16. Magouliotis DE, Tasiopoulou VS, Tzovaras G. One anastomosis gastric bypass versus Roux-en-Y gastric bypass for morbid obesity: an updated meta-analysis. Obes Surg. 2019;29(9):2721–30.
17. O'Brien PE, Hindle A, Brennan L, et al. Long-term outcomes after bariatric surgery: a systematic review and meta-analysis of weight loss at 10 or more years for all bariatric procedures and a single-centre review of 20-year outcomes after adjustable gastric banding. Obes Surg. 2019;29(1):3–14.
18. Moon RC, Kirkpatrick V, Gaskins L, Teixeira AF, Jawad MA. Safety and effectiveness of single-versus double-anastomosis duodenal switch at a single institution. Surg Obes Relat Dis. 2019;15(2):245–52.
19. Smith MD, Patterson E, Wahed AS, et al. Thirty-day mortality after bariatric surgery: independently adjudicated causes of death in the longitudinal assessment of bariatric surgery. Obes Surg. 2011;21(11):1687–92.
20. Stein PD, Matta F. Pulmonary embolism and deep venous thrombosis following bariatric surgery. Obes Surg. 2013;23(5):663–8.
21. Kitahama S, Smith MD, Rosencrantz DR, Patterson EJ. Is bariatric surgery safe in patients who refuse blood transfusion? Surg Obes Relat Dis. 2013;9(3):390–4.
22. Augustin T, Aminian A, Romero-Talamás H, Rogula T, Schauer PR, Brethauer SA. Reoperative surgery for management of early complications after gastric bypass. Obes Surg. 2016;26(2):345–9.
23. Silecchia G, Iossa A. Complications of staple line and anastomoses following laparoscopic bariatric surgery. Ann Gastroenterol. 2018;31(1):56.
24. Kermansaravi M, Shahmiri SS, DavarpanahJazi AH, et al. One anastomosis/mini-gastric bypass (OAGB/MGB) as revisional surgery following primary restrictive bariatric procedures: a systematic review and meta-analysis. Obes Surg. 2020;1-14:370.
25. Abou Rached A, Basile M, El Masri H. Gastric leaks post sleeve gastrectomy: review of its prevention and management. World J Gastroenterol WJG. 2014;20(38):13904.
26. Rosenthal RJ, Panel ISGE. International Sleeve Gastrectomy Expert Panel Consensus Statement: best practice guidelines based on experience of> 12,000 cases. Surg Obes Relat Dis. 2012;8(1):8–19.
27. Vidarsson B, Sundbom M, Edholm D. Incidence and treatment of small bowel leak after Roux-en-Y gastric bypass: a cohort study from the Scandinavian Obesity Surgery Registry. Surg Obes Relat Dis. 2020;16(8):1005–10.
28. Becker DA, Balcer LJ, Galetta SL. The neurological complications of nutritional deficiency following bariatric surgery. J Obes. 2012;2012:1.
29. Leyva-Alvizo A, Arredondo-Saldaña G, Leal-Isla-Flores V, et al. Systematic review of management of gallbladder disease in patients undergoing minimally invasive bariatric surgery. Surg Obes Relat Dis. 2020;16(1):158–64.
30. Chiu S, Birch DW, Shi X, et al. Effect of sleeve gastrectomy on gastro-esophageal reflux disease: a systematic review. Surg Obes Relat Dis. 2011;7:510–5.
31. Pyke O, Yang J, Cohn T, et al. Marginal ulcer continues to be a major source of morbidity over time following gastric bypass. Surg Endosc. 2019;33(10):3451–6.
32. Husain S, Ahmed AR, Johnson J, Boss T, O'Malley W. Small-bowel obstruction after laparoscopic Roux-en-Y gastric bypass: etiology, diagnosis, and management. Arch Surg. 2007;142(10):988–93.
33. Karampinis I, Lion E, Hetjens S, et al. Trocar site HERnias after bariatric laparoscopic surgery (HERBALS): a prospective cohort study. Obes Surg. 2020:1–7.
34. Rebibo L, Hakim S, Dhahri A, Yzet T, Delcenserie R, Regimbeau J-M. Gastric stenosis after laparoscopic sleeve gastrectomy: diagnosis and management. Obes Surg. 2016;26(5):995–1001.
35. Singhal R, Bryant C, Kitchen M, et al. Band slippage and erosion after laparoscopic gastric banding: a meta-analysis. Surg Endosc. 2010;24(12):2980–6.
36. Egberts K, Brown WA, O'Brien PE. Systematic review of erosion after laparoscopic adjustable gastric banding. Obes Surg. 2011;21(8):1272–9.

37. Martin LC, Merkle EM, Thompson WM. Review of internal hernias: radiographic and clinical findings. Am J Roentgenol. 2006;186(3):703–17.
38. Altieri MS, Pryor A, Yang J, et al. The natural history of perforated marginal ulcers after gastric bypass surgery. Surg Endosc. 2018;32(3):1215–22.
39. Pierik AS, Coblijn UK, de Raaff CAL, van Veen RN, van Tets WF, van Wagensveld BA. Unexplained abdominal pain in morbidly obese patients after bariatric surgery. Surg Obes Relat Dis. 2017;13(10):1743–51.
40. Aceto P, Perilli V, Modesti C, Ciocchetti P, Vitale F, Sollazzi L. Airway management in obese patients. Surg Obes Relat Dis. 2013;9(5):809–15.
41. Kassir R, Debs T, Blanc P, et al. Complications of bariatric surgery: presentation and emergency management, vol. 27; 2016. p. 77.
42. Kim J, Azagury D, Eisenberg D, DeMaria E, Campos GM. ASMBS position statement on prevention, detection, and treatment of gastrointestinal leak after gastric bypass and sleeve gastrectomy, including the roles of imaging, surgical exploration, and nonoperative management. Surg Obes Relat Dis. 2015;11(4):739–48.
43. Lim R, Beekley A, Johnson DC, Davis KA. Early and late complications of bariatric operation. Trauma Surg Acute Care Open. 2018;3(1):e000219.
44. Dilauro M, McInnes MDF, Schieda N, et al. Internal hernia after laparoscopic Roux-en-Y gastric bypass: optimal CT signs for diagnosis and clinical decision making. Radiology. 2017;282(3):752–60.
45. Joo MK. Endoscopic approach for major complications of bariatric surgery. Clin Endosc. 2017;50(1):31.
46. Al Hajj G, Chemaly R. Fistula following laparoscopic sleeve gastrectomy: a proposed classification and algorithm for optimal management. Obes Surg. 2018;28(3):656–64.
47. Arterburn DE, Telem DA, Kushner RF, Courcoulas AP. Benefits and risks of bariatric surgery in adults: a review. JAMA. 2020;324(9):879–87.

Gynecological Emergencies

J. L. Kilkenny and M. S. J. Wilson

1   Introduction

General surgeons assess patients with abdominal pain, both male and female, including adults and children. The differential diagnosis is broad, particularly in female patients. Differential diagnoses must be modified when assessing women of all ages, especially those of reproductive age. Gynecological disease processes in pregnant women include ectopic pregnancy, uterine rupture, and threatened abortion. All can present to the general surgeon if presenting atypically. Gynecological disorders in nonpregnant women also present to general surgery as frequent abdominal pain as the primary symptom. These may include adnexal torsion, ovarian cyst complications, pelvic inflammatory disease, and tubo-ovarian abscess. Recognition and awareness of these disease processes and their appropriate investigation are crucial in obtaining optimal and timely outcomes for this patient cohort.

Acute appendicitis is the most common surgical emergency and is also the most common cause of non-gynecological pelvic pain [1, 2]. Gynecological conditions affecting the right adnexa such as pelvic inflammatory disease or a ruptured ovarian cyst can mimic appendicitis. Gynecological causes account for 22–36% of patients who present with right iliac fossa pain, presumed to be appendicitis [3]. Despite vast improvements in imaging in recent times, it may still be difficult to differentiate between gynecologic and non-gynecological causes of pain, and it is therefore imperative that general surgeons understand gynecological disease processes. This chapter aims to provide an overview of the gynecological emergencies that can

J. L. Kilkenny
Craigavon Area Hospital, Portadown, UK

M. S. J. Wilson (✉)
Forth Valley Royal Hospital, Larbert, UK
e-mail: michael.wilson3@nhs.scot

© The Author(s), under exclusive license to Springer Nature Switzerland AG 2023
F. Coccolini et al. (eds.), *Mini-invasive Approach in Acute Care Surgery*,
Hot Topics in Acute Care Surgery and Trauma,
https://doi.org/10.1007/978-3-031-39001-2_22

present as an emergency to general surgery on initial presentation to hospital or encountered during a diagnostic laparoscopy.

1.1 History and Examination

Evaluation of women with abdominal or pelvic pain begins with a complete history. This should include the history of the presenting complaint as well as medical and surgical history (previous pelvic surgery), sexual and contraceptive histories, and date of last menstrual period. A recent study reported that gynecological history taking by general surgeons, in females of reproductive age, was poor, with last menstrual period, contraception use, and sexual activity documented in only 38%, 28%, and 16% of patients, respectively [4]. The same study reported only 61% of eligible patients admitted as an emergency had a documented pregnancy status [4]. A urinary β-hCG should be performed in every woman of reproductive age presenting with abdominal pain principally to rule out ectopic pregnancy. It is also an important factor when considering imaging using ionizing radiation and emergency surgery requiring general anesthetic. The importance of β-hCG levels in ectopic pregnancy is discussed later in the chapter. Physical examination should include a full abdominal examination and a bimanual vaginal examination, where indicated, by an experienced practitioner.

2 Pelvic Inflammatory Disease

2.1 Overview

Pelvic inflammatory disease (PID) is the most common infectious disease that affects young women aged 15–25 years, contributing to 125,000–150,000 hospital admissions each year in the United States [5, 6]. It is an infectious and inflammatory disorder of the upper female genital tract that is almost always a sexually transmitted infection [7]. It encompasses a broad range of diseases including endometritis, salpingitis, salpingo-oophoritis, tubo-ovarian abscess (TOA), and pelvic peritonitis. *Chlamydia trachomatis* is the predominant sexually transmitted organism associated with PID, but less than 50% of cases test positive for sexually transmitted organisms [8]. The risk factors for developing PID are detailed in Table 1 [7]. PID is a major concern due to the long-term implications that include infertility, chronic pelvic pain, and ectopic pregnancy [9].

2.2 Clinical Presentation

A diagnosis of PID should be made on clinical grounds, but its symptoms overlap with other lower abdominal and pelvic conditions causing diagnostic uncertainty and can be easily mistaken for other conditions such as acute appendicitis.

Table 1 Risk factors for pelvic inflammatory disease

Risk factors for pelvic inflammatory disease
Factors relating to sexual behavior
• <25 years old
• Early age of first coitus
• Multiple sexual partners
• Recent new partner (within previous 3 months)
• History of STI in the woman or her partner
Recent instrumentation of the uterus or interruption of the cervical barrier
• Termination of pregnancy
• Insertion of intrauterine device (within the past 4–6 weeks)
• Hysterosalpingography
• In vitro fertilization and intrauterine insemination

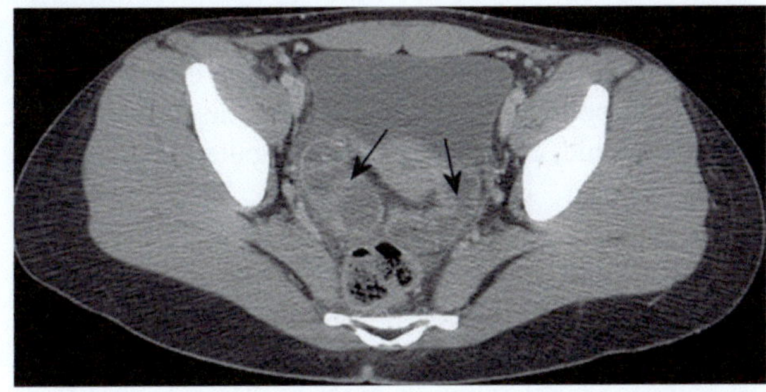

Fig. 1 Contrast-enhanced CT in a 43-year-old woman with advanced PID demonstrates pyosalpinx with dilated, thick-walled, enhancing fallopian tubes containing fluid (*arrow*). (Reproduced from Augustin et al. 2017)

Typical symptoms of PID include lower abdominal pain, typically bilateral but can be unilateral. Fever and vomiting are present in some cases. A thorough gynecological history is vital and can identify symptoms such as new deep dyspareunia and abnormal vaginal bleeding or discharge. Occasionally, PID can present as right upper quadrant pain in the form of Fitz-Hugh-Curtis syndrome [9] (see Sect. 3.4). Physical examination usually reveals bilateral lower abdominal tenderness, adnexal tenderness (with or without a palpable mass), cervical motion tenderness on bimanual examination, abnormal vaginal discharge, and occasionally a fever.

2.3   Investigation

A pregnancy test should be performed in all women of reproductive age. A high vaginal swab should be taken for bacterial vaginosis and candidiasis. Specific testing for *Chlamydia trachomatis*, *Neisseria gonorrhoeae*, and *Mycoplasma genitalium* should be carried out. Ultrasonography is of limited value for uncomplicated PID but is helpful if a tubo-ovarian abscess or hydrosalpinx is suspected [7]. MRI (magnetic resonance imaging) and CT (computed tomography) scanning of the pelvis may be helpful in differentiating PID from alternative diagnoses, but they are not indicated routinely as an initial investigation [7]. An example of CT findings in PID can be seen in Fig. 1.

2.4   Management

Uncomplicated PID is generally treated with oral antibiotics as per local guidelines. The reasons for hospitalization of those with PID include pregnancy, inability to exclude a competing diagnosis, or a tubal abscess.

3   Tubo-ovarian Abscess

3.1   Overview

A tubo-ovarian abscess (TOA) is an infectious mass of the adnexa that generally occurs as a sequela of PID, although it can occur independently [10]. It can encompass adjacent organs including the bowel and bladder. The classical symptoms of TOA include an adnexal mass, fever, elevated white blood cell count, lower abdominal-pelvic pain, and/or vaginal discharge [11]. Clinical presentation can be highly variable, causing it to mimic acute appendicitis.

3.2   Investigation

As discussed previously, ultrasonography, preferably transvaginal, is the investigation of choice to identify complications of PID. CT, likely performed to investigate abdominal pain, will show a clear abscess, with associated fat stranding, as seen in Fig. 2 [12].

3.3   Management

Broad-spectrum antibiotics are the first-line treatment for TOA; however, recent studies suggest early laparoscopic surgical intervention achieves a more rapid recovery, reduces length of hospitalization, and reduces abscess recurrence rates [13, 14]. It also reduces length of operation and blood loss when compared to late

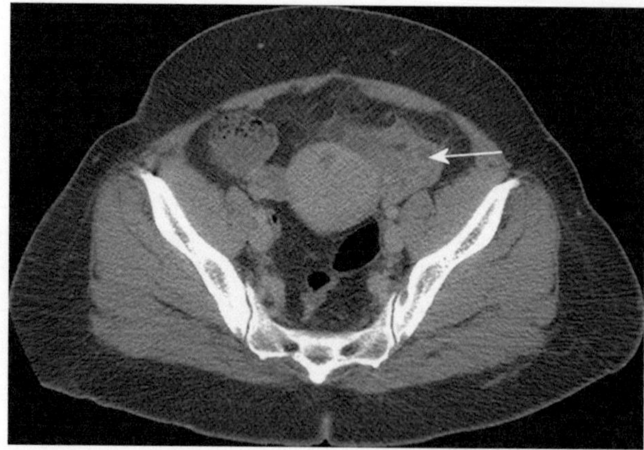

Fig. 2 Advanced PID in a 49-year-old woman with left-sided tubo-ovarian abscess. Contrast-enhanced CT scans demonstrate enlarged ovary with abnormal enhancement and periovarian pelvic edema (*arrow*). (Reproduced from Augustin et al. 2017)

laparoscopy after antibiotic failure [14]. Predicting the success of antibiotic treatment has been the subject of many recent studies. TOA diameter greater than 5.5 cm is a predictor in the failure of antibiotic management and can be used to predict which cases will benefit from early laparoscopy [3, 15–17]. Early laparoscopy should also be considered in postmenopausal women where TOA can be associated with a malignant tumor and in patients who desire to maintain fertility by potentially reducing adhesion formation compared to antibiotic treatment alone [14–18].

3.4 Fitz-Hugh-Curtis Syndrome

The Fitz-Hugh-Curtis syndrome (FHCS) is characterized by perihepatic inflammation and is a chronic manifestation of pelvic inflammatory disease. Microorganisms associated with PID ascend from the endometrium to the fallopian tubes and peritoneal cavity [19]. The possibility of lymphatic and hematogenous spread is discussed in the literature [20, 21]. This results in adhesion formation between the anterior surface of the liver and the abdominal wall and can present as right upper quadrant pain. Pain is exacerbated by movement and deep breathing and can be associated with other symptoms of PID including lower abdominal pain, vaginal discharge, and fever. Typical appearances on CT imaging can be seen in Fig. 3 [12].

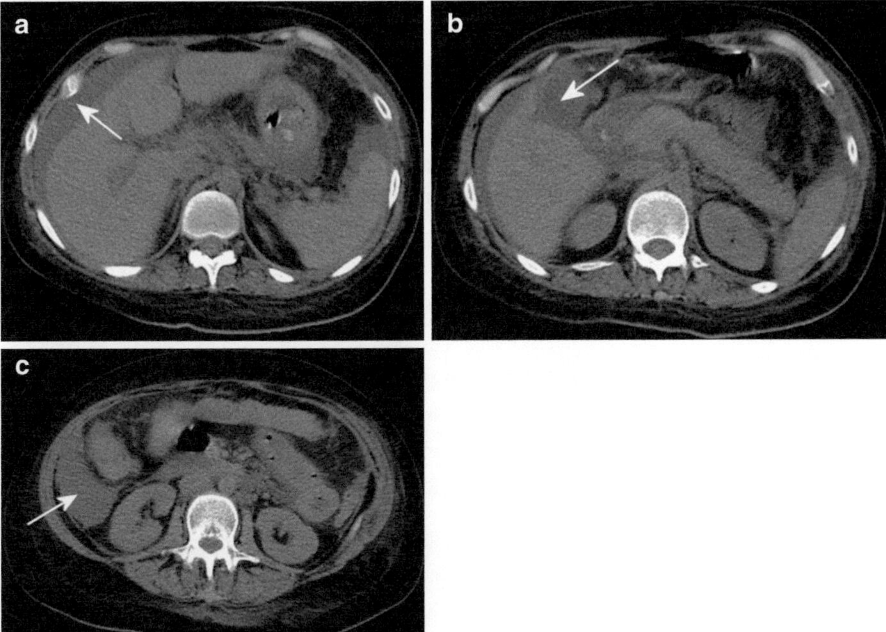

Fig. 3 Fitz-Hugh-Curtis syndrome in a 21-year-old patient with advanced PID. (**a**) Non-contrast CT demonstrating inflammatory stranding and fluid in the perihepatic region (*arrow*); (**b**) pericholecystic inflammatory changes and gallbladder wall thickening (*arrow*); (**c**) fluid along the right paracolic gutter (*arrow*). (Reproduced from Augustin et al. 2017)

Symptomatic relief can be achieved by laparoscopic adhesiolysis (see Fig. 4, e.g., of the adhesions seen on laparoscopy) alongside systemic antibiotic treatment to address the cause [19].

4   Ectopic Pregnancy

4.1   Overview

Like other gynecological emergencies, ectopic pregnancy may mimic other gastrointestinal or urinary conditions and may present to the general surgeon. A high level of suspicion must always be present when assessing a woman of childbearing age. Ectopic pregnancy (EP) occurs when the developing blastocyst becomes implanted at a site other than the endometrium of the uterine cavity [22]. Most cases occur in the fallopian tube, as seen in Fig. 5, with the remainder occurring in various locations, including the ovary, cervix, cesarean section scar, and peritoneal cavity. One to two percent of all pregnancies are ectopic and are the leading cause of maternal death within the first trimester accounting for 75% of first trimester deaths and 9–13% of all pregnancy-related deaths [22, 23]. In developing countries, the incidence is thought to be significantly higher, and it is estimated that 10% of women admitted to hospital with an ectopic pregnancy will ultimately die [24, 25].

Although half of women who have an ectopic pregnancy have no known risk factors, several risk factors for ectopic pregnancy (Table 2) have been identified including tubal damage, pelvic inflammatory disease, history of infertility, and cigarette smoking [26]. One third of all cases of ectopic pregnancy are thought to be due to smoking, either current or past exposure [27]. A recent study suggests that the risk of ectopic pregnancy only returns to that of nonsmokers after >10 years of cessation [22].

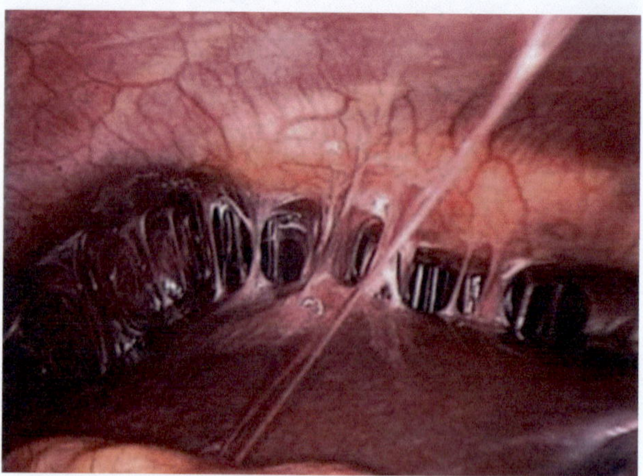

Fig. 4 "Violin-string" adhesions of chronic Fitz-Hugh-Curtis syndrome. (Reproduced from Theofanakis et al. 2011)

Fig. 5 Ectopic pregnancy in the fallopian tube. (Reproduced from Caronia et al. 2015)

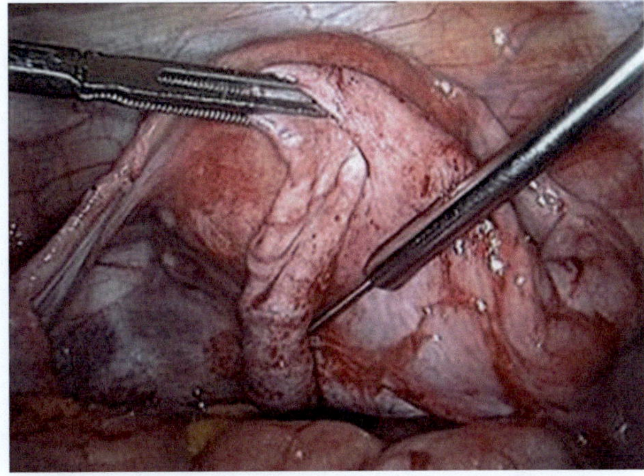

Table 2 Risk factors for ectopic pregnancy (Sivalingam et al. 2011)

Risk factors for ectopic pregnancy
Fallopian tube damage
• Previous tubal surgery (including female sterilization) and pelvic surgery including cesarean section and ovarian cystectomy
• Previous abdominal surgery including appendectomy and bowel surgery
• Confirmed genital infection and pelvic inflammatory disease, commonly caused by chlamydial infection
Infertility
• Documented tubal disease
• Assisted reproductive technology
• Endometriosis
• Unexplained infertility
Contraceptive failure
• Progestogen-only contraception
• Intrauterine contraceptive device
Cigarette smoking
Previous ectopic pregnancy
Age >35

4.2 Clinical Presentation

Ectopic pregnancy usually presents during the first trimester. The clinical presentation can vary from vaginal bleeding with abdominal pain to hemorrhagic shock. The typical presentation is 6–10 weeks' gestational age in a stable patient with pain and bleeding although it has been reported that a third of patients have no clinical signs [28–30]. A ruptured ectopic pregnancy, as seen in Fig. 6, must be considered in any woman with a positive pregnancy test presenting with syncope or signs of hemodynamic shock. Diagnosis is usually confirmed with a combination of transvaginal ultrasonography (TVS) and serum β-hCG concentration.

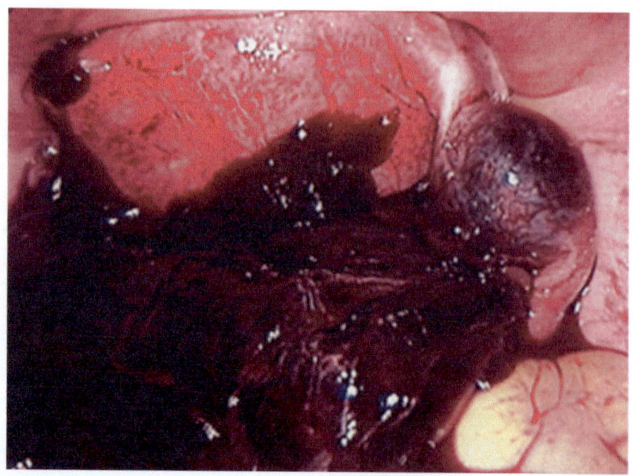

Fig. 6 Bleeding tubal ectopic pregnancy with hemoperitoneum. (Reproduced from M. Jean Uy-Kroh 2015)

4.3 Investigation

TVS should identify the intrauterine gestation sac with almost 100% accuracy at a gestational age of 5.5 weeks. The presence of an intrauterine pregnancy should rule out ectopic pregnancy in most cases except in the rare case of a heterotopic pregnancy where an ectopic pregnancy coexists with an intrauterine pregnancy [31]. In the absence of an intrauterine sac, an ectopic pregnancy can be identified by the presence of a non-cystic adnexal mass, usually visible within the fallopian tube. False negatives (15–35%) can occur with TVS if the ectopic is small or concealed by uterine abnormalities such as fibroids or by the bowel [32]. Repeat ultrasound examination can be carried out and will be guided by the patient's clinical condition. If TVS is inconclusive and clinical suspicion remains, diagnostic laparoscopy is the gold standard investigation for ectopic pregnancy [23].

4.4 Management of Ectopic Pregnancy

4.4.1 Expectant Management

Ectopic pregnancy can resolve spontaneously through regression or tubal abortion. The National Institute for Health and Care Excellence (NICE) guidelines recommend offering expectant management to women who:

- Are clinically stable and pain-free
- Have a tubal pregnancy measuring less that 35 mm with no visible heartbeat on ultrasound scan
- Have serum β-hCG levels of 1000 IU/L or less
- Can easily return for follow-up

As tubal rupture can occur even when β-hCG levels are low, these patients should be closely monitored until β-hCG levels fall below 15 IU/L [29].

4.4.2   Medical Management

Medical treatment can be used in patients with an unruptured tubal ectopic pregnancy who are hemodynamically stable [33]. Methotrexate is the most widely used medication for ectopic pregnancy and is usually delivered intramuscularly in either single dose, two doses, or multidose protocols [32, 34]. NICE guidelines recommend that methotrexate should be the first-line management for women who are able to return for follow up and who have:

- No significant pain
- An unruptured ectopic pregnancy with no visible heartbeat
- Serum β-hCG between 1500 and 5000 IU/L
- No intrauterine pregnancy (as confirmed on ultrasound scan)

Patients in whom surgical intervention is predicted to be difficult, such as multiple previous laparotomies, can be suitable for a trial of medical management if their clinical condition allows. Due to the potential serious side effect profile of methotrexate (hepatotoxicity and bone marrow toxicity), regular full blood count, liver function, and renal function tests are required. Serial assessment of β-hCG levels is also carried out to ensure the level is declining.

4.4.3   Surgical Management

The majority of tubal ectopic pregnancies are managed surgically [35]. Surgical management is necessary for hemodynamically unstable patients and in those for whom expectant or medical management is not deemed suitable. Surgery should be offered to women with an ectopic pregnancy who are unable to return for methotrexate monitoring or who have:

- Significant pain
- Adnexal mass of 35 mm or larger
- Fetal heartbeat visible on ultrasound
- Serum β-hCG level of 5000 IU/L or more [36]

Numerous studies have shown that a laparoscopic approach confers far lower morbidity than laparotomy, by reducing operative time and blood loss, analgesia requirements, need for blood transfusion, less adhesion formation, and length of stay postoperatively [35, 37–39]. The surgical options for a tubal ectopic pregnancy are salpingectomy or salpingotomy. If the contralateral tube if healthy, a salpingectomy should be performed, where the fallopian tube is removed [35, 36]. In women with fertility-reducing factors such as previous ectopic pregnancy, contralateral tubal damage, or previous pelvic inflammatory disease, a salpingotomy should be performed where the ectopic pregnancy is dissected out of the fallopian tube, leaving the tube in situ [35, 36]. One in five women may need further treatment after salpingotomy which may include methotrexate and/or salpingectomy [36].

5 Ovarian Cysts

5.1 Overview

Ovarian cysts are an important differential diagnosis to consider in the management of women presenting with lower abdominal pain. Ovarian cysts are most common in women of reproductive age with the mean age of diagnosis ranging from 27 to 30 years, with a reported 4% of women being admitted to hospital with an ovarian cyst [40–43]. The majority are functional cysts including corpus luteum cysts and follicular cysts, but endometrioma or "chocolate cysts" and dermoid cysts can also present acutely, but rarely.

5.2 Cyst Rupture and Hemorrhage

Ovarian cyst rupture and hemorrhage are essentially physiological events during the ovarian cycle involving the corpus luteum or the follicle. *Mittelschmerz* is the term to describe the physiologic rupture of a corpus luteum cyst during ovulation which often causes sudden-onset localized unilateral pain as fluid is spilled into the peritoneal cavity and tends to resolve within 48 h [40, 43]. Ovarian cyst rupture most commonly occurs on the right side and therefore may be difficult to differentiate from acute appendicitis [41, 43].

5.2.1 Clinical Presentation

Sudden-onset, acute abdominal pain is the most frequent presenting symptom of a hemorrhagic or ruptured ovarian cyst, but symptoms such as vaginal bleeding, vomiting, and syncope have also been reported [40]. Generally, most women remain systemically well but may have some peritoneal irritation although it is not usually associated with pyrexia, tachycardia, or raised inflammatory markers [43]. Rupture of a large hemorrhagic cyst can result in hemorrhagic shock.

5.2.2 Investigation

The diagnosis of an ovarian cyst accident is made clinically with the use of blood tests and imaging. TVS is the preferred imaging modality in adults and transabdominal in children. Many women develop physiological cysts that are found incidentally, and therefore, clinical correlation is required, as the presence of an ovarian cyst does not always mean it will be the cause of presenting symptoms. Similarly, free fluid in the pouch of Douglas can indicate a ruptured cyst, but 40% of women will have some sonographically detected free fluid in the pouch of Douglas during normal ovulation [43]. A full overview of investigations for ovarian cyst accidents can be seen in Table 3 [43].

Table 3 Investigations for suspected ovarian cyst accidents (Bottomley et al. 2009)

Investigations for suspected ovarian cyst accidents
A urinary pregnancy test must always be performed in women of reproductive age with abdominal pain
Full blood count, urea and electrolytes, and possibly liver function and coagulation screen (depending on the clinical situation) should be taken
The white cell count may be raised in torsion but also with appendicitis, infection, and a pelvic abscess
Urine dipstick to rule out urinary infection or calculus
Triple swabs for infection should be taken if PID is a possible differential diagnosis from the history and examination
Transvaginal ultrasound examination (transabdominal in children) should be arranged preferably at the time of presentation
Transabdominal ultrasound or CT scan to examine the appendix or other abdominal causes if the adnexae appear normal on TVS and clinical concern remains
Ca125 should not usually be taken as it is particularly nonspecific in the acute setting

5.2.3 Management

Ovarian cysts can be managed conservatively with analgesia and observation. Simple cysts can be expectantly managed if asymptomatic up to 10 cm in the adult but carry a risk of torsion. Surgical intervention is indicated for patients who have [44]:

- No relief of symptoms within 48 h of presentation
- Signs of worsening hemorrhage
- Diagnostic uncertainty or possibility of torsion [40, 43]

Laparoscopic ovarian cystectomy is the preferred surgical intervention, combined with a copious washout. Where there is uncontrollable hemorrhage, oophorectomy may be indicated. Laparotomy should be reserved for cases in which laparoscopy is unsafe or not feasible.

5.3 Other Ovarian Cysts

5.3.1 Endometriotic Cysts

Endometriosis corresponds to the ectopic endometrial glands and stroma outside the uterine cavity. Endometriotic cysts/endometriomas generally occur within the ovaries and are the result of repeated cyclic hemorrhage within a deep implant [41]. Surgery is generally avoided where possible in patients with endometriosis due to the risk of damage to adjacent organs, adhesion formation, lack of improvement in pain, or recurrence of disease/pain. Rupture of these cysts is relatively rare, but emergency surgical intervention may be indicated to reduce the dissemination of endometriotic cyst fluid, prevent adhesions, and preserve fertility [45].

5.3.2 Dermoid Cysts

Approximately 20–25% of all ovarian neoplasms are germ cell tumors, and over 95% of these are benign mature teratomas or dermoid cysts [46]. Dermoid cysts present with symptoms such as abdominal pain, nausea, and vomiting, and signs can include abdominal tenderness and a palpable mass. Most dermoid cysts are diagnosed by ultrasonography [47]. They should be referred to gynecology and laparoscopically excised due to the risk of ovarian torsion, spontaneous rupture, or malignancy.

5.3.3 Ovarian Cysts in Postmenopausal Women

Special consideration must be given to the management of ovarian cysts in post-menopausal women due to the higher risk of malignancy. A full history including risk factors and family history should be obtained. Serum cancer antigen 125 (CA125) and TVS are the initial investigations of choice [48]. The findings of these investigations will be used to calculate the risk of malignancy index (RMI), triaging women into low and high risk of malignancy groups. Where the initial imaging was a CT scan, an ultrasound scan should be obtained in order to correctly calculate the score [48].

6   Adnexal Torsion

6.1   Overview

Adnexal torsion is an uncommon gynecological emergency, representing approximately 3% of emergency presentations [40, 49, 50]. Adnexal torsion is defined as a partial or complete twisting of the uterine adnexa around its vascular pedicle, including the infundibulopelvic ligament and tubo-ovarian ligament [40]. Torsion results in a mechanical impairment to vascular and lymphatic flow which can result in arterial compromise and ovarian necrosis. Adnexal torsion occurs more commonly in the right adnexa, possibly due to the longer utero-ovarian ligament and the resulting hypermobility [40]. The left adnexa has decreased mobility likely due to the presence of the sigmoid colon [51]. In adults, adnexal torsion is commonly associated with an adnexal mass such as a cyst or neoplasm, which provides a fixed point around which the adnexa might twist [1]. In children and adolescents, however, as many as 46% of cases involve an ovary without an associated mass and are thought to be due to con-genitally long ovarian ligaments, excessive laxity of the pelvic ligaments, or a rela-tively small uterus that allows more space for the adnexa to twist [52, 53]. Patients who have undergone previous pelvic surgery are at an increased risk for adnexal torsion, possibly due to the presence of pelvic adhesions around which the adnexa may twist [54, 55]. Other risk factors are detailed in Table 4.

6.2   Clinical Presentation

The preoperative diagnosis of adnexal torsion is challenging because of its nonspe-cific clinical presentation. It typically presents with sudden-onset severe unilateral pain in the lower abdomen with associated nausea and/or vomiting [60–63]. Pain can be intermittent, waxing, and waning, which may indicate intermittent torsion.

Table 4 Risk factors for adnexal torsion

Risk factors for adnexal torsion
Previous adnexal torsion [56]
Assisted conception and ovarian hyperstimulation syndrome
• Ovulation induction leads to increase size and weight of ovary [57]
Successful pregnancy
• Enlarged corpus luteal cysts increase rate of torsion in the first trimester [58]
Benign adnexal masses and cysts
Polycystic ovarian syndrome
Previous tubal ligation [59]

On examination, abdominal tenderness is the main finding but rebound tenderness and guarding may be present. An abdominal mass is palpable in 24% of cases [63]. If necrosis has developed, a fever and leukocytosis may be present.

6.3 Investigation

The diagnosis of adnexal torsion is clinical, but investigations can be used to generate a differential diagnosis. β-hCG testing must be performed. Urinalysis may show blood and/or leukocytes, but positive urine cultures are not common [63, 64]. Mild elevations in white blood cell counts are seen in 20–62% of women, but surgery should not be delayed for results of inflammatory markers if there is high clinical suspicion [52, 53, 64–66].

Ultrasound is the gold standard imaging choice for adnexal torsion as it can evaluate ovarian anatomy and blood flow [59]. Transabdominal ultrasonography has a sensitivity of 92% and a specificity of 96% in detecting adnexal torsion and is the imaging of choice in pediatric and adolescent patients [67]. In adults, TVS should be used wherever possible but transabdominal imaging is acceptable [59]. Doppler ultrasound can confirm arterial flow to the ovary; however, preserved arterial flow can be seen in cases of early torsion [68]. Computed tomography has a low sensitivity of 42.2% at identifying adnexal torsion so should not be used as a first-line investigation [63, 67]. CT is commonly used in the assessment of lower abdominal pain, and if adnexal torsion is reported, no further investigations are required prior to surgical management. Magnetic resonance imaging does not offer improved sensitivity compared with ultrasound. It may be helpful, however, when torsion is suspected during pregnancy because of its ability to better characterize the adnexal mass [68]. Typical findings of adnexal torsion on imaging are shown in Table 5 [52, 53, 68, 69].

6.4 Management

Urgent surgical intervention is indicated when adnexal torsion is suspected because ovarian viability decreases with increased time from onset of pain to time of surgery [53]. The duration of vascular compromise to produce irreversible

Table 5 Appearances of adnexal torsion on imaging

Appearances of adnexal torsion on imaging	
Ultrasound	Increased ovarian size
	Abnormal location of the adnexa compared to the uterus
	Free fluid
	Peripheral distribution of follicles
	Absent Doppler arterial flow (can be preserved)
	Whirlpool sign (coiled vascular pedicle)
Computed tomography	Asymmetric ovarian enlargement
	Peripheral follicle distribution
	Whirlpool sign
	Fallopian tube thickening
	Inflammatory fat stranding
	Free fluid
	Uterine deviation toward torsion
Magnetic resonance	Asymmetric ovarian enlargement
	Peripheral follicle distribution
	Stromal edema
	Coiled pedicle

damage is unknown, and normal ovarian function has been reported up to 72 h after torsion [53, 64]. A 10-year retrospective study showed that girls with suspected adnexal torsion waited twice as long for imaging and surgical intervention compared to boys with suspected testicular torsion [70].

The standard management of adnexal torsion is laparoscopy and detorsion with salvage of the adnexa [54, 55]. The appearance of the ovary at laparoscopy is not a reliable indicator of ovarian viability, with multiple studies reporting future ovarian function despite a grossly ischemic appearance at the time of surgery [71–73]. A blue/black ovary may appear not to improve after detorsion, but relook laparoscopy at 36 h can show near normal-appearing ovaries [50]. If a cyst is present, a cystectomy can be performed. Oophoropexy is a procedure used to fix the ovary in position, limiting its range of movement. The indications for oophoropexy are repeated torsion or an absent contralateral ovary [74, 75]. Oophorectomy or adnexectomy should be reserved for cases of severe vascular compromise, necrosis, peritonitis, or an ovarian mass [40].

7   Summary

There are many indications for laparoscopy in women with gynecologic emergencies. Often, these diseases can be encountered by a general surgeon. The use of laparoscopy in these instances has the same benefit as laparoscopy in other surgical specialties and, when allowable, should be utilized.

References

1. Vandermeer FQ, Wong-You-Cheong JJ. Imaging of acute pelvic pain. Clin Obstet Gynecol. 2009;52:2–20.
2. Karam AR, Birjawi GA, Sidani CA, Haddad MC. Alternative diagnoses of acute appendicitis on helical CT with intravenous and rectal contrast. Clin Imaging. 2007;31:77–86.
3. McCartan DP, Fleming FJ, Grace PA. The management of right iliac fossa pain—is timing everything? Surgeon. 2010;8:211–7.
4. Wilson MSJ, Powell-Bowns M, Robertson AG, et al. Results of a national multicenter audit assessment of gynecologic history in surgical patients. Int J Gynecol Obstet. 2017;139:197–201.
5. Ramphal SR, Moodley J. Emergency gynaecology. Best Pract Res Clin Obstet Gynaecol. 2006;20:729–50.
6. Ness RB, Smith KJ, Chang C-CH, Schisterman EF, Bass DC. Prediction of pelvic inflammatory disease among young, single, sexually active women. Sex Transm Dis. 2006;33:137–42.
7. Ross J, Guaschino S, Cusini M, Jensen J. 2017 European guideline for the management of pelvic inflammatory disease. Int J STD AIDS. 2018;29:108–14.
8. Laboratory-confirmed gonorrhea and/or chlamydia rates in clinically diagnosed pelvic inflammatory disease and cervicitis. https://reference.medscape.com/medline/abstract/22030186. Accessed 15 Apr 2021.
9. Brunham RC, Gottlieb SL, Paavonen J. Pelvic inflammatory disease. N Engl J Med. 2015;372:2039–48.
10. Granberg S, Gjelland K, Ekerhovd E. The management of pelvic abscess. Best Pract Res Clin Obstet Gynaecol. 2009;23:667–78.
11. Livengood CH. Tubo-ovarian abscess. Contemp Ob-Gyn. 1999;44:108.
12. Augustin G, Prutki M. Pelvic inflammatory disease. Cham: Springer; 2018. p. 199–206.
13. DeWitt J, Reining A, Allsworth JE, Peipert JF. Tuboovarian abscesses: is size associated with duration of Hospitalization & Complications? Obstet Gynecol Int. 2010;2010:1–5.
14. Jiang X, Shi M, Sui M, Wang T, Yang H, Zhou H, Zhao K. Clinical value of early laparoscopic therapy in the management of tubo-ovarian or pelvic abscess. Exp Ther Med. 2019;18:1115–22.
15. Topçu HO, Kokanali K, Güzel AI, Tokmak A, Erkilinç S, Ümit C, Doĵanay M. Risk factors for adverse clinical outcomes in patients with tubo-ovarian abscess. J Obstet Gynaecol (Lahore). 2015;35:699–702.
16. Akselim B, Karaşin SS, Demirci A, Üstünyurt E. Can antibiotic treatment failure in tubo-ovarian abscess be predictable? Eur J Obstet Gynecol Reprod Biol. 2021;258:253–7.
17. Kinay T, Unlubilgin E, Cirik DA, Kayikcioglu F, Akgul MA, Dolen I. The value of ultrasonographic tubo-ovarian abscess morphology in predicting whether patients will require surgical treatment. Int J Gynecol Obstet. 2016;135:77–81.
18. Rosen M, Breitkopf D, Waud K. Tubo-ovarian abscess management options for women who desire fertility. Obstet Gynecol Surv. 2009;64:681–9.
19. Theofanakis CP, Kyriakidis AV. Fitz-Hugh-Curtis syndrome. https://doi.org/10.1007/s10397-010-0642-8.
20. Lopez-Zeno JA, Keith LG, Berger GS. The Fitz-Hugh-Curtis syndrome revisited. Changing perspectives after half a century. J Reprod Med. 1985;30:567–82.
21. Banerjee B, Rennison A, Boyes BE. Sonographic features in a case of Fitz-Hugh-Curtis syndrome masquerading as malignancy. Br J Radiol. 1992;65:342–4.
22. Gaskins AJ, Missmer SA, Rich-Edwards JW, Williams PL, Souter I, Chavarro JE. Demographic, lifestyle, and reproductive risk factors for ectopic pregnancy. Fertil Steril. 2018;110:1328–37.
23. Sivalingam VN, Duncan WC, Kirk E, Shephard LA, Horne AW. Diagnosis and management of ectopic pregnancy. J Fam Plan Reprod Heal Care. 2011;37:231–40.
24. Goyaux N, Leke R, Keita N, Thonneau P. Ectopic pregnancy in African developing countries. Acta Obstet Gynecol Scand. 2003;82:305–12.

25. Leke RJ, Goyaux N, Matsuda T, Thonneau PF. Ectopic pregnancy in Africa: a population-based study. Obstet Gynecol. 2004;103:692–7.
26. Barnhart KT, Sammel MD, Gracia CR, Chittams J, Hummel AC, Shaunik A. Risk factors for ectopic pregnancy in women with symptomatic first-trimester pregnancies. Fertil Steril. 2006;86:36–43.
27. Ankum WM, Mol BW, Van der Veen F, Bossuyt PM. Risk factors for ectopic pregnancy: a meta-analysis. Fertil Steril. 1996;65:1093–9.
28. Walker JJ. Ectopic pregnancy. Clin Obstet Gynecol. 2007;50:89–99.
29. Tay JI. Regular review: ectopic pregnancy. BMJ. 2000;320:916–9.
30. Kaplan BC, Dart RG, Moskos M, Kuligowska E, Chun B, Hamid MA, Northern K, Schmidt J, Kharwadkar A. Ectopic pregnancy: prospective study with improved diagnostic accuracy. Ann Emerg Med. 1996;28:10–7.
31. Ahmed AA, Tom BDM, Calabrese P. Ectopic pregnancy diagnosis and the pseudo-sac. Fertil Steril. 2004;81:1225–8.
32. Levine D. Ectopic pregnancy. Radiology. 2007;245:385–97.
33. Mukul LV, Teal SB. Current Management of Ectopic Pregnancy. Obstet Gynecol Clin N Am. 2007;34:403–19.
34. Murray H, Baakdah H, Bardell T, Tulandi T. Diagnosis and treatment of ectopic pregnancy. CMAJ. 2005;173:905–12.
35. Elson CJ, Salim R, Potdar N, Chetty M, Ross JA, Kirk EJ. Diagnosis and management of ectopic pregnancy. BJOG Int J Obstet Gynaecol. 2016;123:e15–55.
36. National Institute for Health and Clinical Excellence. Ectopic pregnancy and miscarriage: diagnosis and initial management. NICE Guideline CG154. 2012:1–34.
37. San Lazaro Campillo IS, Meaney S, O'Donoghue K, Corcoran P. Ectopic pregnancy hospitalisations: a national population-based study of rates, management and outcomes. Eur J Obstet Gynecol Reprod Biol. 2018;231:174–9.
38. Lundorff P, Thorburn J, Hahlin M, Källfelt B, Lindblom B. Laparoscopic surgery in ectopic pregnancy: a randomized trial versus laparotomy. Acta Obstet Gynecol Scand. 1991;70:343–8.
39. Gray DT, Thorburn J, Lundorff P, Strandell A, Lindblom B. A cost-effectiveness study of a randomised trial of laparoscopy versus laparotomy for ectopic pregnancy. Lancet. 1995;345:1139–43.
40. Boyd CA, Riall TS. Unexpected gynecologic findings during abdominal surgery. Curr Probl Surg. 2012;49:195–251.
41. Lee YR. CT imaging findings of ruptured ovarian endometriotic cysts: emphasis on the differential diagnosis with ruptured ovarian functional cysts. Korean J Radiol. 2011;12:59–65.
42. Choi NJ, Rha SE, Jung SE, Choi BG, Oh SN, Byun JY, Kim MR. Ruptured endometrial cysts as a rare cause of acute pelvic pain: can we differentiate them from ruptured corpus luteal cysts on CT scan? J Comput Assist Tomogr. 2011;35:454–8.
43. Bottomley C, Bourne T. Diagnosis and management of ovarian cyst accidents. Best Pract Res Clin Obstet Gynaecol. 2009;23:711–24.
44. American College of Obstetricians and Gynecologists' Committee on Practice Bulletins—Gynecology. Practice Bulletin No. 174: evaluation and management of adnexal masses. Obstet Gynecol. 2016;128:e210–26.
45. Evangelinakis N, Grammatikakis I, Salamalekis G, Tziortzioti V, Samaras C, Chrelias C, Kassanos D. Prevalence of acute hemoperitoneum in patients with endometriotic ovarian cysts: a 7-year retrospective study. Clin Exp Obstet Gynecol. 2009;36:254–5.
46. Savasi I, Lacy JA, Gerstle JT, Stephens D, Kives S, Allen L. Management of Ovarian Dermoid Cysts in the pediatric and adolescent population. J Pediatr Adolesc Gynecol. 2009;22:360–4.
47. Rogers EM, Allen L, Kives S. The recurrence rate of ovarian dermoid cysts in pediatric and adolescent girls. J Pediatr Adolesc Gynecol. 2014;27:222–6.
48. Royal College of Obstretician and Gynaecologist. The management of ovarian cysts in postmenopausal women. 2016.
49. Balci O, Icen MS, Mahmoud AS, Capar M, Colakoglu MC. Management and outcomes of adnexal torsion: a 5-year experience. Arch Gynecol Obstet. 2011;284:643–6.

50. Adnexal torsion in adolescents: ACOG Committee Opinion No, 783. Obstet Gynecol. 2019;134:E56–E63.
51. Valsky DV, Esh-Broder E, Cohen SM, Lipschuetz M, Yagel S. Added value of the gray-scale whirlpool sign in the diagnosis of adnexal torsion. Ultrasound Obstet Gynecol. 2010;36:630–4.
52. Kives S, Gascon S, Dubuc É, Van Eyk N. No. 341-diagnosis and management of adnexal torsion in children, adolescents, and adults. J Obstet Gynaecol Canada. 2017;39:82–90.
53. Adeyemi-Fowode O, McCracken KA, Todd NJ. Adnexal torsion. J Pediatr Adolesc Gynecol. 2018;31:333–8.
54. Houry D, Abbott JT. Ovarian torsion: a fifteen-year review. Ann Emerg Med. 2001;38:156–9.
55. Lo LM, Chang SD, Horng SG, Yang TY, Lee CL, Liang CC. Laparoscopy versus laparotomy for surgical intervention of ovarian torsion. J Obstet Gynaecol Res. 2008;34:1020–5.
56. Asfour V, Varma R, Menon P. Clinical risk factors for ovarian torsion. J Obstet Gynaecol (Lahore). 2015;35:721–5.
57. Graziano A, Monte GL, Engl B, Marci R. Recurrent ovarian torsion in a pregnancy complicated by ovarian hyperstimulation syndrome. J Minim Invasive Gynecol. 2014;21(5):723–4.
58. Ginath S, Shalev A, Keidar R, et al. Differences between adnexal torsion in pregnant and non-pregnant women. J Minim Invasive Gynecol. 2012;19:708.
59. Ssi-Yan-Kai G, Rivain AL, Trichot C, Morcelet MC, Prevot S, Deffieux X, De Laveaucoupet J. What every radiologist should know about adnexal torsion. Emerg Radiol. 2018;25:51–9.
60. Aziz D, Davis V, Allen L, Langer JC. Ovarian torsion in children: is oophorectomy necessary? J Pediatr Surg. 2004;39:750–3.
61. Appelbaum H, Abraham C, Choi-Rosen J, Ackerman M. Key clinical predictors in the early diagnosis of adnexal torsion in children. J Pediatr Adolesc Gynecol. 2013;26:167–70.
62. Karaman E, Beger B, Çetin O, Melek M, Karaman Y. Ovarian torsion in the normal ovary: a diagnostic challenge in postmenarchal adolescent girls in the emergency department. Med Sci Monit. 2017;23:1312–6.
63. Rey-Bellet Gasser C, Gehri M, Joseph J-M, Pauchard J-Y. Is it ovarian torsion? A systematic literature review and evaluation of prediction signs. Pediatr Emerg Care. 2016;32:256–61.
64. Poonai N, Poonai C, Lim R, Lynch T. Pediatric ovarian torsion: case series and review of the literature. Can J Surg. 2013;56:103–8.
65. Oelsner G, Shashar D. Adnexal torsion. Clin Obstet Gynecol. 2006;49(3):459–63.
66. Tsafrir Z, Azem F, Hasson J, et al. Risk factors, symptoms, and treatment of ovarian torsion in children: the twelve-year experience of one center. J Minim Invasive Gynecol. 2012;19:29–33.
67. Bronstein ME, Pandya S, Snyder CW, Shi Q, Muensterer OJ. A meta-analysis of b-mode ultrasound, Doppler ultrasound, and computed tomography to diagnose pediatric ovarian torsion. Eur J Pediatr Surg. 2015;25:82–6.
68. Lourenco AP, Swenson D, Tubbs RJ, Lazarus E. Ovarian and tubal torsion: imaging findings on US, CT, and MRI. Emerg Radiol. 2014;21:179–87.
69. Wilkinson C, Sanderson A. Adnexal torsion—a multimodality imaging review. Clin Radiol. 2012;67:476–83.
70. Piper H, Oltmann S, Xu L, et al. Ovarian torsion: diagnosis of inclusion mandates earlier intervention. J Pediatr Surg. 2012;47:2071–6.
71. Göçmen A, Karaca M, Sari A. Conservative laparoscopic approach to adnexal torsion. Arch Gynecol Obstet. 2008;277:535–8.
72. Galinier P, Carfagna L, Delsol M, Ballouhey Q, Lemasson F, Le Mandat A, Moscovici J, Guitard J, Pienkowski C, Vaysse P. Ovarian torsion. Management and ovarian prognosis: a report of 45 cases. J Pediatr Surg. 2009;44:1759–65.
73. Wang JH, Wu DH, Jin H, Wu YZ. Predominant etiology of adnexal torsion and ovarian outcome after detorsion in premenarchal girls. Eur J Pediatr Surg. 2010;20:298–301.
74. Fuchs N, Smorgick N, Tovbin Y, Ben Ami I, Maymon R, Halperin R, Pansky M. Oophoropexy to prevent adnexal torsion: how, when, and for whom? J Minim Invasive Gynecol. 2010;17:205–8.
75. Comeau IM, Hubner N, Kives SL, Allen LM. Rates and technique for Oophoropexy in pediatric ovarian torsion: a single-institution case series. J Pediatr Adolesc Gynecol. 2017;30:418–21.

Role of Emergency Laparoscopy in Pediatric Patients

Robert B. Laverty and Margaret E. Gallagher

1   Background

Since its advent, minimally invasive surgery has slowly replaced open surgery to become the favored approach for many pediatric procedures, even in the acute care setting. An estimated 80,000 of these procedures are performed annually in the USA, 40% of which are performed in adult hospitals [1, 2]. Given the relative shortage of pediatric surgeons, especially in rural areas, many of these surgeries are being performed by dedicated general surgeons. Studies have shown equivalent outcomes among both pediatric-trained and general surgeons for commonly performed general surgery procedures (e.g., appendectomies, small bowel obstructions, and cholecystectomies), while superior outcomes were shown in less commonly performed general surgery procedures (e.g., pyloromyotomy) when done by a pediatric-trained surgeon [3, 4]. This chapter seeks to prepare acute care surgeons to manage these types of urgent pediatric cases.

R. B. Laverty
Department of Surgery, Brooke Army Medical Center, Fort Sam Houston, TX, USA
e-mail: Robert.b.laverty.mil@health.mil

M. E. Gallagher (✉)
Department of Surgery, Brooke Army Medical Center, Fort Sam Houston, TX, USA

Department of Surgery, Blanchfield Army Community Hospital, Fort Campbell, KY, USA

Department of Pediatric Surgery, Vanderbilt University Medical Center, Nashville, TN, USA
e-mail: margaret.e.gallagher@vumc.org; margaret.e.gallagher23.mil@health.mil

2 General Considerations

The advantages of laparoscopic surgery when compared to open approaches are well known and hold true for pediatric patients: decreased pain, shorter hospital length of stay, fewer wound infections, and lower overall morbidity [5]. The same principles of laparoscopic surgery for adult patients also apply in this population. Differences in body habitus, however, often mandate smaller equipment and slight variations in technique.

Just as it is in adults, gaining access to the abdomen is one of the most critical steps of these procedures. Prior to the start of an operation, providers should have a foley catheter placed or use the Credé's maneuver in infants (manual pressure exerted externally on the bladder) to decompress the bladder. This is especially important given that the bladder is intra-abdominally located in the younger patient. The open Hasson technique is the most commonly employed, typically through or around the umbilical ring. During the first few years of life, the abdomen can be entered through the umbilical ring prior to closure. To do so, one should elevate the umbilical skin using a toothed forceps and make a vertical incision with a scalpel. A hemostat can then be used to bluntly enter the abdomen through the natural opening, and the ring can then be extended safely to the appropriate size needed for the trocar. A Veress access may also be employed acknowledging the decreased distance between the skin and major vessels. If a surgeon is not knowledgeable in the Veress approach, then this technique should not be used in a young child.

In infants, special care must be taken to avoid cannulating the umbilical vein with the trocar. Insufflation into such can result in a massive air embolus and cardiopulmonary collapse. To decrease this risk, once the trocar is placed through the umbilicus, the camera can be inserted prior to insufflation to ensure intra-abdominal and not intravenous trocar insertion has been achieved. Additionally, the trocar should be aimed superiorly during insertion to avoid injury to the aortic bifurcation, iliac vessels, and bladder.

Ports usually range from 3 to 5 mm in size, though most toddlers will be able to tolerate a 12 mm port. Whereas adult length trocars are 10–15 cm in length, pediatric ones are 6 cm long. As mentioned, pediatric instruments are typically shorter and smaller as well. A comparison of the 5 mm and 3 mm instrument heads is seen in Fig. 1 [6]. For insufflation in neonates and infants, lower pressure (8–10 mmHg) and flow rates (3–5 L/min) should be used as compared to larger children and adults [7]. The lowest pressure possible should be used to achieve adequate working space.

Fig. 1 Comparison of 3
and 5 mm laparoscopic
instrument heads

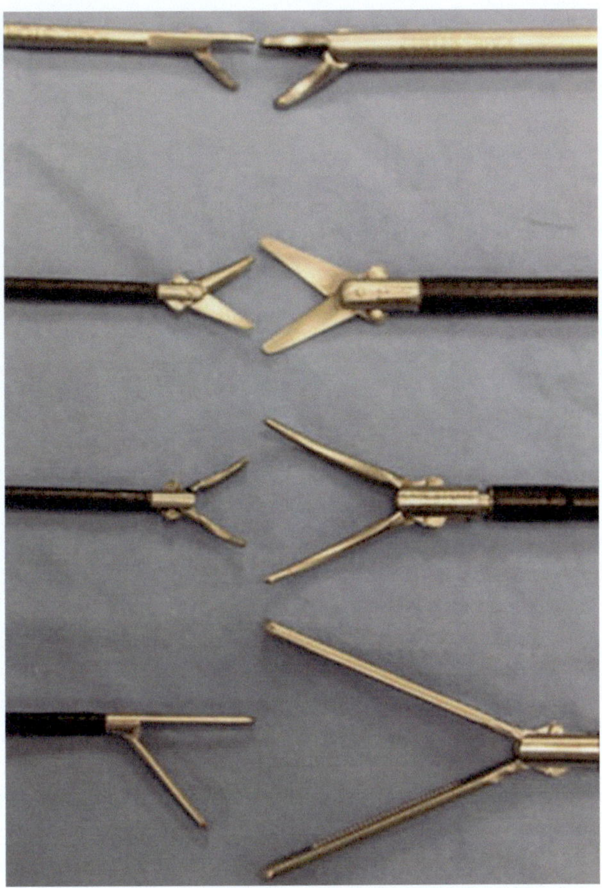

3   Appendicitis

Appendicitis is the most common pediatric diagnosis requiring urgent surgery in the USA [1]. For uncomplicated appendicitis, the three-port standard laparoscopic appendectomy (SLA) remains the typical treatment for this disease process and is well described throughout the literature [8]. During SLA, providers are not limited to endoscopic staplers for transection of the appendiceal base. Hem-o-lok clips and endoloop closure devices have been demonstrated to be safe and cost-effective alternatives [9, 10]. These are placed at the base of the appendix, which is then transected distal to these closure devices.

The single-incision laparoscopic appendectomy (SILA), however, has gained popularity in recent years due to technological advancements and to further enhance cosmesis [11]. The SILA is performed through a transumbilical incision. Upon entering the peritoneum, a 10 mm, 0° operative scope with a 5 mm working channel is placed. Pneumoperitoneum is then established, and the

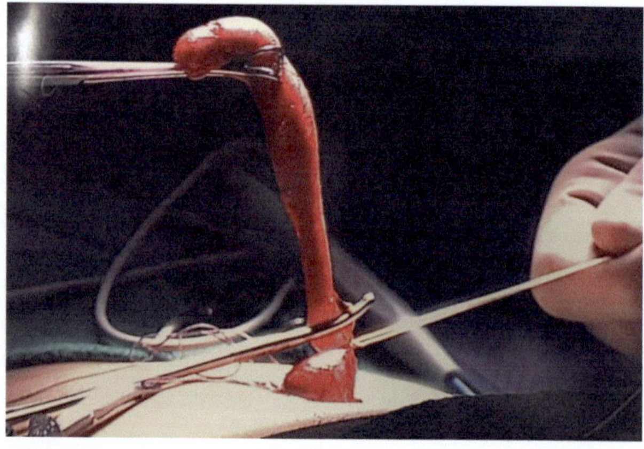

Fig. 2 The appendix has been brought out through the transumbilical port site in a single-incision laparoscopic appendectomy. The mesoappendix has been divided and the base of the appendix is about to be transected

appendix is grasped and exteriorized through the umbilical port site. Mobilization of the cecum may be required which can be accomplished through blunt or sharp dissection using instruments or finger sweeps. The appendix is resected extracorporeally in a similar fashion to an open appendectomy, as seen in Fig. 2. The stump can be inverted with a purse-string suture, and the cecum is returned to the abdominal cavity [12]. Interestingly, compared to SLA, SILA has been associated with shorter hospital stays, lower cost, and better wound cosmesis [13–15].

Multi-institutional trials are ongoing to more definitively answer the question regarding the efficacy of medical management alone in uncomplicated appendicitis. Previous studies have shown this to be associated with a 1-year success rate of greater than 70%, decreased disability days, and lower cost [16–18]. The management of complicated appendicitis—with the known presence of a phlegmon or abscess—is more controversial. Nonoperative management of complicated appendicitis is most commonly used in patients with long duration of symptoms, at least 3 days, as long as there is no diffuse peritonitis, obstruction, or mass [19]. In these patients, if there is a drainable fluid collection, a drain should be placed into the discrete, walled-off abscesses and maintained until their output is minimal. However, recent studies have shown improvement in return to normal activity and decreased complications when early appendectomy is performed (within 24 h of admission) for perforated appendicitis [20]. Patients with concern for ongoing sepsis due to appendicitis should undergo source control through open or minimally invasive means.

4   Inguinal Hernia

Inguinal hernias are common in the pediatric patient population, with an estimated incidence of 1–5% in full-term infants [21]. The vast majority of these are indirect and arise from a patent processus vaginalis (or canal of Nuck in females). In males, the small intestines are the most commonly herniated intra-abdominal contents, whereas the ovaries are more common in females [22]. Patients will typically present with a lump or swelling in the groin area. Upon initial examination, providers should attempt to reduce the hernia. Gentle pressure should be applied superiorly and laterally at the superficial inguinal ring using one's thumb and index finger to direct the hernia toward the internal ring. Providers should use circular motion and additional, gradual pressure to help coax it back into the abdominal cavity. Displacement of the scrotum medially and gentle tension on the testicle may also facilitate reduction [23].

In the setting of strangulated or irreducible inguinal hernias, urgent surgical repair is warranted. Benefits to laparoscopic repair include decreased postoperative morbidity (e.g., scrotal edema, testicular atrophy, and wound infection), avoidance of the edematous groin, the ability to inspect both the bowel for viability, and the ability to inspect the contralateral side for the presence of a bilateral hernia [24]. There are multiple different techniques for laparoscopic inguinal hernia repair in children; one can be seen in Fig. 3. All techniques include a high ligation of the hernia sac [25]. Mesh is typically not placed in pediatric repairs.

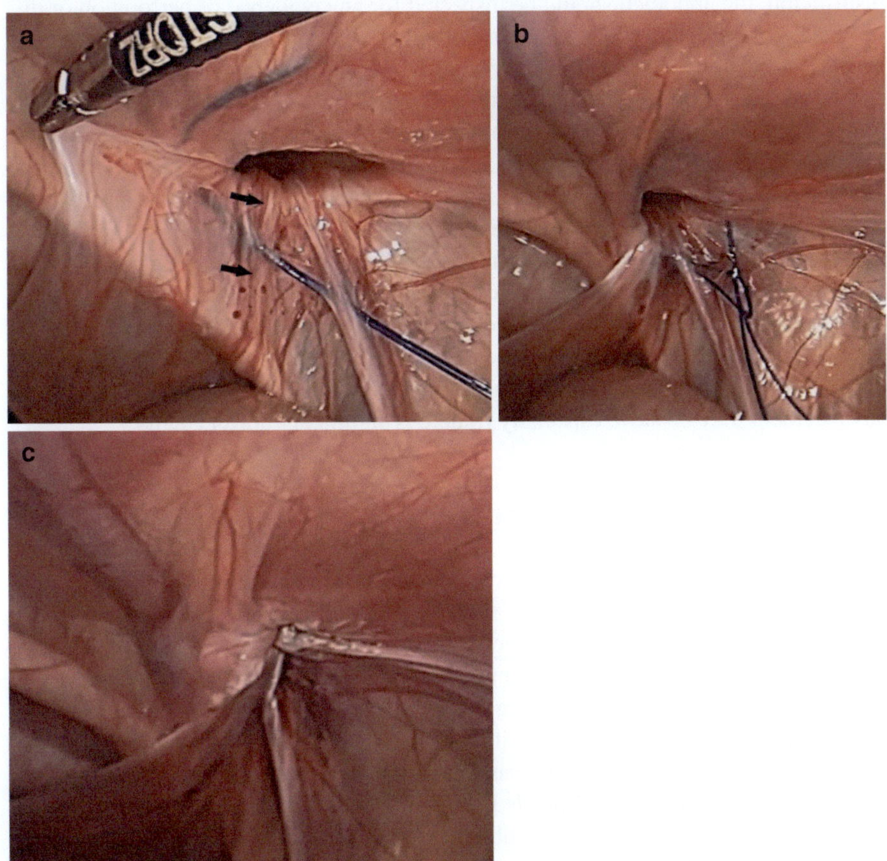

Fig. 3 In this view of a right inguinal hernia, the large indirect hernia is seen (**a**), and a suture has been passed using a Tuohy needle through the peritoneum after passing between the peritoneum and the vas deferens (arrow) and testicular vessels. The double loop technique is seen (**b**) with complete closure of the ring in (**c**)

5   Intussusception

Intussusception is a frequent cause of bowel obstructions in pediatric patients. This is defined as an invagination of a proximal portion of the bowel into a distal section of the bowel, usually in the setting of a lead point (children older than 5) or enlarged lymphoid tissue (age less than 5). Intussusception most frequently occurs before the age of two. Peak incidence is between 5 and 10 months of age [19]. Radiographic reduction with pneumatic or hydrostatic enemas remains the first-line treatment in the pediatric population with success rates reported in up to 90% of patients [26]. In the setting of failure of conservative management, multiple recurrences, or suspicion of a pathologic lead point, operative intervention is indicated. Laparoscopy has been demonstrated to be a safe and effective approach in these settings [27].

Generally, three ports are placed, although a single-incision technique may also be employed. Initial port placement should be a periumbilical or umbilical incision. After insufflation, the abdomen should be inspected for any evidence of perforation or disseminated disease. After identification of the intussusception, two other ports should be placed to allow triangulation for visualization and manipulation of the bowel. In order to then perform reduction, gentle tension or traction should be applied to the intussusceptum (the proximal bowel), while pressure is applied on the edge of the intussuscipiens (the distal bowel). This combination of tension and pressure has been avoided in the open approach but has been shown to be safe and effective laparoscopically [19]. The intussusceptum is then carefully reduced. Once reduced, the bowel should be inspected for viability and to identify any potential pathologic lead points. If there is failure to reduce the intussusception or bowel is not viable upon reduction, then one can proceed with a bowel resection through a transumbilical incision or right lower quadrant incision. Laparoscopic reduction has an approximate success rate of 85% [28]. Patients can be started on a liquid diet and advanced as tolerated. Diet advancement may be slow, especially if there is significant bowel edema.

6   Meckel's Diverticulum

A Meckel's diverticulum is a true diverticulum that typically arises from the antimesenteric portion of the ileum as a result of the incomplete obliteration of the vitelline, or omphalomesenteric, duct. When symptomatic, these can present as a gastrointestinal bleed (due to the presence of ectopic gastric mucosa), a bowel obstruction from a volvulus or internal hernia, or as a lead point in an intussusception. A Meckel's may also present similarly to appendicitis, as diverticulitis or perforation. When a normal appendix is encountered during a surgery for suspected appendicitis, the small bowel needs to be ran at least 2 ft back from the ileocecal valve to ensure a Meckel's diverticulitis isn't causing the child's symptoms. When discovered incidentally in a pediatric patient, there is still debate surrounding whether to proceed with resection. Many studies state that the lifetime risk of a serious complication from the Meckel's outweighs the risk of the operation, specifically in children less than 8 years of age [29]. A 4% lifetime likelihood of bleeding, obstruction, diverticulitis, or perforation has been previously reported [30]. This

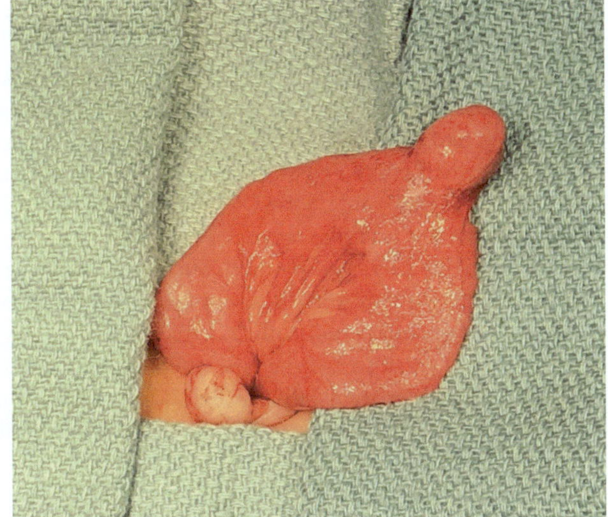

Fig. 4 A Meckel's diverticulum has been brought through the umbilical incision along with the adjacent ileum in order for a segmental bowel resection to be performed

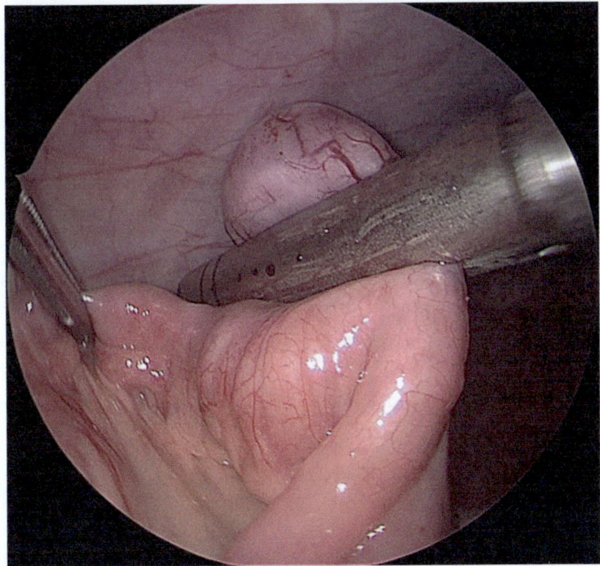

Fig. 5 Laparoscopic diverticulectomy is performed for a bleeding Meckel's, ensuring adequate diameter of the adjacent ileum

resection can be accomplished laparoscopically either via segmental small bowel resection or with a stapled diverticulectomy. If a segmental bowel resection is performed, this can be completed through the umbilical incision as seen in Fig. 4. The laparoscopic diverticulectomy-only approach has been shown to reduce hospital length of stay and operative time as compared to segmental resection. Complete, margin-free resection of the gastric mucosa has been demonstrated via diverticulectomy when these are taken at the base with endoscopic stapling devices [31]. When performing a diverticulectomy, as seen in Fig. 5, care needs to be taken to ensure there is no narrowing of the adjacent small bowel.

7   Pyloric Stenosis

Frequently seen in 2–10-week-old infants, pyloric stenosis is another common pediatric diagnosis requiring acute surgical care. This can be fatal if left untreated as dehydration and malnutrition can occur from this gastric outlet obstructive process. The surgery itself is not an emergency, but the resuscitation of the child is. A recent retrospective review of ACS NSQIP data revealed that the management of this process by minimally invasive means has increased in recent years. The authors demonstrated that laparoscopic pyloromyotomy, as compared to open pyloromyotomy, was associated with a shorter hospital length of stay, decreased rates of surgical site infection, and overall complications without a difference in rates of reoperation [32].

After diagnosis of pyloric stenosis, close attention should be paid to the patient's fluid and electrolyte status. Hypokalemia, hypochloremia, and metabolic alkalosis are common and need to be corrected prior to taking the patient to the operating room. Access to the abdominal cavity can be typically performed directly through the umbilicus with a 3 or 5 mm port. After insufflation, usually only to a set pressure of 8 mmHg, a 3 mm nontraumatic bowel grasper or pyloric (Geiger) clamp is placed laterally in the right upper quadrant through a stab incision, and a third 3 mm incision is made in the left upper quadrant. The proximal duodenum or pylorus should then be grasped gently and retracted to expose the hypertrophic pylorus from under the edge of the liver. Using Bovie monopolar energy on cutting mode or a pyloromyotomy knife, an incision is then made from the duodenal side of the pylorus to the stomach carrying it through the serosa and underlying muscle fibers while keeping the submucosal layer intact. A bowel grasper or pyloric muscle spreader can then be used to spread and further separate the pyloric musculature. The two sides of the divided pyloric muscle should be able to move independently from one another, and the submucosa should bulge into the myotomy site. Figure 6 shows the laparoscopic view of a hypertrophic pylorus and a completed pyloromyotomy with bulging submucosa. At the conclusion of the case, a leak test should be performed.

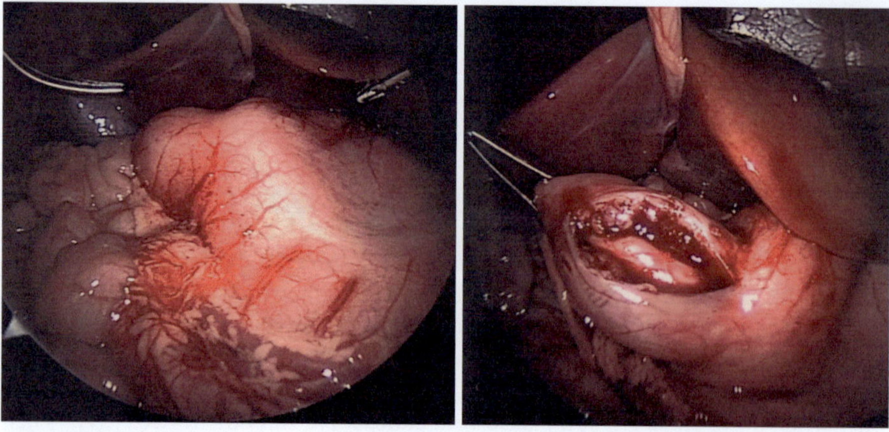

Fig. 6 Laparoscopic view of the hypertrophic pylorus and completed myotomy

As mentioned above, a systematic review of patient outcomes following pyloro-myotomy when performed by different surgical specialties demonstrated improved overall morbidity when treated by pediatric surgeons or general surgeons with oper-ative volumes of over four cases per year [3]. Acute care general surgeons should be prepared to handle these types of cases, though, and recognize their limitations when doing so. This should only be considered if adequate volume per year is expected, patient has access to a children's unit, and there is appropriate pediatric anesthetic and medical care available. The learning curve for laparoscopic pyloro-myotomy is believed to be 35 cases, at which time there is a decline in the rate of incomplete myotomies or mucosal perforations [33]. As with all surgeries that can be performed laparoscopically or open, a surgeon should do which operation they are most comfortable with.

8   Ovarian Pathology

Ovarian cysts, neoplasms, and torsion can occur in the female pediatric population. In these patients, prompt diagnosis and treatment of these conditions are of the utmost importance to minimize complications and risk of infertility. Minimally invasive approaches are acceptable for each of these diseases.

Treatment options for ovarian cysts include aspiration or resection, fenestration, unroofing, cysto-ovariectomy, and cysto-adnexectomy, the choice of which depends on the size and character of the cyst, ability to preserve ovarian tissue, and operator experience [34]. Benign neoplasms should be removed via ovarian-sparing tech-niques. If a malignant process is suspected, consideration should be given to trans-fer to a pediatric subspecialist.

While ultrasonography is typically used for diagnosis of ovarian torsion, diag-nostic laparoscopy may be required in the setting of unclear patient presentations and/or imaging. Tenets of these operations include ovarian and fertility preservation and oophorectomy should be avoided if possible. The black-blue appearance of ovaries in the setting of torsion can be deceptive and does not always indicate irre-versible ischemia. Ovarian detorsion should be performed if the diagnosis is con-firmed. In the setting of concomitant ovarian pathology, these should also be addressed in the same operation to prevent recurrence.

9   Conclusion

With further technologic advances and increased evidence of efficacy, the use of laparoscopy in the pediatric population for surgical emergencies will likely continue to grow. Appendicitis, inguinal hernias, intussusception, Meckel's diverticulum, pyloric stenosis, and select ovarian pathology are examples of surgical problems that may be managed through minimally invasive means. Surgeons should be aware of these management options and techniques.

References

1. Uribe-Leitz TMA, Sturgeon DJ, et al. Defining the national burden of pediatric emergency general surgery. J Am Coll Surg. 2018;227(4):S143.
2. Somme S, Bronsert M, Morrato E, Ziegler M. Frequency and variety of inpatient pediatric surgical procedures in the United States. Pediatrics. 2013;132(6):e1466–72. https://doi.org/10.1542/peds.2013-1243.
3. Evans C, van Woerden HC. The effect of surgical training and hospital characteristics on patient outcomes after pediatric surgery: a systematic review. J Pediatr Surg. 2011;46(11):2119–27. https://doi.org/10.1016/j.jpedsurg.2011.06.033.
4. Judhan RJ, Silhy R, Statler K, Khan M, Dyer B, Thompson S, et al. The integration of adult acute care surgeons into pediatric surgical care models supplements the workforce without compromising quality of care. Am Surg. 2015;81(9):854–8.
5. Buia A, Stockhausen F, Hanisch E. Laparoscopic surgery: a qualified systematic review. World J Methodol. 2015;5(4):238–54. https://doi.org/10.5662/wjm.v5.i4.238.
6. Krpata DM, Ponsky TA. Needlescopic surgery: what's in the toolbox? Surg Endosc. 2013;27(3):1040–4. https://doi.org/10.1007/s00464-012-2548-1.
7. Hunter JG, Spight DH, Sandone C, Fairman JE. Atlas of minimally invasive surgical operations. New York, NY: McGraw-Hill Education; 2018.
8. Semm K. Endoscopic appendectomy. Endoscopy. 1983;15(2):59–64. https://doi.org/10.1055/s-2007-1021466.
9. Al-Temimi MH, Berglin MA, Kim EG, Tessier DJ, Johna SD. Endostapler versus hem-O-Lok clip to secure the appendiceal stump and mesoappendix during laparoscopic appendectomy. Am J Surg. 2017;214(6):1143–8. https://doi.org/10.1016/j.amjsurg.2017.08.031.
10. White C, Hardman C, Parikh P, Ekeh AP. Endostapler vs Endoloop closure of the appendiceal stump in laparoscopic appendectomy: which has better outcomes? Am J Surg. 2020;222:413. https://doi.org/10.1016/j.amjsurg.2020.12.047.
11. Rispoli G, Armellino MF, Esposito C. One-trocar appendectomy. Surg Endosc. 2002;16(5):833–5. https://doi.org/10.1007/s00464-001-9107-5.
12. Hernandez-Martin S, Ayuso L, Molina AY, Pison J, Martinez-Bermejo MA, Perez-Martinez A. Transumbilical laparoscopic-assisted appendectomy in children: is it worth it? Surg Endosc. 2017;31(12):5372–80. https://doi.org/10.1007/s00464-017-5618-6.
13. Perea L, Peranteau WH, Laje P. Transumbilical extracorporeal laparoscopic-assisted appendectomy. J Pediatr Surg. 2018;53(2):256–9. https://doi.org/10.1016/j.jpedsurg.2017.11.012.
14. Binet A, Braïk K, Lengelle F, Laffon M, Lardy H, Amar S. Laparoscopic one port appendectomy: evaluation in pediatric surgery. J Pediatr Surg. 2018;53(11):2322–5. https://doi.org/10.1016/j.jpedsurg.2017.12.018.
15. Aly OE, Black DH, Rehman H, Ahmed I. Single incision laparoscopic appendicectomy versus conventional three-port laparoscopic appendicectomy: a systematic review and meta-analysis. Int J Surg. 2016;35:120–8. https://doi.org/10.1016/j.ijsu.2016.09.087.
16. Minneci PC, Mahida JB, Lodwick DL, Sulkowski JP, Nacion KM, Cooper JN, et al. Effectiveness of patient choice in nonoperative vs surgical management of pediatric uncomplicated acute appendicitis. JAMA Surg. 2016;151(5):408–15. https://doi.org/10.1001/jamasurg.2015.4534.
17. Tanaka Y, Uchida H, Kawashima H, Fujiogi M, Takazawa S, Deie K, et al. Long-term outcomes of operative versus nonoperative treatment for uncomplicated appendicitis. J Pediatr Surg. 2015;50(11):1893–7. https://doi.org/10.1016/j.jpedsurg.2015.07.008.
18. Svensson JF, Patkova B, Almström M, Naji H, Hall NJ, Eaton S, et al. Nonoperative treatment with antibiotics versus surgery for acute nonperforated appendicitis in children: a pilot randomized controlled trial. Ann Surg. 2015;261(1):67–71. https://doi.org/10.1097/SLA.0000000000000835.

19. Pepper VK, Stanfill AB, Pearl RH. Diagnosis and management of pediatric appendicitis, intussusception, and Meckel diverticulum. Surg Clin North Am. 2012;92(3):505–26, vii. https://doi.org/10.1016/j.suc.2012.03.011.

20. Blakely ML, Williams R, Dassinger MS, Eubanks JW, Fischer P, Huang EY, et al. Early vs interval appendectomy for children with perforated appendicitis. Arch Surg. 2011;146(6):660–5. https://doi.org/10.1001/archsurg.2011.6.

21. Weaver KL, Poola AS, Gould JL, Sharp SW, St Peter SD, Holcomb GW. The risk of developing a symptomatic inguinal hernia in children with an asymptomatic patent processus vaginalis. J Pediatr Surg. 2017;52(1):60–4. https://doi.org/10.1016/j.jpedsurg.2016.10.018.

22. Panabokke G, Clifford ID, Craig SS, Nataraja RM. Reduction of paediatric inguinal hernias. Emerg Med Australas. 2016;28(2):224–7. https://doi.org/10.1111/1742-6723.12549.

23. Yeap E, Nataraja RM, Pacilli M. Inguinal hernias in children. Aust J Gen Pract. 2020;49(1):38–43. https://doi.org/10.31128/ajgp-08-19-5037.

24. Esposito C, St Peter SD, Escolino M, Juang D, Settimi A, Holcomb GW. Laparoscopic versus open inguinal hernia repair in pediatric patients: a systematic review. J Laparoendosc Adv Surg Tech A. 2014;24(11):811–8. https://doi.org/10.1089/lap.2014.0194.

25. Smith A, Speck K. Pediatric laparoscopic inguinal hernia repair: a review of techniques. https://www.sages.org/wiki/pediatric-laparoscopic-inguinal-hernia-repair-a-review-of-techniques/.

26. Huppertz HI, Soriano-Gabarró M, Grimprel E, Franco E, Mezner Z, Desselberger U, et al. Intussusception among young children in Europe. Pediatr Infect Dis J. 2006;25(1 Suppl):S22–9. https://doi.org/10.1097/01.inf.0000197713.32880.46.

27. Apelt N, Featherstone N, Giuliani S. Laparoscopic treatment of intussusception in children: a systematic review. J Pediatr Surg. 2013;48(8):1789–93. https://doi.org/10.1016/j.jpedsurg.2013.05.024.

28. Burjonrappa SC. Laparoscopic reduction of intussusception: an evolving therapeutic option. JSLS. 2007;11(2):235–7.

29. Onen A, Ciğdem MK, Oztürk H, Otçu S, Dokucu AI. When to resect and when not to resect an asymptomatic Meckel's diverticulum: an ongoing challenge. Pediatr Surg Int. 2003;19(1–2):57–61. https://doi.org/10.1007/s00383-002-0850-z.

30. Soltero MJ, Bill AH. The natural history of Meckel's diverticulum and its relation to incidental removal. A study of 202 cases of diseased Meckel's diverticulum found in King County, Washington, over a fifteen year period. Am J Surg. 1976;132(2):168–73. https://doi.org/10.1016/0002-9610(76)90043-x.

31. Robinson JR, Correa H, Brinkman AS, Lovvorn HN. Optimizing surgical resection of the bleeding Meckel diverticulum in children. J Pediatr Surg. 2017;52(10):1610–5. https://doi.org/10.1016/j.jpedsurg.2017.03.047.

32. Kethman WC, Harris AHS, Hawn MT, Wall JK. Trends and surgical outcomes of laparoscopic versus open pyloromyotomy. Surg Endosc. 2018;32(7):3380–5. https://doi.org/10.1007/s00464-018-6060-0.

33. Oomen M, Bakx R, Peeters B, Boersma D, Wijnen M, Heij H. Laparoscopic pyloromyotomy, the tail of the learning curve. Surg Endosc. 2013;27(10):3705–9. https://doi.org/10.1007/s00464-013-2951-2.

34. Raźnikiewicz A, Korlacki W, Grabowski A. The role of laparoscopy in paediatric and adolescent gynaecology. Wideochir Inne Tech Maloinwazyjne. 2020;15(3):424–36. https://doi.org/10.5114/wiitm.2020.97817.

Minimally Invasive Surgery for Emergency General Surgery in Elderly

Kenji Okumura, Matthew McGuirk, and Rifat Latifi

1   Introduction

Emergency general surgery (EGS) and emergent trauma surgeries represent a large proportion of hospital utilization in the United States. It has been reported that 20% of the inpatient population in 2019 were EGS with an estimated inpatient cost of $341 billion [1]. Scott et al. reported the seven most common EGS procedures to be partial colectomy, small bowel resection, cholecystectomy, peptic ulcer disease (PUD), lysis of adhesions, appendectomy, and laparotomy. These seven procedures accounted for 80% of all EGS procedures [2]. Emergency surgery has been associated with a 1.2–2.4-fold risk for morbidity and mortality, and elderly patients have been associated with high complications including mortality [2].

The elderly population is rapidly increasing around the world. In the United States alone in 2015, there were 47.8 million people aged 65 or older, and the population is projected to be more than double to 98 million by 2060 [3]. The number of patients requiring an operation has outpaced even this expansive growth in the aging population [4], and it is expected to grow further.

The role of minimally invasive surgery (MIS) has been growing in all surgical specialties. Whereas surgery has traditionally required large incisions sufficient to allow the surgeon to introduce his/her hands into the body and to allow sufficient light to see the structures being operated on, innovations in MIS have allowed the surgeon to perform complex procedures with small incisions but great visualization.

K. Okumura · M. McGuirk
Department of Surgery, Westchester Medical Center, Valhalla, NY, USA
e-mail: Kenji.Okumura@wmchealth.org; Matthew.McGuirk@wmchealth.org

R. Latifi (✉)
Department of Surgery, Westchester Medical Center, Valhalla, NY, USA

Department of Surgery, New York Medical College, Valhalla, NY, USA
e-mail: Rifat.Latifi@wmchealth.org

© The Author(s), under exclusive license to Springer Nature Switzerland AG 2023
F. Coccolini et al. (eds.), *Mini-invasive Approach in Acute Care Surgery*,
Hot Topics in Acute Care Surgery and Trauma,
https://doi.org/10.1007/978-3-031-39001-2_24

The MIS approach in EGS has increased, and the outcomes of a MIS approach have shown significant improvement in the EGS [5].

Although there are limitations for MIS in EGS [6], such as hemodynamic instability and severe abdominal distention, the role of MIS in EGS has been well established. In this chapter, we discuss the role of MIS for the elderly in the several general surgery settings.

2 Esophagus

Esophageal perforation (Boerhaave's syndrome) is a rare but life-threatening spontaneous perforation and is associated with significant morbidity and mortality, especially in the elderly. Historically, thoracotomy has been the mainstay of treatment; however, it is associated with high morbidity and pain [7–9]. Minimally invasive surgical approaches have been reported with promising outcomes in terms of morbidity, length of stay, and postoperative pain [8, 9]. However, the management of Boerhaave's syndrome remains a significant challenge. Early diagnosis and prompt treatment are the keys to manage this challenge successfully. Since the survival rate is significantly decreased when diagnostic delay is longer than 24 h [10], the best, most prompt approach needs to be selected. Endoscopic approach has also been another mainstay of the treatment for esophageal perforation for the selected population [11, 12]. Due to the complexity of this selecting process, Abbas et al. proposed a perforation severity score [13] which correlates with the severity of the illness. Although the application of a MIS approach is debated in the setting of patients with early presentation and stable vital signs, MIS seems the promising and feasible approach [8]. The definite management algorithm to adopt MIS is lacking, but MIS techniques, particularly the use of robotic approach, would be one of the great treatment tools for esophageal perforation.

3 Stomach and Peptic Ulcer Disease

The incidence and prevalence of peptic ulcer disease (PUD) in developed countries, including in the United States, have declined over the years, which also shows a decrease in hospitalization and mortality related to PUD [14]. Even through the evolution of the medical treatment for PUD, surgery is the gold standard treatment for perforated PUD for elderly population. Patients requiring surgery for PUD tend to be elderly with associated comorbidities [15]. Emergency surgery for perforated PUD has been shown to have a mortality of 6–30% [16]; however, the elderly has a higher mortality. In the emergent setting, the procedure of choice for perforated PUD is determined based on the general patient's condition and location of perforation. Simple patch closure (Graham patch repair) [17] of the perforation should be considered in the setting of shock, delayed presentation, and significant medical comorbidities, especially in the elderly. MIS approaches have been widely used in the setting of perforated duodenal ulcer [18]. The outcome of MIS showed significant decrease to the length of hospital stay, wound infection, and decreased incisional hernias [19]. Compared to open procedures, laparoscopic repair of perforated PUD has a longer operating time; however, it is found to have similar postoperative results to the open approach [20–22]. Some authors warn to use a MIS approach for ages over 70 and more than 24 h of symptoms, both of which lead to high morbidity and mortality [23]. When the perforation of PUD is located in the stomach, a biopsy to rule out malignancy should be performed, and the surgeon should consider converting to laparotomy in the situations when hemodynamic instability, a large ulcer (more than 20 mm), or a perforation located at posterior wall are present [24, 25]. Currently, the literature regarding the robotic surgery approach for PUD is lacking; however, robotic surgery would be a good treatment option for PUD due to the ergonomics of robotic surgery.

4 Hepato-Pancreato-Biliary System

Pyogenic liver abscess is a rare but life-threating disease. Historically, the treatment of choice for pyogenic liver abscess has been an open surgical approach, although with the advancement of minimally invasive therapy such as image-guided percutaneous needle aspiration or catheter drainage and the availability of broad-spectrum antibiotics, patients with pyogenic liver abscess rarely require surgical interventions [26]. Surgical drainage is indicated for abscess of biliary origin; intra-abdominal collections secondary to surgery, or in cases where percutaneous drainage is contraindicated or expected to fail due to the presence of multi-loculated abscess; biliary communication; elevated urea; and creatinine and total bilirubin levels [27, 28]. In these cases, a minimally invasive approach such as a laparoscopic or robotic approach would be a reasonable option as alternative to conventional open surgery, but further studies must be conducted to support the assumption.

Over the years, laparoscopic cholecystectomy has become the standard approach for cholecystectomy. Historically, laparoscopic cholecystectomy was limited for elective settings due to increasing the risk of common bile duct injury and other morbidities. However, currently, laparoscopic cholecystectomy is one of the most common MIS procedures, even in the acute setting [29]. The outcomes of MIS include decreased pain, recovery time, morbidity, and mortality when compared to open cholecystectomy. Despite these benefits, the surgical community has been reluctant to implement the laparoscopic approach in elderly patients [30]. With advanced surgical techniques and improvement of perioperative management, early cholecystectomy is safe for the elderly [31]. Others have suggested a delayed cholecystectomy for severely ill elderly patients [31, 32]. We submit to early rather than late cholecystectomy in the elderly.

The prevalence of hospitalizations for acute pancreatitis has increased significantly in the United States since the prevalence of gallstone-related disorders and metabolic syndrome increased [33, 34]. The incidence of acute pancreatitis has increased, and the incidence of pancreatic cyst/pseudocyst has also increased in the elderly. A minimally invasive "step-up" approach was proposed in 2006 for the management of severe/necrotizing pancreatitis [35]. The initial treatment of necrotizing pancreatitis is conservative, and once peripancreatic necrosis becomes infected, mortality increases significantly [36]. Open necrosectomy was performed as treatment; however, it was associated with high mortality and morbidity [37]. The "step-up" approach consists of less invasive approaches such as percutaneous catheter drainage, endoscopic transgastric procedures, and minimally invasive necrosectomy. These procedures were started as initial treatment instead of laparotomy/necrosectomy for infected necrotizing pancreatitis (Fig. 1) [35]. The PANTER-study was conducted in the randomized setting to investigate the usefulness of this "step-up" approach; the PANTER trial conveyed the benefits in the randomized setting [38], and it has now been widely accepted [39]. With this minimally invasive "step-up" approach and improvement of critical care, the outcomes of necrotizing pancreatitis have been improving recently.

5   Small Bowel Obstruction and Hernias

Small bowel obstruction (SBO) continues to be a significant cause of morbidity and mortality in the United States. The most common causes of intestinal obstruction in developed countries are adhesions, which continue to increase as the number of surgical procedures and population of elderly increase [40, 41]. SBO in the elderly is challenging. Sakari et al. reported about half of patients with small bowel obstruction are elderly with comorbidities which predispose to postoperative complications and mortality [42]. MIS has been associated with less formation of adhesions and reduced the event of SBO [43]. While the postoperative outcomes of MIS for SBO showed better outcomes regarding the length of stay and complications, the MIS approach is challenging, especially in the setting of SBO. SBO causes dilated small bowel, which associates with the risk of bowel injury during initial access and limits the working space for surgeons. However, previous laparotomy causes adhesions,

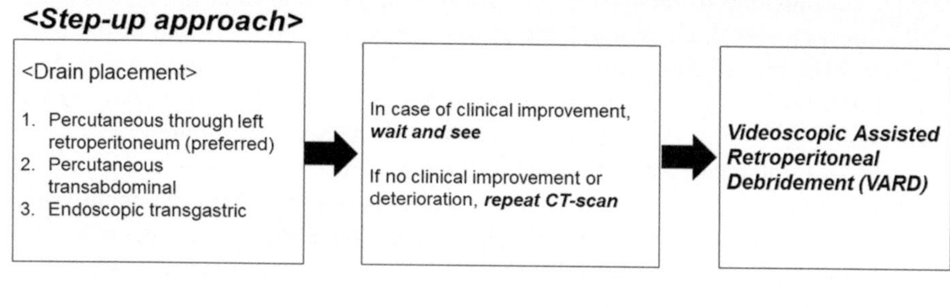

Fig. 1 Step-up approach vs. traditional approach to the management of necrotizing pancreatitis

and the MIS approach is not universally applied, but it is beneficial to perform MIS on the elderly.

Incarcerated hernia is also a surgical emergency, and the incidence of developing a hernia increases with aging [44, 45]. In the elective setting, MIS is prevalent and shows better outcomes regarding postoperative pain, incidence of postoperative complications, and length of hospital stay. In emergent situations, the open approach is still common and standard; however, some patients would benefit from a laparoscopic approach, especially in simple lysis of adhesions. Pei et al. has shown that a laparoscopic approach for SBO increased 1.6% per year and 28.7% in 2013 [46]. MIS is applied more and more in developed countries, especially in semi-elective settings. In emergent situations, the MIS approach can also be applied; however, if the chance of bowel necrosis requiring small bowel resection is high, the open approach is recommended since the laparoscopic approach requires mesh repair. The usage of synthetic mesh for emergent setting requiring bowel resection is controversial [47, 48], and biologic mesh has been supported as alternative choice for hernia repair [49, 50]. We use non-cross-linked acellular porcine dermal matrix (Strattice™) in all patients with contaminated fields requiring small bowel resection [51, 52]. We reported that elderly patients undergoing complex abdominal wall hernia repair with biologic mesh experienced similar outcomes to non-elderly patients when using propensity matching [52].

6   Appendicitis in Elderly

The incidence of acute appendicitis decreases in the elderly population, and the epidemiology and the outcomes of acute appendicitis in the elderly differ greatly from the non-elderly population [53]. In general, the risk of morbidity and mortality with appendicitis in the elderly is greater than in the younger population. Elderly patients tend to be associated with high comorbidities and experience complicated appendicitis with perforation. In a meta-analysis done in 2018, Jaschinski et al. studied the differences between laparoscopic and open appendectomy. Laparoscopic appendectomy has lower postoperative pain and less wound infections [54, 55], shorter length of stay, and a shorter time until they were able to return to normal activities. Initially, the disadvantage of laparoscopic appendectomy was reported to be a higher association of intra-abdominal abscesses [54, 56, 57]. However, after the last few decades, the outcomes became similar, and current evidence shows that there are no differences between open and laparoscopic appendectomy in intra-abdominal abscess [54, 55].

Delayed diagnosis of appendicitis is common in elderly, and this is associated with higher perforation and intra-abdominal abscess. Managing elderly with perforated appendicitis and intra-abdominal abscesses is challenging, although patients who undergo laparoscopic appendectomy have a shorter length of stay and less complications than patients who underwent open appendectomies [58]. The rate of laparoscopic surgery for perforated appendicitis has been increasing [59]. Though the laparoscopic approach is both safe and effective, there is still controversy surrounding the use of peritoneal lavage or leaving intra-abdominal drains. St. Peter et al. reported that there was no advantage to irrigating the peritoneal cavity over just suction alone [60]; they performed a randomized study for irrigation versus suction only for perforated appendicitis. They did not display any advantage to irrigation of the peritoneal cavity over suction alone [60]. Hajibandeh et al. performed a systematic review and meta-analysis and concluded that irrigation with normal saline during laparoscopic appendectomy does not provide additional benefits compared with suction alone [61]. The placement of abdominal drainage after appendectomy is a controversial matter of debate. Allemann et al. reported that the routine use of drainage was associated with longer hospital stay and higher complication rate, with a similar abdominal abscess rate [62]. There are also studies showing that leaving a drain can both decrease abscesses and lead to longer length of stay and higher wound infections [53, 63].

7   Colon and Rectum

The minimally invasive approach for colorectal surgery has been well established; however, the evidence of MIS for emergency colorectal surgery is limited [64]. In the emergent setting, laparoscopy is mainly used for a diagnostic approach, depending on the skills of the surgeon. Exploratory laparoscopy has a significantly lower morbidity and mortality compared with exploratory laparotomy in the emergency setting [65]. Depending on the findings and surgeons' skills, selected patients will be able to receive laparoscopic procedures such as repairs, resections, diversions, or ostomy creations.

With an increased number of colonoscopies, the incidence of iatrogenic colon perforation is rare, but surgeons still face the risk of iatrogenic perforation [66, 67]. Once the diagnosis of perforation is confirmed, the decision between surgical and nonoperative treatments will depend on the type of injury, the quality of the bowel perforation, the underlying colonic pathology, and the clinical condition of the patient [66, 67]. The emergent surgery approach is reasonable and safe [67]; however, select patients that experience localized pain, free air without diffuse free fluids in radiographs, hemodynamic stability, an absence of fever, and no signs of inflammation might be appropriate for nonoperative management initially; nevertheless, elderly patient require extra cautions [66–68]. In the case of failure of endoscopic treatment or signs of peritonitis, laparoscopic exploration should be considered. Early diagnosis is the key to success for treatment and lowering the risk of complication.

Sigmoid volvulus is also considered a surgical emergency, and endoscopic therapy is the first line of the treatment in the cases without signs of bowel necrosis and perforation. In selective patients, the laparoscopic approach might be considered. Halabi et al. reported that laparoscopic techniques were applied for 3.7% of patients with volvulus and most of them for relatively younger patients with lower comorbidity scores [69].

Diverticular disease of the colon is a major cause of hospital admission, and acute diverticulitis is one of the common diseases requiring emergent treatment. Most patients with diverticulitis are treated conservatively; however, patients with complicated diverticulitis require surgical treatment, particularly Hinchey grade III and IV classification. While most patients with freely perforated diverticulitis require surgery, the choice of techniques largely depends on the extent of contamination. The laparoscopic approach for acute complicated diverticulitis is controversial. O'Sullivan et al. proposed laparoscopic lavage for the management of perforated diverticulitis in 1996 [70]. Several studies were performed in Europe and these results showed ambivalent results [71–73]. Select patients with Hinchey III diverticulitis might benefit from laparoscopy as a bridge to elective colectomy [74].

8 MIS for Traumatic Intra-abdominal Surgical Emergencies

Laparoscopic surgery for abdominal trauma, both penetrating and blunt, has been shown to be safe and effective. Similar to for EGS, it is important for patients to be hemodynamically stable prior to undergoing MIS approaches; otherwise, a laparotomy is mandatory. MIS for trauma has been associated with shorter operating time, lower blood loss, faster return to diet, and shorter length of stay with no significant differences in mortality [6, 75]. In the geriatric population, evidence regarding MIS for trauma remains lacking. MIS for a penetrating injury is a good indication to explore the injury [76, 77]. Due to this, the mechanism of the injuries occurring in the geriatric population is mainly blunt trauma [78]. Laparoscopic surgery for both blunt and penetrating trauma in the elderly is also an effective tool for hemodynamically stable patients with low conversion rates, reduced morbidity, and decreased lengths of stay [79–81].

9 Laparoscopic vs. Robotically Assisted Emergency Surgery

Minimally invasive surgery has rapidly evolved from the one novel laparoscopic approach to robotic surgery. In the past few decades, robotic systems have gone from systems which were significantly limited to full-fledged platforms featuring 3D vision, articulated instruments, and even the latest wireless connectivity as standard [82]. The use of robotic procedures has recently started to increase in general surgery [83]. General surgeons are getting familiar to using the recent robotic technology. Currently, most robotic procedures are used for the elective setting. Most surgeons in general surgery are using robotic technology for acute appendectomy, hernia repair, and cholecystectomy.

Presently, the utility for robotic technique is limited, especially in the elderly population and in emergent situations. Recent technological progress with robotic devices and platforms for general surgery will lead to use for elderly patients. Since robotic surgery has shown positive outcomes, further studies are needed to evaluate the benefits and disadvantages for the elderly population. Nonetheless, robotic surgery supports the ergonomics of a surgeon and reduces work-related musculoskeletal disorders [84–86]. Based on these facts, we expect that robotic platforms will be utilized for any setting including emergent situations.

References

1. Knowlton LM, Minei J, Tennakoon L, Davis KA, Doucet J, Bernard A, et al. The economic footprint of acute care surgery in the United States: implications for systems development. J Trauma Acute Care Surg. 2019;86:609–16.
2. Scott JW, Olufajo OA, Brat GA, Rose JA, Zogg CK, Haider AH, et al. Use of National Burden to define operative emergency general surgery. JAMA Surg. 2016;151:e160480.
3. Subject: Profile of Older Americans: 2016 | ACL Administration for Community Living. https://acl.gov/news-and-events/announcements/subject-profile-older-americans-2016. Accessed 13 Jul 2021.
4. Etzioni DA, Liu JH, Maggard MA, Ko CY. The aging population and its impact on the surgery workforce. Ann Surg. 2003;238:170–7.
5. Arnold M, Elhage S, Schiffern L, Lauren Paton B, Ross SW, Matthews BD, et al. Use of minimally invasive surgery in emergency general surgery procedures. Surg Endosc. 2020;34:2258–65.
6. Trejo-Ávila ME, Valenzuela-Salazar C, Betancourt-Ferreyra J, Fernández-Enríquez E, Romero-Loera S, Moreno-Portillo M. Laparoscopic versus open surgery for abdominal trauma: a case-matched study. J Laparoendosc Adv Surg Tech A. 2017;27:383–7.
7. Pickering O, Pucher PH, De'Ath H, Abuawwad M, Kelly J, Underwood TJ, et al. Minimally invasive approach in Boerhaave's syndrome: case series and systematic review. J Laparoendosc Adv Surg Tech A. 2020;31:1254.
8. Aiolfi A, Micheletto G, Guerrazzi G, Bonitta G, Campanelli G, Bona D. Minimally invasive surgical management of Boerhaave's syndrome: a narrative literature review. J Thorac Dis. 2020;12:4411–7.
9. Elliott JA, Buckley L, Albagir M, Athanasiou A, Murphy TJ. Minimally invasive surgical management of spontaneous esophageal perforation (Boerhaave's syndrome). Surg Endosc. 2019;33:3494–502.
10. Cameron JL, Kieffer RF, Hendrix TR, Mehigan DG, Baker RR. Selective nonoperative management of contained intrathoracic esophageal disruptions. Ann Thorac Surg. 1979;27:404–8.
11. Gurwara S, Clayton S. Esophageal perforations: an endoscopic approach to management. Curr Gastroenterol Rep. 2019;21:57.
12. Watkins JR, Farivar AS. Endoluminal therapies for esophageal perforations and leaks. Thorac Surg Clin. 2018;28:541–54.
13. Abbas G, Schuchert MJ, Pettiford BL, Pennathur A, Landreneau J, Landreneau J, et al. Contemporaneous management of esophageal perforation. Surgery. 2009;146:749–56.
14. Lanas A, Chan FKL. Peptic ulcer disease. Lancet. 2017;390:613–24.
15. Wang YR, Richter JE, Dempsey DT. Trends and outcomes of hospitalizations for peptic ulcer disease in the United States, 1993 to 2006. Ann Surg. 2010;251:51–8.
16. Svanes C, Lie RT, Svanes K, Lie SA, Søreide O. Adverse effects of delayed treatment for perforated peptic ulcer. Ann Surg. 1994;220:168–75.
17. Graham R. The treatment of perforated duodenal ulcers. Surg Gyneco Obste. 1937;64:235–8.
18. Quah GS, Eslick GD, Cox MR. Laparoscopic repair for perforated peptic ulcer disease has better outcomes than open repair. J Gastrointest Surg. 2019;23:618–25.
19. Lagoo S, McMahon RL, Kakihara M, Pappas TN, Eubanks S. The sixth decision regarding perforated duodenal ulcer. JSLS. 2002;6:359–68.

20. Miserez M, Eypasch E, Spangenberger W, Lefering R, Troidl H. Laparoscopic and conventional closure of perforated peptic ulcer. A comparison Surg Endosc. 1996;10:831–6.
21. Lau WY, Leung KL, Kwong KH, Davey IC, Robertson C, Dawson JJ, et al. A randomized study comparing laparoscopic versus open repair of perforated peptic ulcer using suture or sutureless technique. Ann Surg. 1996;224:131–8.
22. Søreide K, Thorsen K, Søreide JA. Strategies to improve the outcome of emergency surgery for perforated peptic ulcer. Br J Surg. 2014;101:e51–64.
23. Bertleff MJOE, Lange JF. Laparoscopic correction of perforated peptic ulcer: first choice? A review of literature. Surg Endosc. 2010;24:1231–9.
24. Druart ML, Van Hee R, Etienne J, et al. Laparoscopic repair of perforated duodenal ulcer. A prospective multicenter clinical trial. Surg Endosc. 1997;11:1017–20.
25. Katkhouda N, Mavor E, Mason RJ, Campos GM, Soroushyari A, Berne TV. Laparoscopic repair of perforated duodenal ulcers: outcome and efficacy in 30 consecutive patients. Arch Surg. 1999;134:845–8; discussion 849–850.
26. Ng S-S-M. Role and outcome of conventional surgery in the treatment of pyogenic liver abscess in the modern era of minimally invasive therapy. WJG. 2008;14:747.
27. Mezhir JJ, Fong Y, Jacks LM, Getrajdman GI, Brody LA, Covey AM, et al. Current Management of Pyogenic Liver Abscess: surgery is now second-line treatment. J Am Coll Surg. 2010;210:975–83.
28. Tan L, Zhou HJ, Hartman M, Ganpathi IS, Madhavan K, Chang S. Laparoscopic drainage of cryptogenic liver abscess. Surg Endosc. 2013;27:3308–14.
29. Gutt CN, Encke J, Köninger J, et al. Acute cholecystitis: early versus delayed cholecystectomy, a multicenter randomized trial (ACDC study, NCT00447304). Ann Surg. 2013;258:385–93.
30. Antoniou SA, Antoniou GA, Koch OO, Pointner R, Granderath FA. Meta-analysis of laparoscopic vs open cholecystectomy in elderly patients. World J Gastroenterol. 2014;20:17626–34.
31. Loozen CS, van Ramshorst B, van Santvoort HC, Boerma D. Early cholecystectomy for acute cholecystitis in the elderly population: a systematic review and meta-analysis. Dig Surg. 2017;34:371–9.
32. Joliat G-R, Longchamp G, Du Pasquier C, Denys A, Demartines N, Melloul E. Delayed cholecystectomy for acute cholecystitis in elderly patients treated primarily with antibiotics or percutaneous drainage of the gallbladder. J Laparoendosc Adv Surg Tech. 2018;28:1094–9.
33. Krishna SG, Kamboj AK, Hart PA, Hinton A, Conwell DL. The changing epidemiology of acute pancreatitis hospitalizations: a decade of trends and the impact of chronic pancreatitis. Pancreas. 2017;46:482–8.
34. Gapp J, Hall AG, Walters RW, Jahann D, Kassim T, Reddymasu S. Trends and outcomes of hospitalizations related to acute pancreatitis: epidemiology from 2001 to 2014 in the United States. Pancreas. 2019;48:548–54.
35. Members of the Dutch Acute Pancreatitis Study Group, Besselink MG, van Santvoort HC, et al. Minimally invasive "step-up approach" versus maximal necrosectomy in patients with acute necrotising pancreatitis (PANTER trial): design and rationale of a randomised controlled multicenter trial [ISRCTN13975868]. BMC Surg. 2006;6:6.
36. Banks PA, Freeman ML. The practice parameters Committee of the American College of gastroenterology. Practice guidelines in acute pancreatitis. Am J Gastroenterol. 2006;101:2379–400.
37. Nieuwenhuijs VB, Besselink MGH, van Minnen LP, Gooszen HG. Surgical management of acute necrotizing pancreatitis: a 13-year experience and a systematic review. Scand J Gastroenterol. 2003;38:111–6.
38. van Santvoort HC, Besselink MG, Bakker OJ, et al. A step-up approach or open necrosectomy for necrotizing pancreatitis. N Engl J Med. 2010;362:1491–502.
39. IAP/APA evidence-based guidelines for the management of acute pancreatitis. Pancreatology. 2013;13:e1–e15.
40. Magidson PD, Martinez JP. Abdominal pain in the geriatric patient. Emerg Med Clin North Am. 2016;34:559–74.

41. Behman R, Nathens AB, Mason S, Byrne JP, Hong NL, Pechlivanoglou P, et al. Association of Surgical Intervention for adhesive small-bowel obstruction with the risk of recurrence. JAMA Surg. 2019;154:413.
42. Sakari T, Christersson M, Karlbom U. Mechanisms of adhesive small bowel obstruction and outcome of surgery; a population-based study. BMC Surg. 2020;20:62.
43. Ha GW, Lee MR, Kim JH. Adhesive small bowel obstruction after laparoscopic and open colorectal surgery: a systematic review and meta-analysis. Am J Surg. 2016;212:527–36.
44. Compagna R, Rossi R, Fappiano F, Bianco T, Accurso A, Danzi M, et al. Emergency groin hernia repair: implications in elderly. BMC Surg. 2013;13:S29.
45. List of Elderly Risk Assessment and Surgical Outcome (ERASO) Collaborative Study Group endorsed by SICUT, ACOI, SICG, SICE, and Italian Chapter of WSES, Ceresoli M, Carissimi F, Nigro A, Fransvea P, et al. Emergency hernia repair in the elderly: multivariate analysis of morbidity and mortality from an Italian registry. Hernia. 2020;26(1):165–75. https://doi.org/10.1007/s10029-020-02269-5.
46. Pei KY, Asuzu D, Davis KA. Will laparoscopic lysis of adhesions become the standard of care? Evaluating trends and outcomes in laparoscopic management of small-bowel obstruction using the American College of Surgeons National Surgical Quality Improvement Project Database. Surg Endosc. 2017;31:2180–6.
47. Argudo N, Pereira JA, Sancho JJ, Membrilla E, Pons MJ, Grande L. Prophylactic synthetic mesh can be safely used to close emergency laparotomies, even in peritonitis. Surgery. 2014;156:1238–44.
48. Sakamoto T, Fujiogi M, Ishimaru M, Matsui H, Fushimi K, Yasunaga H. Comparison of postoperative infection after emergency inguinal hernia surgery with enterectomy between mesh repair and non-mesh repair: a national database analysis. Hernia. 2021;26:217. https://doi.org/10.1007/s10029-021-02439-z.
49. Nissen NN, Menon V, Bresee C, Tran TT, Annamalai A, Poordad F, et al. Recurrent hepatocellular carcinoma after liver transplant: identifying the high-risk patient. HPB (Oxford). 2011;13:626–32.
50. Slater NJ, van der Kolk M, Hendriks T, van Goor H, Bleichrodt RP. Biologic grafts for ventral hernia repair: a systematic review. Am J Surg. 2013;205:220–30.
51. Latifi R, Samson D, Haider A, Azim A, Iftikhar H, Joseph B, et al. Risk-adjusted adverse outcomes in complex abdominal wall hernia repair with biologic mesh: a case series of 140 patients. Int J Surg. 2017;43:26–32.
52. Gogna S, Latifi R, Policastro A, Prabhakaran K, Anderson P, Con J, et al. Complex abdominal wall hernia repair with biologic mesh in elderly: a propensity matched analysis. Hernia. 2020;24:495–502.
53. Fugazzola P, Ceresoli M, Agnoletti V, et al. The SIFIPAC/WSES/SICG/SIMEU guidelines for diagnosis and treatment of acute appendicitis in the elderly (2019 edition). World J Emerg Surg 2020;15:19.
54. Jaschinski T, Mosch CG, Eikermann M, Neugebauer EA, Sauerland S. Laparoscopic versus open surgery for suspected appendicitis. Cochrane Database Syst Rev. 2018;11:CD001546.
55. Jaschinski T, Mosch C, Eikermann M, Neugebauer EA. Laparoscopic versus open appendectomy in patients with suspected appendicitis: a systematic review of meta-analyses of randomised controlled trials. BMC Gastroenterol. 2015;15:48.
56. Sporn E, Petroski GF, Mancini GJ, Astudillo JA, Miedema BW, Thaler K. Laparoscopic appendectomy—is it worth the cost? Trend analysis in the US from 2000 to 2005. J Am Coll Surg. 2009;208:179–185.e2.
57. Brügger L, Rosella L, Candinas D, Güller U. Improving outcomes after laparoscopic appendectomy: a population-based, 12-year trend analysis of 7446 patients. Ann Surg. 2011;253:309–13.
58. Ball CG, Kortbeek JB, Kirkpatrick AW, Mitchell P. Laparoscopic appendectomy for complicated appendicitis: an evaluation of postoperative factors. Surg Endosc. 2004;18:969–73.
59. Masoomi H, Mills S, Dolich MO, Ketana N, Carmichael JC, Nguyen NT, et al. Comparison of outcomes of laparoscopic versus open appendectomy in adults: data from the Nationwide Inpatient Sample (NIS), 2006-2008. J Gastrointest Surg. 2011;15:2226–31.

60. St Peter SD, Adibe OO, Iqbal CW, et al. Irrigation versus suction alone during laparoscopic appendectomy for perforated appendicitis: a prospective randomized trial. Ann Surg. 2012;256:581–5.
61. Hajibandeh S, Hajibandeh S, Kelly A, Shah J, Khan RMA, Panda N, et al. Irrigation versus suction alone in laparoscopic appendectomy: is dilution the solution to pollution? A systematic review and meta-analysis. Surg Innov. 2018;25:174–82.
62. Allemann P, Probst H, Demartines N, Schäfer M. Prevention of infectious complications after laparoscopic appendectomy for complicated acute appendicitis—the role of routine abdominal drainage. Langenbeck's Arch Surg. 2011;396:63–8.
63. Lin H-F, Lai H-S, Lai I-R. Laparoscopic treatment of perforated appendicitis. World J Gastroenterol. 2014;20:14338–47.
64. Chand M. Systematic review of emergent laparoscopic colorectal surgery for benign and malignant disease. WJG. 2014;20:16956.
65. O'Malley E, Boyle E, O'Callaghan A, Coffey JC, Walsh SR. Role of laparoscopy in penetrating abdominal trauma: a systematic review. World J Surg. 2013;37:113–22.
66. de'Angelis N, Di Saverio S, Chiara O, et al. WSES guidelines for the management of iatrogenic colonoscopy perforation. World J Emerg Surg. 2017;2018(13):5.
67. Panteris V, Haringsma J, Kuipers E. Colonoscopy perforation rate, mechanisms and outcome: from diagnostic to therapeutic colonoscopy. Endoscopy. 2009;41:941–51.
68. Fatima H, Rex DK. Minimizing endoscopic complications: colonoscopic polypectomy. Gastrointest Endosc Clin N Am. 2007;17:145–56.
69. Halabi WJ, Jafari MD, Kang CY, Nguyen VQ, Carmichael JC, Mills S, et al. Colonic volvulus in the United States: trends, outcomes, and predictors of mortality. Ann Surg. 2014;259:293–301.
70. O'Sullivan GC, Murphy D, O'Brien MG, Ireland A. Laparoscopic management of generalized peritonitis due to perforated colonic diverticula. Am J Surg. 1996;171:432–4.
71. Vennix S, Musters GD, Mulder IM, et al. Laparoscopic peritoneal lavage or sigmoidectomy for perforated diverticulitis with purulent peritonitis: a multicentre, parallel-group, randomised, open-label trial. Lancet. 2015;386:1269–77.
72. Angenete E, Thornell A, Burcharth J, et al. Laparoscopic lavage is feasible and safe for the treatment of perforated diverticulitis with purulent peritonitis: the first results from the randomized controlled trial DILALA. Ann Surg. 2016;263:117–22.
73. Schultz JK, Yaqub S, Wallon C, Blecic L, Forsmo HM, Folkesson J, et al. Laparoscopic lavage vs primary resection for acute perforated diverticulitis: the SCANDIV randomized clinical trial. JAMA. 2015;314:1364.
74. Biffl WL, Moore FA, Moore EE. What is the current role of laparoscopic lavage in perforated diverticulitis? J Trauma Acute Care Surg. 2017;82:810–3.
75. Gao Y, Li S, Xi H, et al. Laparoscopy versus conventional laparotomy in the management of abdominal trauma: a multi-institutional matched-pair study. Surg Endosc. 2020;34:2237–42.
76. Koto MZ, Matsevych OY, Mosai F, Patel S, Aldous C, Balabyeki M. Laparoscopy for blunt abdominal trauma: a challenging endeavor. Scand J Surg. 2019;108:273–9.
77. Menegozzo CAM, Damous SHB, Alves PHF, Rocha MC, Collet E, Silva FS, Baraviera T, et al. "Pop in a scope": attempt to decrease the rate of unnecessary nontherapeutic laparotomies in hemodynamically stable patients with thoracoabdominal penetrating injuries. Surg Endosc. 2020;34:261–7.
78. Gioffrè-Florio M. Trauma in elderly patients: a study of prevalence, comorbidities and gender differences. GHIR. 2018;39:35.
79. Huscher CGS, Mingoli A, Sgarzini G, Brachini G, Ponzano C, Di Paola M, et al. Laparoscopic treatment of blunt splenic injuries: initial experience with 11 patients. Surg Endosc. 2006;20:1423–6.
80. Bain K, Meytes V, Chang GC, Timoney MF. Laparoscopy in penetrating abdominal trauma is a safe and effective alternative to laparotomy. Surg Endosc. 2019;33:1618–25.
81. Uranues S, Popa DE, Diaconescu B, Schrittwieser R. Laparoscopy in penetrating abdominal trauma. World J Surg. 2015;39:1381–8.

82. Rojas A, Gachabayov M, Abouezzi Z, Bergamaschi R, Latifi R. Current robotic platforms in surgery and the road ahead. Surg Technol Int. 2021;38:39–46.
83. Leal Ghezzi T, Campos Corleta O. 30 years of robotic surgery. World J Surg. 2016;40:2550–7.
84. Catanzarite T, Tan-Kim J, Whitcomb EL, Menefee S. Ergonomics in surgery: a review. Female Pelvic Med Reconstr Surg. 2018;24:1–12.
85. Andolfi C, Umanskiy K. Current trends and perspectives in robotic surgery. J Laparoendosc Adv Surg Tech. 2019;29:127–8.
86. Ruhle BC, Ferguson Bryan A, Grogan RH. Robot-assisted endocrine surgery: indications and drawbacks. J Laparoendosc Adv Surg Tech. 2019;29:129–35.

Role of Emergency Laparoscopy in Surgical and Endoscopic Complications

Aleix Martínez-Pérez (iD), Carmen Payá-Llorente,
Álvaro Pérez-Rubio, and Nicola de'Angelis

1 Introduction

Post-procedural complications are inherently linked with any surgical or endoscopic procedure. The reported incidence rates are highly varying and depend mostly on the type of the index intervention and the definitions adopted for each complication [1]. Postoperative adverse events increase in-hospital costs up to five times when compared with similar operations without complications [2]. Explorative laparoscopy is an alternative to conventional laparotomy for patients with suspected early abdominal complications. It can be especially useful when the physical examination and the radiologic tests are inconclusive. A primary or a repeated laparoscopic procedure can be both used to obtain a prompt and definitive diagnosis and to treat most of these complications, especially when control of a septic focus is needed [3, 4]. Compared with the performance of a standard laparotomy, the use of laparoscopy in the emergency setting reduces the postoperative pain, time to recovery, wound infections, ileus, and incisional hernia rates while also improving cosmesis [4]. A

A. Martínez-Pérez (✉)
Department of General and Digestive Surgery, Hospital Universitario Doctor Peset, Valencia,
Spain

Faculty of Health Sciences, Valencian International University (VIU), Valencia, Spain

C. Payá-Llorente · Á. Pérez-Rubio
Department of General and Digestive Surgery, Hospital Universitario Doctor Peset, Valencia,
Spain

N. de'Angelis
Unit of Colorectal and Digestive Surgery, DIGEST Department, Beaujon University Hospital,
AP-HP, University of Paris Cité, Clichy, France

© The Author(s), under exclusive license to Springer Nature Switzerland AG 2023   343
F. Coccolini et al. (eds.), *Mini-invasive Approach in Acute Care Surgery*,
Hot Topics in Acute Care Surgery and Trauma,
https://doi.org/10.1007/978-3-031-39001-2_25

mini-invasive approach also has less operative trauma and a lower systemic stress response [5]. Even if the prior approach was open, performing a second-look evaluation using laparoscopy has demonstrated to be safe and effective [6].

However, up to 25% of the re-laparoscopies are negative [7]; so a significant number of patients are subjected to an unnecessary surgical risk. Certain situations should preclude surgeons from creating a pneumoperitoneum, such as the presence of hemodynamic instability or severe respiratory failure [8]. Moreover, other conditions hinder the application of minimally invasive therapies but are not considered absolute contraindications. They are (1) severe bowel dilatation, (2) multiple and firm adhesions (the "frozen abdomen"), (3) diffuse peritonitis, (4) massive hemorrhage, and (5) extensive mesenteric ischemia [9]. The risk of iatrogenic injury to abdominal organs is the major drawback of emergency laparoscopy. This is facilitated by the intense inflammation of the tissues and the presence of multiple adhesions, which hampers the proper identification of the anatomical structures.

Laparoscopic reinterventions are most frequently undertaken to manage early postoperative complications after colorectal surgical procedures like anastomotic leak, bowel obstruction, or bleeding [4]. Postoperative hemorrhage following abdominal surgery is a potentially life-threatening complication. The use of laparoscopy is a reasonable option in stable patients, but in hemodynamically unstable patients, a laparotomy would be mandatory. When a bleeding source is not found laparoscopically, a prompt conversion to an open approach minimizes the risk for future adverse events. To localize the origin of the hemorrhage can be hazardous if dense clots or severe inflammation are present, but success rates are promising if the surgery is carried on by expert teams [10].

A mechanical bowel obstruction is an infrequent condition in the early postoperative period following laparoscopic surgery. Trocar site hernias are the most common cause [11]. They can be managed through the trocar site, by a re-laparoscopy, or by laparotomy. Diagnostic laparoscopy allows evaluation of the intestine in cases with suspected Richter's hernia, avoiding the need of a laparotomy [12]. Laparoscopic adhesiolysis after an open procedure could be an option for surgeons, but few series have been reported [4]. This approach is not recommended in cases with massive abdominal distension or in those presenting with signs of peritonitis [13].

2 Complications After Colorectal Surgery

2.1 Incidence and Risk Factors

Colorectal resections are associated with high postoperative complication rates; they can be detected in up to 50% of the patients [14]. The most important within them are anastomotic leak (AL), surgical site infection, bleeding, hollow viscus perforation, intestinal obstruction, ischemia, and urologic injuries [15]. AL is the main cause of reoperation following colorectal surgery; its incidence ranges within 3–30% depending on the series [16]. In 2010, the International Study Group of Rectal Cancer graded AL in a three-tiered system based on the aggressiveness of the treatment needed: (a) AL requiring no active therapeutic intervention, (b) AL requiring active therapeutic intervention but manageable without a relaparotomy, and (c) AL requiring a re-laparotomy [17]. Years ago, nearly all ALs were treated through a laparotomy. However, surgeons have been continuously improving their laparoscopic skills, and the indications to operate on colorectal postoperative complications using a laparoscopic approach have increased.

2.2   Anastomotic Leaks

Depending on the type of procedure and the anastomosis initially performed, different mini-invasive surgical operations could be performed when AL is suspected or detected. For ileocolic AL, the laparoscopic approach is rarely used, since these cases are usually accompanied by severe septic conditions. However, in small leaks without extensive contamination, an explorative laparoscopy, anastomosis repair, and proper lavage and drainage of the abdominal cavity could be an affordable option. If a wide anastomotic defect is found, redoing the anastomosis would be mandatory. A diverting ileostomy can be also performed depending on the patient's characteristics and the clinical status. Colorectal AL presenting with a wide defect causing diffuse peritonitis and/or colonic ischemia usually requires the resection of the anastomosis and the performance of a terminal colostomy (i.e., a Hartmann's procedure). This should be accompanied by a profuse lavage and drainage of the cavity. However, in smaller defects, surgeons should make the choice between fixing or redoing the anastomoses. In the latest years, with the rise of trans-anal minimally invasive surgery (TAMIS), a new tool has emerged to evaluate and to repair colorectal AL located between 5 cm and 15 cm from the anal verge. The procedure would consist of the debridement of the leak edges and then re-suturing through the TAMIS access. The technique has shown to be safe and effective, especially if it is undertaken during the first five postoperative days [18]. A coloanal anastomosis can be similarly repaired under direct visualization or using a conventional anoscope [6]. If not performed at the first operation, a diverting ileostomy can be helpful to shorten the time to resume the oral intake.

2.3   Other Complications

Different teams have demonstrated that a laparoscopic approach can be useful to treat other complications like (a) bowel injuries with a primary repair; (b) complete ureteric transections by end-to-end anastomosis; (c) bowel obstructions by either lysis of adhesions or reducing internal hernias; and (d) hemostasis by coagulation, endo-loop application, clipping, suturing, or using hemostatic agents [19].

In these particular situations, the use of laparoscopy provides a faster resumption of oral intake and an earlier stoma function [20]. Its use may also shorten the intensive care unit (ICU) and hospital stays [21]. Moreover, the number of stomas that can be definitively reconnected after a laparoscopic emergency management is higher than for open surgery [22]. Sometimes, the technical difficulty does not allow to complete the reoperation by laparoscopy, and conversion is required. Such a conversion is related with more severe postoperative pain, longer hospital stays, and higher rates of ileus and wound infection [10]. Even so, an initial minimally invasive approach permits some progress of control of the complication which could prevent larger incisions if conversion is required. Finally, while the diagnosis and treatment of these complications using a laparoscopic approach are often technically feasible, the surgeons should make the choice to undergo reoperative laparoscopy depending on the experience of the whole surgical team and the availability of the different technologic resources, thus individualizing each singular case.

3 Complications After Other Surgical Procedures

3.1 Upper Gastrointestinal Surgery

Anastomotic leaks after upper gastrointestinal resections are associated with high morbidity and mortality. For small controlled leaks, a conservative treatment based on broad-spectrum antibiotics and percutaneous drainage with or without endoscopic stenting are the ideal choice [23]. Literature reports focusing on the use of minimally invasive surgical approaches in these situations have been anecdotal to date. Laparoscopic washout followed by the placement of a percutaneous trans-anastomotic suction tube has been described [24]. The laparoscopic repair also constitutes an alternative for iatrogenic gastric perforations that occurred during other laparoscopic operations [5, 10]. Similarly, early complications after laparoscopic anti-reflux surgery can be treated by the same mini-invasive approach. If the complication is early, such as paraesophageal herniation or severe dysphagia, a laparoscopic revision of the anti-reflux procedure would be an option, ideally within the first seven days [25, 26].

3.2 Hepatobiliary Surgery

Minimally invasive reinterventions after cholecystectomy are frequently due to postoperative bleeding or bile duct injuries. Bleeding after cholecystectomy or liver resection can be managed laparoscopically [27, 28]. Bile duct injury is the most feared complication of cholecystectomy; they are classified according to the system proposed by Strasberg [29]. Percutaneous drainage and endoscopic stenting are usually the first steps to treat biliary and cystic leaks (Strasberg A, C and D) [30]. In selected cases, a postoperative laparoscopy can be undertaken to confirm the diagnosis, to achieve sepsis control, or to perform a definitive repair. A re-laparoscopy to gain sepsis control with extensive abdominal washout and drain placement has been performed in small injuries and minor leaks from the cystic stump or small accessory ducts from the gallbladder bed (Luschka's) [31, 32]. Although few cases are found in the literature, a laparoscopic reconstruction after major bile duct injuries is feasible for highly experienced teams [33, 34]. Robot-assisted, traditional laparoscopic, and open Roux-en-Y hepaticojejunostomy has been proposed as an alternative to repair complex injuries [35].

3.3 Appendectomy

Laparoscopic surgery in post-appendectomy complications has been used to drain intra-abdominal abscesses, to extract retained fecaliths, and to manage stump appendicitis or postoperative bleeding. The most common treatment for the first of them is to administer intravenous antibiotics, adding or not a percutaneous drainage of the fluid collections. If failure of the previous, or in those patients presenting with multiple abscesses, a laparoscopic exploration could be an alternative to laparotomy [36]. Different teams have evaluated the role of early laparoscopic washout in these situations. They considered it to provide an earlier resolution of the sepsis, when compared with the percutaneous or open approaches [37]. It has been proposed that a re-laparoscopy is the first choice for abscesses detected within the first seven days after the index procedure [38], especially if the sepsis cannot be controlled by drainage and antibiotics alone. Stump appendicitis is an infrequent complication following appendectomy. A new laparoscopic exploration would be the best chance to confirm the diagnosis and to complete the removal of the appendix [39].

3.4 Urologic Surgery

The role of re-laparoscopy after minimally invasive urologic procedures is very limited; the largest case series only included 12 patients [40]. Redo-laparoscopy due to bleeding is the most frequently performed procedure [41].

4 Iatrogenic Perforations During Colonoscopy

4.1 Background

Colorectal perforations complicating lower gastrointestinal endoscopic procedures are deleterious events associated with important morbidity and mortality. Iatrogenic colonoscopy perforations (ICP) can be produced at both therapeutic and diagnostic procedures. The sigmoid colon is the most common site of perforation, but the presentation differs depending on several factors [42]. Half of the ICP are detected by the endoscopy operator during the procedure, and they are usually located intraperitoneally. Blunt trauma is considered the most frequent etiologic factor for ICP, producing larger perforations often located at the sigmoid colon. Conversely, excessive insufflation produces linear lacerations usually at the cecal region. Therapeutic procedures, such as mucosal/submucosal dissections, stricture dilatation, or stenting, present significant rates of ICP. Thermal injuries are linked with small and delayed ischemic perforations. The symptoms of ICP commonly start within 48 h after the endoscopic procedure. To obtain an early diagnosis is critical for the patient's behavior, as delays greater than 24 h have been associated with the need for more invasive treatments [43]. The presence of extra-colonic free air at radiologic explorations confirms the diagnosis of ICP.

4.2 Surgical Management

The endoscopic closure is a useful option for ICP detected intra-procedurally. This should be followed by conservative treatment that consists of serial clinical and imaging monitoring with bowel rest, intravenous fluids, and broad-spectrum antibiotics. Close observation is required to detect the early development of peritonitis and/or sepsis indicating that the endoscopic repair may have failed. A similar approach can be used in patients with small and sealed-off perforations seen on CT scan. The failure of the conservative approach has been reported in up to 20% of the cases [46]. Therefore, the early success of a nonoperative management should not preclude close follow-up. Indications of surgery for ICP include the development of sepsis, signs of diffuse peritonitis, or in presence of large perforations not suitable to endoscopic closure. Surgery can be initially justified also in the presence of certain concomitant pathologies (e.g., unresected polyps with suspicion of carcinoma) [44, 45].

4.3 Role of Laparoscopy

Laparoscopic exploration has been increasingly used for ICP management. The intraoperative findings observed during a careful inspection of the whole peritoneal cavity would determine the choice between the different surgical alternatives. Surgeons should consider the characteristics of the perforation (e.g., size, degree of contamination, timing, mechanism) and the patient's features (e.g., comorbidities, general and sepsis status, presence of underlying lesions). Large perforations or associating mesocolon avulsions or unresected lesions should lead one to perform a colonic resection (with or without stoma formation). If no suspicious lesion remains after the endoscopy, and the ICP consists of a small tear in a healthy colon, a laparoscopic primary repair can be safely performed (Fig. 1). The World Society of Emergency Surgery (WSES) guidelines for the management of ICP, recently published, proposed that an explorative laparoscopy in the setting of ICP would be useful with diagnostic or therapeutic intention, depending on the surgeon's skills, the local resources, and the potential risks for definitive surgical procedures. Moreover, it can be applied also in cases of doubtful diagnosis, to rule out the need of further treatments (e.g., laparotomy) or if the endoscopic/conservative treatment is unfeasible or fails (e.g., sepsis or peritonitis development). Conversely, an

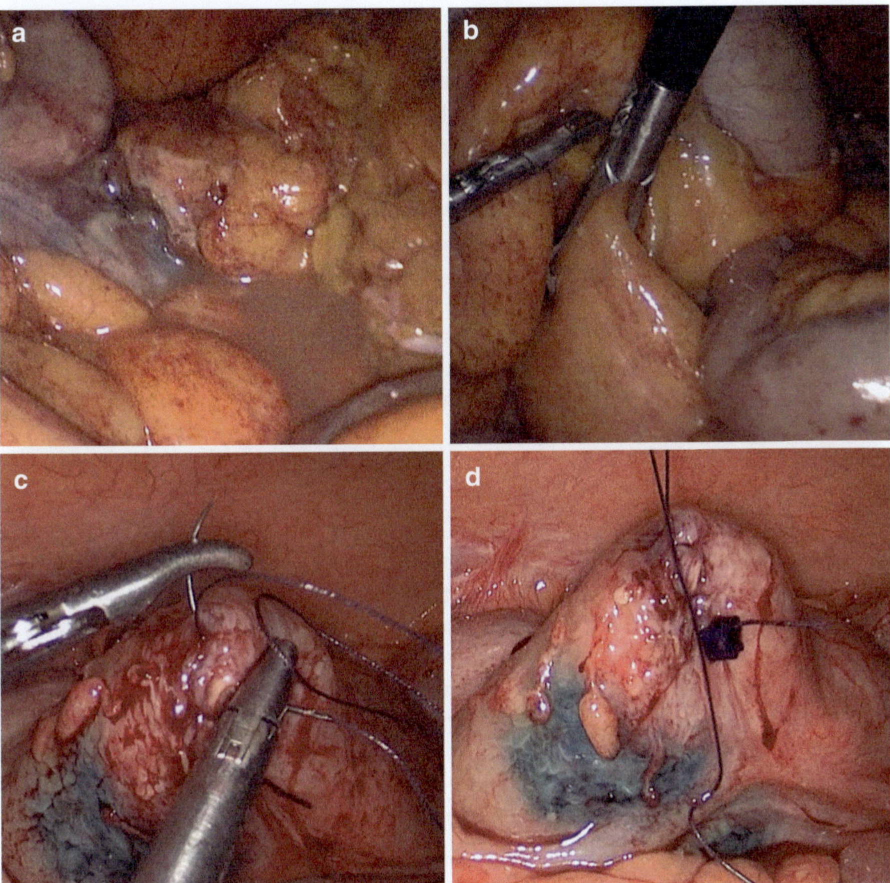

Fig. 1 (**a**, **b**) ICP perforation located in the right colon. Laparoscopic right hemicolectomy was performed. (**c**, **d**) Endoscopy-related cecal perforation treated with laparoscopic primary closure

explorative laparoscopy may not be indicated if the patient is hemodynamically unstable, if there is a potential risk for anesthesia-related complications, or if there are any contraindications for surgery in general (e.g., coagulopathy). Relative contraindications for this approach would be (1) recent laparotomy or more than four previous abdominal surgeries with extensive adhesions and high risk of iatrogenic injury, (2) massive bowel dilatation, and (3) aortoiliac aneurysmatic disease [42]. The most frequent causes of conversion are (1) the experience of the surgical team, (2) adverse surgical field conditions precluding the success of a laparoscopic procedure (e.g., contamination, large defects, inflammation, advanced cancer), and (3) patient's hemodynamic destabilization.

A recent systematic review with a meta-analysis including six studies published between 2008 and 2016 concluded that the laparoscopic approach appears to provide better postoperative results than open surgery in selected patients undergoing surgical management of ICP [46]. Overall, 90 patients underwent laparoscopic procedures due to ICP, with a conversion rate of 10%. Complications were observed in 18.2% of patients who underwent laparoscopy and in 53.5% of patients who underwent open procedures ($p < 0.001$). LOS was five days shorter for patients receiving less invasive procedures ($p < 0.001$). Noteworthy, the six included studies were considered to be at high risk of bias, and therefore, the quality of the evidence was judged to be low [47–52].

5 Iatrogenic Perforations During Upper Digestive Endoscopy

5.1 Esophageal Perforations

Iatrogenic harm is the most common cause of esophageal perforation. When they are secondary to diagnostic explorations, they are typically located at the upper portions. When they are due to sudden pressure increases, they are commonly found at the distal esophagus. Like ICP, nonoperative management can be undertaken in stable patients presenting with small perforations with minor contamination [53]. Explorative laparoscopy/thoracoscopy would be the first step in the surgical procedure depending on the surgical team skills and the available technological resources.

The minimally invasive repair of any esophageal perforations is technically hazardous in almost all possible scenarios. Therefore, it should be reserved to situations in which highly specialized expertise is available [54]. The surgical procedure should include the control of the sepsis with local debridement and the drainage of any collections. The primary closure of the defect could be attempted, but to assure adequate enteral support, feeding tube placement (e.g., nasogastric tube, gastrostomy, jejunostomy) is critical [53].

5.2 Complications Following Endoscopic and Percutaneous Gastrostomy

Gastric leak is a typical complication of patients with a gastrostomy. The laparoscopic repair of leaks following percutaneous or endoscopic gastrostomy has been

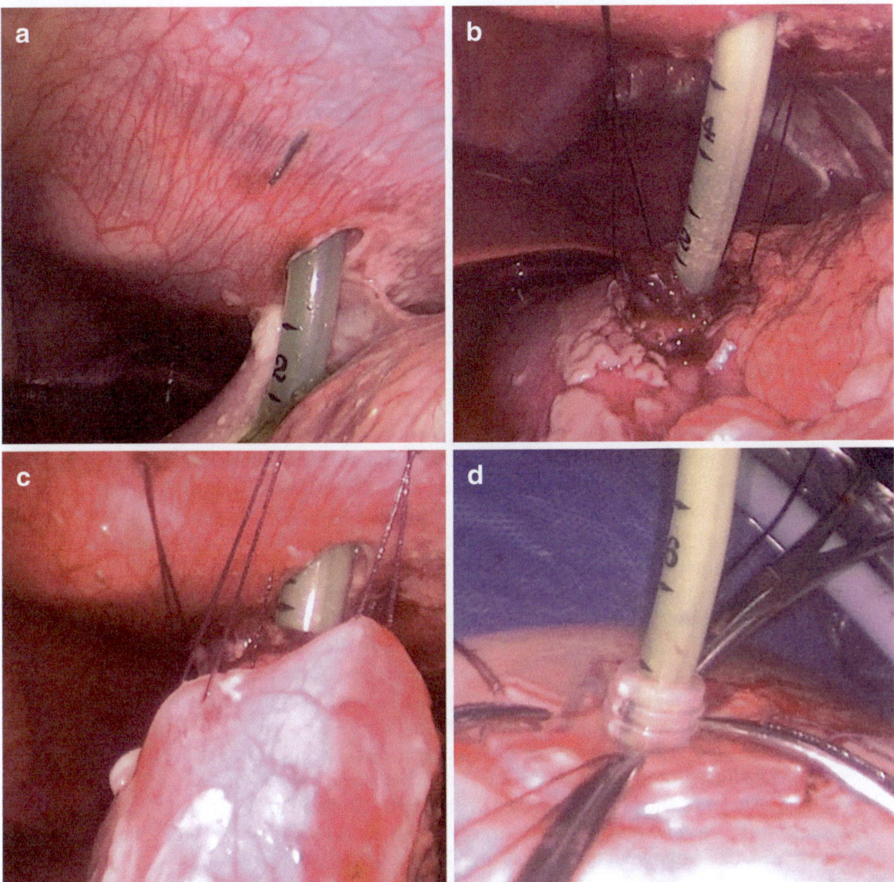

Fig. 2 (**a**) Percutaneous gastrostomy leakage as evidenced during explorative laparoscopy. (**b, c**) Laparoscopic gastropexy. (**d**) New external fixation of the plate

reported [5, 55]. This approach allows the surgeon to explore the entire abdominal cavity and to attach the stomach to the abdominal wall (Fig. 2). Another adverse event related to percutaneous gastrostomy is the buried bumper syndrome. This is an infrequent problem in which the internal bumper of the gastrostomy migrates into the stomach or the abdominal wall. Pediatric series have reported successful cases treated by laparoscopy [56].

6 Summary

Minimally invasive techniques can be employed in most cases of surgical or endoscopic complications. Early recognition and treatment are paramount, but there is a role for endoscopic correction of leaks or perforation. On the other hand, patients who are unstable, who have difficult abdomens, or who present important comorbidities, like a coagulopathy, should be managed in the most expeditious way, which typically means an open technique. If the situation can be handled with laparoscopy, the patients will usually have fewer complications.

References

1. Pearse R, Dawson D, Fawcett J, Rhodes A, Grounds RM, Bennett ED. Early goal-directed therapy after major surgery reduces complications and duration of hospital stay. A randomised, controlled trial [ISRCTN38797445]. Crit Care. 2005;9(6):R687–93.
2. Vonlanthen R, Slankamenac K, Breitenstein S, Puhan MA, Muller MK, Hahnloser D, et al. The impact of complications on costs of major surgical procedures: a cost analysis of 1200 patients. Ann Surg. 2011;254(6):907–13.
3. Kirshtein B, Roy-Shapira A, Domchik S, Mizrahi S, Lantsberg L. Early relaparoscopy for management of suspected postoperative complications. J Gastrointest Surg. 2008;12(7):1257–62.
4. Rosin D, Zmora O, Khaikin M, Bar Zakai B, Ayalon A, Shabtai M. Laparoscopic management of surgical complications after a recent laparotomy. Surg Endosc. 2004;18(6):994–6.
5. Kirshtein B, Domchik S, Mizrahi S, Lantsberg L. Laparoscopic diagnosis and treatment of postoperative complications. Am J Surg. 2009;197(1):19–23.
6. Seshadri PA, Poulin EC, Mamazza J, Schlachta CM. Simplified laparoscopic approach to "second-look" laparotomy: a review. Surg Laparosc Endosc Percutan Tech. 1999;9(4):286–9.
7. Vennix S, Abegg R, Bakker OJ, van den Boezem PB, Brokelman WJ, Sietses C, et al. Surgical re-interventions following colorectal surgery: open versus laparoscopic management of anastomotic leakage. J Laparoendosc Adv Surg Tech A. 2013;23(9):739–44.
8. Hori Y. Diagnostic laparoscopy guidelines: this guideline was prepared by the SAGES guidelines committee and reviewed and approved by the Board of Governors of the Society of American Gastrointestinal and Endoscopic Surgeons (SAGES), November 2007. Surg Endosc. 2008;22(5):1353–83.
9. Feigel A, Sylla P. Role of minimally invasive surgery in the reoperative abdomen or pelvis. Clin Colon Rectal Surg. 2016;29(2):168–80.
10. Agrusa A, Frazzetta G, Chianetta D, Di Giovanni S, Gulotta L, Di Buno G, et al. "Relaparoscopic" management of surgical complications: the experience of an emergency center. Surg Endosc. 2016;30(7):2804–10.
11. Duron JJ, Hay JM, Msika S, Gaschard D, Domergue J, Gainant A, et al. Prevalence and mechanisms of small intestinal obstruction following laparoscopic abdominal surgery: a retrospective multicenter study. French Association for Surgical Research. Arch Surg. 2000;135(2):208–12.
12. Boughey JC, Nottingham JM, Walls AC. Richter's hernia in the laparoscopic era: four case reports and review of the literature. Surg Laparosc Endosc Percutan Tech. 2003;13(1):55–8.
13. McCormick JT, Simmang CL. Reoperation following minimally invasive surgery: are the "rules" different? Clin Colon Rectal Surg. 2006;19(4):217–22.
14. Sheikh L, Croft R, Harmston C. Counting the costs of complications in colorectal surgery. N Z Med J. 2019;132(1497):32–6.
15. Corcione F, Cuccurullo D, Pirozzi F, Sciuto A, La Barbera C, Mandalà S. The role of laparoscopy in emergency treatment of complications after laparoscopic and endoscopic procedures. The role of laparoscopy in emergency abdominal surgery. Milano: Springer Milan; 2012. p. 175–87.

16. Kingham TP, Pachter HL. Colonic anastomotic leak: risk factors, diagnosis, and treatment. J Am Coll Surg. 2009;208(2):269–78.

17. Rahbari NN, Weitz J, Hohenberger W, Heald RJ, Moran B, Ulrich A, et al. Definition and grading of anastomotic leakage following anterior resection of the rectum: a proposal by the International Study Group of Rectal Cancer. Surgery. 2010;147(3):339–51.

18. Chen WT, Bansal S, Ke TW, Chang SC, Huang YC, Kato T, et al. Combined repeat laparoscopy and transanal endolumenal repair (hybrid approach) in the early management of postoperative colorectal anastomotic leaks: technique and outcomes. Surg Endosc. 2018;32(11):4472–80.

19. Cuccurullo D, Pirozzi F, Sciuto A, Bracale U, La Barbera C, Galante F, et al. Relaparoscopy for management of postoperative complications following colorectal surgery: ten years experience in a single center. Surg Endosc. 2015;29(7):1795–803.

20. Wind J, Koopman AG, van Berge Henegouwen MI, Slors JF, Gouma DJ, Bemelman WA. Laparoscopic reintervention for anastomotic leakage after primary laparoscopic colorectal surgery. Br J Surg. 2007;94(12):1562–6.

21. Fransvea P, Costa G, D'Agostino L, Sganga G, Serao A. Redo-laparoscopy in the management of complications after laparoscopic colorectal surgery: a systematic review and meta-analysis of surgical outcomes. Tech Coloproctol. 2021;25(4):371–83.

22. Lee CM, Huh JW, Yun SH, Kim HC, Lee WY, Park YA, et al. Laparoscopic versus open reintervention for anastomotic leakage following minimally invasive colorectal surgery. Surg Endosc. 2015;29(4):931–6.

23. Gong W, Li J. Combat with esophagojejunal anastomotic leakage after total gastrectomy for gastric cancer: a critical review of the literature. Int J Surg. 2017;47:18–24.

24. Bui T, Chan S. Laparoscopic approach for esophagojejunal anastomotic leak in patients requiring re-look intervention: how we do it. Surg Case Rep. 2021;4(3):3.

25. Watson DI, de Beaux AC. Complications of laparoscopic antireflux surgery. Surg Endosc. 2001;15(4):344–52.

26. Yau P, Watson DI, Devitt PG, Game PA, Jamieson GG. Early reoperation following laparoscopic antireflux surgery. Am J Surg. 2000;179(3):172–6.

27. Dagher I, Proske JM, Carloni A, Richa H, Tranchart H, Franco D. Laparoscopic liver resection: results for 70 patients. Surg Endosc. 2007;21(4):619–24.

28. Dexter SP, Miller GV, Davides D, Martin IG, Sue Ling HM, Sagar PM, et al. Relaparoscopy for the detection and treatment of complications of laparoscopic cholecystectomy. Am J Surg. 2000;179(4):316–9.

29. Strasberg SM, Hertl M, Soper NJ. An analysis of the problem of biliary injury during laparoscopic cholecystectomy. J Am Coll Surg. 1995;180(1):101–25.

30. Dumonceau JM, Tringali A, Papanikolaou IS, Blero D, Mangiavillano B, Schmidt A, et al. Endoscopic biliary stenting: indications, choice of stents, and results: European Society of Gastrointestinal Endoscopy (ESGE) clinical guideline—updated October 2017. Endoscopy. 2018;50(9):910–30.

31. Wills VL, Jorgensen JO, Hunt DR. Role of relaparoscopy in the management of minor bile leakage after laparoscopic cholecystectomy. Br J Surg. 2000;87(2):176–80.

32. Barband AR, Kakaei F, Daryani A, Fakhree MB. Relaparoscopy in minor bile leakage after laparoscopic cholecystectomy: an alternative approach? Surg Laparosc Endosc Percutan Tech. 2011;21(4):288–91.

33. Palermo M, Trelles N, Gagner M. Laparoscopic revisional hepaticojejunostomy for biliary stricture after open repair following common bile duct injury: a case report. Surg Innov. 2011;18(1):105–9.

34. Cuendis-Velázquez A, Morales-Chávez C, Aguirre-Olmedo I, Torres-Ruiz F, Rojano-Rodríguez M, Fernández-Álvarez L, et al. Laparoscopic hepaticojejunostomy after bile duct injury. Surg Endosc. 2016;30(3):876–82.

35. Giulianotti PC, Quadri P, Durgam S, Bianco FM. Reconstruction/repair of iatrogenic biliary injuries: is the robot offering a new option? Short clinical report. Ann Surg. 2018;267(1):e7–9.

36. Laxague F, Schlottmann F, Piatti JM, Sadava EE. Minimally invasive step-up approach for the management of postoperative intraabdominal abscess after laparoscopic appendectomy. Surg Endosc. 2021;35(2):787–91.
37. Allaway MGR, Clement K, Eslick GD, Cox MR. Early laparoscopic washout may resolve persistent intra-abdominal infection post-appendicectomy. World J Surg. 2019;43(4):998–1006.
38. Leister I, Becker H. [Relaparoscopy as an alternative to laparotomy for laparoscopic complications]. Chirurg. 2006;77(11):986–97.
39. Casas MA, Laxague F, Schlottmann F, Sadava EE. Re-laparoscopy for the treatment of complications after laparoscopic appendectomy: is it possible to maintain the minimally invasive approach? Updates Surg. 2020;73:2199.
40. Wszolek Matthew F, Sorcini A, Moinzadeh A, Tuerk Ingolf A. RELAPAROSCOPY FOR THE DETECTION AND TREATMENT OF COMPLICATIONS OF LAPAROSCOPIC UROLOGIC SURGERY. J Urol. 2009;181(4S):277–8.
41. Vitagliano G, Castilla R, Fernandez Long JG. Relaparoscopy in the treatment of complications after laparoscopic urological procedures. Arch Esp Urol. 2013;66(2):215–20.
42. de'Angelis N, Di Saverio S, Chiara O, Sartelli M, Martinez-Perez A, Patrizi F, et al. WSES guidelines for the management of iatrogenic colonoscopy perforation. World J Emerg Surg. 2017;2018(13):5.
43. Kim HH, Kye BH, Kim HJ, Cho HM. Prompt management is most important for colonic perforation after colonoscopy. Ann Coloproctol. 2014;30(5):228–31.
44. Damore LJ 2nd, Rantis PC, Vernava AM 3rd, Longo WE. Colonoscopic perforations. Etiology, diagnosis, and management. Dis Colon Rectum. 1996;39(11):1308–14.
45. Panteris V, Haringsma J, Kuipers EJ. Colonoscopy perforation rate, mechanisms and outcome: from diagnostic to therapeutic colonoscopy. Endoscopy. 2009;41(11):941–51.
46. Martinez-Perez A, de'Angelis N, Brunetti F, Le Baleur Y, Paya-Llorente C, Memeo R, et al. Laparoscopic vs. open surgery for the treatment of iatrogenic colonoscopic perforations: a systematic review and meta-analysis. World J Emerg Surg. 2017;12:8.
47. Schloricke E, Bader FG, Hoffmann M, Zimmermann M, Bruch HP, Hildebrand P. [Open surgical versus laparoscopic treatment of iatrogenic colon perforation—results of a 13-year experience]. Zentralbl Chir. 2013;138(3):257–61.
48. Bleier JI, Moon V, Feingold D, Whelan RL, Arnell T, Sonoda T, et al. Initial repair of iatrogenic colon perforation using laparoscopic methods. Surg Endosc. 2008;22(3):646–9.
49. Kim J, Lee GJ, Baek JH, Lee WS. Comparison of the surgical outcomes of laparoscopic versus open surgery for colon perforation during colonoscopy. Ann Surg Treat Res. 2014;87(3):139–43.
50. Coimbra C, Bouffioux L, Kohnen L, Deroover A, Dresse D, Denoel A, et al. Laparoscopic repair of colonoscopic perforation: a new standard? Surg Endosc. 2011;25(5):1514–7.
51. Rotholtz NA, Laporte M, Lencinas S, Bun M, Canelas A, Mezzadri N. Laparoscopic approach to colonic perforation due to colonoscopy. World J Surg. 2010;34(8):1949–53.
52. Shin DK, Shin SY, Park CY, Jin SM, Cho YH, Kim WH, et al. Optimal methods for the management of iatrogenic colonoscopic perforation. Clin Endosc. 2016;49(3):282–8.
53. Chirica M, Kelly MD, Siboni S, Aiolfi A, Riva CG, Asti E, et al. Esophageal emergencies: WSES guidelines. World J Emerg Surg. 2019;14:26.
54. Ivatury RR, Moore FA, Biffl W, Leppeniemi A, Ansaloni L, Catena F, et al. Oesophageal injuries: position paper, WSES, 2013. World J Emerg Surg. 2014;9(1):9.
55. Backus CL, Muscoriel SJ, Iannitti DA, Heniford BT. Laparoscopic repair of the leaking percutaneous endoscopic gastrostomy. J Laparoendosc Adv Surg Tech A. 2000;10(2):105–9.
56. Singh RR, Eaton S, Cross KM, Curry JI, De Coppi P, Kiely EM, et al. Management of a complication of percutaneous gastrostomy in children. Eur J Pediatr Surg. 2013;23(1):76–9.

Role of Bedside Laparoscopy

Rhiannon Bradshaw, Heather M. Grossman Verner,
Rachel Krzeczowski, and Michael S. Truitt

1   Target Patient Populations and Indications

The target patient populations and indications for bedside laparoscopy (BL) are diverse. In general, BL is helpful for patients who cannot be reliably examined, such as patients who are intubated, sedated, obtunded, or demented. In addition, it can be useful to evaluate a patient who is unable to be transported to the OR secondary to maximal hemodynamic or respiratory requirements. It can be used among trauma, general surgery, burn [1, 2], and post-cardiac surgery patient populations [3]. Common indications for BL include unexplained abdominal pain and the need to rule out acute acalculous cholecystitis, intestinal ischemia, or a perforated hollow viscus [3]. Less commonly, it has been used to assess for an aorto-aortic anastomotic leak after an open aortic repair [4].

BL can be used, in lieu of diagnostic peritoneal lavage, to assess fascial violation in penetrating trauma or to rule out diaphragmatic injury in trauma patients [1]. In blunt trauma, especially patients with a positive seatbelt sign, BL can evaluate the presence of hemoperitoneum and associated mesenteric injury [5]. This may shorten hospital length of stay by avoiding the need for serial abdominal exams.

BL can serve both diagnostic and therapeutic purposes. For example, in a patient with concern for a bowel perforation, a negative BL can potentially help avoid both a trip to the OR and a negative exploratory laparotomy. Similarly, in a vented patient with concern for acute acalculous cholecystitis who cannot communicate or give a reliable abdominal exam, BL can be used to confirm this diagnosis [1]. On the

R. Bradshaw · M. S. Truitt (✉)
Department of Surgery, Methodist Dallas Medical Center, Dallas, TX, USA
e-mail: RhiannonBradshaw@mhd.com

H. M. Grossman Verner · R. Krzeczowski
Clinical Research Institute, Methodist Health System, Dallas, TX, USA
e-mail: HeatherGrossmanVerner@mhd.com; RachelKrzeczowski@mhd.com

© The Author(s), under exclusive license to Springer Nature Switzerland AG 2023   355
F. Coccolini et al. (eds.), *Mini-invasive Approach in Acute Care Surgery*,
Hot Topics in Acute Care Surgery and Trauma,
https://doi.org/10.1007/978-3-031-39001-2_26

therapeutic side, BL in acute acalculous cholecystitis allows for simultaneous placement of a drainage catheter [5]. Likewise, BL can be used for placement, reassessment, and/or revision of gastrostomy tubes and peritoneal dialysis catheters [6].

BL is particularly useful in acute mesenteric ischemia (AMI). In this diagnostically challenging disease, the exam is unreliable, there are no definitive laboratory values, and computed tomography (CT) scans can be inconclusive. Bergamini et al. recently demonstrated that BL allowed them to avoid unnecessary laparotomies in post-cardiac surgery ICU patients with AMI and nonocclusive mesenteric ischemia [7].

2 Benefits

BL can be used to confirm or rule out the presence of intra-abdominal pathologies in patients who are too unstable for transport to radiology for diagnostic imaging. Additionally, CT is unreliable for some conditions, namely, diaphragmatic injuries [8, 9], hollow viscus injuries [10, 11], or intestinal ischemia in the absence of perforation; in these cases, laparoscopy may be necessary to make a diagnosis. As noted by Rehm, "the abdomen is a notorious *black hole*" for these problems [5].

BL not only reduces the incidence of nontherapeutic laparotomies [12] but also reduces morbidity [13, 14]. The morbidity from a negative laparotomy varies between 5 and 43% [15]. Possible short-term complications include wound infection [16], skin/fascial dehiscence, evisceration, or prolonged ileus. Long-term complications including incisional hernia or adhesive small bowel obstruction are common [17, 18].

BL can help avoid a positive, but futile, laparotomy in patients with an intra-abdominal catastrophe. For example, Peris et al. reported diffuse intestinal hypoperfusion in 2 of 32 patients in whom diagnostic BL was performed [3]. The BLs avoided what is colloquially known as a "peek and shriek" type of operation—a laparotomy in which most bowel is noted to be nonviable and the patient is closed without further intervention. Gagne et al. similarly found extensive intestinal necrosis in 3 of 19 patients. This allowed them to have informed discussions with the family and avoid further futile interventions [19].

BL is often more expeditious than a trip to the OR, as it can be completed and a diagnosis obtained very quickly. Often, all that is necessary is a single 5 or 10 mm trocar for the camera (Table 1). Additional trocars can be added as needed.

Gagne et al. demonstrated the feasibility of a mini-BL using a 3 mm camera and instruments [19]. These mini-laparoscopies took an average of 21 min [19]. Traditional BL procedure times have been reported between 20 and 40 min [3, 20, 21]. Compared to diagnostic peritoneal lavage in the ICU, BL took only 5 min longer: 14 min vs. 19 min [22].

BL can be performed with local anesthesia (e.g., lidocaine or bupivacaine), conscious sedation (e.g., intravenous midazolam, fentanyl, or propofol), or both, avoiding the need for and risks of general anesthesia. Successful cases performed in ICU patients without the use of endotracheal intubation have also been reported [19, 20].

Table 1 Suggested surgical equipment

Minimum required equipment
Laparoscopic tower (insufflation, light source, camera, monitor)
5 or 10 mm laparoscope
Two trocars (Hasson or Veress needle)
Blunt laparoscopic grasper
Basic laparoscopic surgical tray (scalpel, sponges, forceps)
Fascial suture and needle driver
Closing equipment (skin glue and/or subcuticular suture)
Sterile drapes, prep
Suggested additional equipment
Additional laparoscopic instruments (ultrasonic dissector, multiple graspers)
Laparoscopic suction/irrigation
Additional trocars

The series reported by Gagne et al. did not require anesthesia providers and were completed with a surgeon and one assistant. Laparoscopy can be done with carbon dioxide or nitrous oxide insufflation to avoid hypercapnia or acidosis [19]. In most cases, insufflation to pressures of 8–10 mm Hg are sufficient, avoiding potential cardiovascular effects.

Early reports of diagnostic laparoscopy were performed only in patients without previous surgery [1]. Subsequent reports found prior abdominal surgery to not be a contraindication for BL and a recent laparotomy is not an absolute contraindication. Pecoraro et al. reported a series in which 7 of 11 patients had a recent laparotomy [20].

3   Potential Disadvantages

There are some drawbacks to BL. For example, transportation of the laparoscopic equipment to the bedside may be inconvenient, may be cumbersome, and may result in excessive wear/tear. Unfamiliarity, poor lighting, and lack of standard procedural instruments may decrease the efficacy of BL. Should additional equipment be required, it may not be readily available at the bedside. The ICU or ER bed is also wider than an OR bed. Moving the ICU or ER bed into different positions may not be possible, making some surgical movements more difficult or less precise than they would be in the OR. Lastly, identification or definitive management of an intra-abdominal pathology may still require a trip to the OR.

BL has further disadvantages when compared to traditional laparotomy. For instance, laparoscopy is inherently limited in its evaluation of retroperitoneal structures. There are also patients who have a hostile abdomen not well suited to laparoscopy. Prior abdominal surgery, while not a contraindication to laparoscopy, may cause adhesive disease that makes laparoscopy more difficult. Pregnancy may limit intra-abdominal volume and therefore working space. Abdominal wall compliance may be limited by carcinomatosis, tuberculous peritonitis [23], or "cocoon abdomen" secondary to sclerosing peritonitis. Together, these factors must be fully considered prior to utilization of BL.

There are risks inherent to laparoscopy as a modality, whether at the bedside or in the OR. Chief among these are the physiologic changes secondary to abdominal insufflation and its effect on multiple systems, including cardiovascular (e.g., decreased preload, increased central venous pressure, increased myocardial oxygen consumption, possible hyper-/hypotension, arrhythmia, and myocardial infarction), pulmonary (e.g., decreased lung volume, decreased compliance, potential for hypercarbia) [24], renal (e.g., decreased perfusion and urine output) [25], and neurologic (e.g., increased intracranial pressure) [26]. Additionally, intraoperative decreased venous return from the lower extremities may lead to deep vein thrombosis and pulmonary embolism [27]. Entering the abdomen is not without risk and may lead to inadvertent hollow viscus injury, vascular injury to epigastric vessels and major intra-abdominal vessels (e.g., the aorta or inferior vena cava), or solid organ injury [5].

4   Conclusions and Future Directions

Current data has been unable to establish if BL may reduce overall cost of care. It seems likely the reduction of required equipment, personnel, and time would significantly reduce the estimated $36–37 USD per minute costs associated with more traditional exploratory laparotomy [28]. More research is needed to quantify the financial benefit of BL.

BL is a useful tool in the surgeon's armamentarium for the diagnosis of intra-abdominal pathology. It can be used in a wide range of patients and is especially useful for the unstable patient who would otherwise require a potentially morbid negative laparotomy. BL is efficient, requires minimal equipment and ancillary staff, and may reduce the cost of care.

References

1. Bender JS, Talamini MA. Diagnostic laparoscopy in critically ill intensive-care-unit patients. Surg Endosc. 1992;6(6):302–4. https://doi.org/10.1007/bf02498865.
2. Brandt CP, Priebe PP, Eckhauser ML. Diagnostic laparoscopy in the intensive care patient. Avoiding the nontherapeutic laparotomy. Surg Endosc. 1993;7(3):168–72. https://doi.org/10.1007/bf00594100.
3. Peris A, Matano S, Manca G, Zagli G, Bonizzoli M, Cianchi G, et al. Bedside diagnostic laparoscopy to diagnose intraabdominal pathology in the intensive care unit. Crit Care. 2009;13(1):R25. https://doi.org/10.1186/cc7730.
4. Ceribelli C, Adami EA, Mattia S, Benini B. Bedside diagnostic laparoscopy for critically ill patients: a retrospective study of 62 patients. Surg Endosc. 2012;26(12):3612–5. https://doi.org/10.1007/s00464-012-2383-4.
5. Rehm CG. Bedside laparoscopy. Crit Care Clin. 2000;16(1):101–12. https://doi.org/10.1016/s0749-0704(05)70099-3.
6. Sackier JM. Laparoscopy in the emergency setting. World J Surg. 1992;16(6):1083–8. https://doi.org/10.1007/bf02067065.

7. Bergamini C, Alemanno G, Giordano A, Pantalone D, Fontani G, Di Bella AM, et al. The role of bed-side laparoscopy in the management of acute mesenteric ischemia of recent onset in post-cardiac surgery patients admitted to ICU. Eur J Trauma Emerg Surg. 2020;48(1):87–96. https://doi.org/10.1007/s00068-020-01500-3.

8. Ghumman Z, Monteiro S, Mellnick V, Coates A, Engels P, Patlas M. Accuracy of preoperative MDCT in patients with penetrating abdominal and pelvic trauma. Can Assoc Radiol J. 2020;71(2):231–7. https://doi.org/10.1177/0846537119888375.

9. İlhan M, Bulakçı M, Bademler S, Gök AF, Azamat İF, Ertekin C. The diagnostic efficacy of computed tomography in detecting diaphragmatic injury secondary to thoracoabdominal penetrating traumas: a comparison with diagnostic laparoscopy. Ulus Travma Acil Cerrahi Derg. 2015;21(6):484–90. https://doi.org/10.5505/tjtes.2015.94389.

10. Bhagvan S, Turai M, Holden A, Ng A, Civil I. Predicting hollow viscus injury in blunt abdominal trauma with computed tomography. World J Surg. 2013;37(1):123–6. https://doi.org/10.1007/s00268-012-1798-3.

11. Mothes H, Mueller-Mau V, Lehmkuhl L, Lehmann T, Settmacher U, Teichgräber U, et al. The role of computed tomography in the diagnostic pathway of acute mesenteric ischemia: a nested case-control study. Acta Radiol. 2020;61(11):1444–51. https://doi.org/10.1177/0284185120905086.

12. Cocco AM, Bhagvan S, Bouffler C, Hsu J. Diagnostic laparoscopy in penetrating abdominal trauma. ANZ J Surg. 2019;89(4):353–6. https://doi.org/10.1111/ans.15140.

13. Xie M, Qi Q, Xu Y, Wang H, Ge S, Luo P. [Comparison of laparoscopic exploration and exploratory laparotomy in the diagnosis and treatment of abdominal open trauma]. Zhonghua Wei Zhong Bing Ji Jiu Yi Xue. 2019;31(2):178–81. https://doi.org/10.3760/cma.j.issn.2095-4352.2019.02.011.

14. Uranüs S, Dorr K. Laparoscopy in abdominal trauma. Eur J Trauma Emerg Surg. 2010;36(1):19–24. https://doi.org/10.1007/s00068-010-9219-5.

15. Schnüriger B, Lam L, Inaba K, Kobayashi L, Barbarino R, Demetriades D. Negative laparotomy in trauma: are we getting better? Am Surg. 2012;78(11):1219–23.

16. Durbin S, DeAngelis R, Peschman J, Milia D, Carver T, Dodgion C. Superficial surgical infections in operative abdominal trauma patients: a trauma quality improvement database analysis. J Surg Res. 2019;243:496–502. https://doi.org/10.1016/j.jss.2019.06.101.

17. Hathaway E, Glaser J, Cardarelli C, Dunne J, Elster E, Safford S, et al. Exploratory laparotomy for proximal vascular control in combat-related injuries. Mil Med. 2016;181(5 Suppl):247–52. https://doi.org/10.7205/milmed-d-15-00155.

18. Hanna K, Asmar S, Ditillo M, Chehab M, Khurrum M, Bible L, et al. Readmission with major abdominal complications after penetrating abdominal trauma. J Surg Res. 2021;257:69–78. https://doi.org/10.1016/j.jss.2020.07.060.

19. Gagné DJ, Malay MB, Hogle NJ, Fowler DL. Bedside diagnostic minilaparoscopy in the intensive care patient. Surgery. 2002;131(5):491–6. https://doi.org/10.1067/msy.2002.122607.

20. Pecoraro AP, Cacchione RN, Sayad P, Williams ME, Ferzli GS. The routine use of diagnostic laparoscopy in the intensive care unit. Surg Endosc. 2001;15(7):638–41. https://doi.org/10.1007/s004640000371.

21. Jaramillo EJ, Treviño JM, Berghoff KR, Franklin ME Jr. Bedside diagnostic laparoscopy in the intensive care unit: a 13-year experience. JSLS. 2006;10(2):155–9.

22. Walsh RM, Popovich MJ, Hoadley J. Bedside diagnostic laparoscopy and peritoneal lavage in the intensive care unit. Surg Endosc. 1998;12(12):1405–9. https://doi.org/10.1007/s004649900869.

23. Geis WP, Kim HC. Use of laparoscopy in the diagnosis and treatment of patients with surgical abdominal sepsis. Surg Endosc. 1995;9(2):178–82. https://doi.org/10.1007/bf00191962.

24. Atkinson TM, Giraud GD, Togioka BM, Jones DB, Cigarroa JE. Cardiovascular and ventilatory consequences of laparoscopic surgery. Circulation. 2017;135(7):700–10. https://doi.org/10.1161/circulationaha.116.023262.

25. Dunn MD, McDougall EM. Renal physiology. Laparoscopic considerations. Urol Clin North Am. 2000;27(4):609–14. https://doi.org/10.1016/s0094-0143(05)70110-5.
26. Kamine TH, Papavassiliou E, Schneider BE. Effect of abdominal insufflation for laparoscopy on intracranial pressure. JAMA Surg. 2014;149(4):380–2. https://doi.org/10.1001/jamasurg.2013.3024.
27. Stein PD, Matta F, Sabra MJ. Pulmonary embolism and deep venous thrombosis following laparoscopic cholecystectomy. Clin Appl Thromb Hemost. 2014;20(3):233–7. https://doi.org/10.1177/1076029613502255.
28. Childers CP, Maggard-Gibbons M. Understanding costs of care in the operating room. JAMA Surg. 2018;153(4):e176233. https://doi.org/10.1001/jamasurg.2017.6233.

Anesthesia Considerations for MIS in Emergency and Trauma Surgery

Hillary Prince and Michael W. Cripps

1   Introduction

The benefits of minimally invasive surgery (MIS) have been well documented in elective surgery cases. Today, MIS approaches are rapidly replacing open surgical techniques as the standard of care, including several urgent and emergent operations; however, the minimally invasive approach to thoracic or abdominal pathology can have a significant, and potentially deleterious, effect on the patient's physiology.

Regardless of the surgical approach, trauma and emergency general surgery patients pose a great challenge to anesthesiologists; little may be known about the patient's baseline physiology and comorbidities, and the need for emergent intervention typically obviates a thorough preoperative workup. The move toward a minimally invasive approach in these patients adds additional layers of complexity that must be considered, including intraoperative decompensation, and the anesthetic plan must afford preparation for such an event. Careful planning and communication between the anesthesia and surgical team are essential to the safety of the patient and to providing the best chance at successful completion of a minimally invasive approach.

H. Prince
Department of Surgery, University of Texas Southwestern Medical Center at Dallas, Dallas, TX, USA
e-mail: hillary.prince@utsouthwestern.edu

M. W. Cripps (✉)
Department of Surgery, University of Colorado Anschutz Medical Center, Aurora, CO, USA
e-mail: michael.cripps@cuanschutz.edu

2 Decision-Making for Using MIS in the Emergency General Surgery and Trauma Setting

The general principles of resuscitation of any trauma or emergency surgery patient must always be followed. Confirmation of a secure airway, reversal of hypoxia, management of hemorrhagic shock or sepsis, correction of acidosis or coagulopathy, and maintenance of normothermia must be prioritized.

2.1 Emergency General Surgery

The range of pathologies with which an emergency general surgery patient may present is important to appreciate, as is the spectrum of severity of illness. This large spectrum of disease type and inflammation combined with various surgical approaches can have a significant impact on anesthesia planning.

Acute appendicitis and cholecystitis account for an extremely large proportion of emergency general surgery operations. For many patients with early disease, there is a minimal inflammatory response, and the operations are very straightforward, with the patients being discharged to home from the recovery unit. However, there is increasing data codifying the severity of illness in these two common operations that show how the inflammatory sepctrum can effect critically ill and septic patients. Although intuitive, there is now clear data that demonstrates that increased severity of inflammation has significant effect on time in the OR, hospital length of stay, conversion to open, and complications [1].

Madni et al. demonstrated that patients with high-grade cholecystitis (Parkland Grading Scale 4 or 5) have significantly increased OR time and risk of conversion to open [1]. This grading of severity can be done early in the operation and can assist in anesthesia planning.

Open operative approaches have been the main interventional modality for emergency general surgery. However, there is increasing use of laparoscopy in other emergency general surgery cases, such as perforated peptic ulcer disease and diverticulitis. These disease processes also have significant spectrum of severity; historically, only those patients with minimal to no physiologic derangements would undergo laparoscopic repair. However, with increasing data suggesting improved outcomes in these patients with less invasive approaches, and the increased comfort level of surgeons utilizing minimally invasive techniques, a trend toward greater use of laparoscopy in more severely ill patients is to be expected [2].

Similarly, patients with bowel obstruction can present quite variably, from single-band adhesive disease to segments of necrotic bowel. Like the above descriptions, these patients will have diametrically opposite physiologic responses that must be taken into consideration. Specific considerations in these patients include increased abdominal pressure resulting from dilated bowel that can become significantly increased during insufflation; this increased abdominal pressure can have an untoward effect on tidal volume and peak airway pressures. Additionally, if there is a closed-loop obstruction that is reduced, there can be an increase in inflammatory cytokines resulting in altered physiology. Careful observation of the progress of the operation and communication with the operative team is critical.

For the septic patient in need of operative intervention, initial management should focus on Surviving Sepsis guidelines, with a focus on the Hour-1 Bundle of Care Elements—obtaining a lactate level and blood/urine cultures, administering broad-spectrum antibiotics, crystalloid resuscitation of 30 mL/kg for hypotension (mean arterial pressure [MAP] <65) or lactate >4, and addition of vasopressors if hypotension is refractory [3]. The importance of early recognition and initiation of therapy cannot be understated; for each hour that antibiotic administration is delayed, for example, the mortality increases by 3–6% [4]. Achieving source control with surgical intervention, while taking into account the hemodynamic instability of the patient, often cannot be delayed. It is important to note that this instability does not necessarily preclude a minimally invasive approach.

With all abdominal emergency general surgery cases, there is a potential for conversion to an open operation. Fortunately, conversion to an open procedure in the abdomen should have no effect on positioning of the patient, and any physiologic effect of the pneumoperitoneum is immediately resolved on opening the abdomen.

2.2 Trauma Surgery

Trauma patients who present in hemorrhagic shock can pose a significant problem to all providers, as the body's compensatory mechanisms can often mask significant volume loss. This pattern of physiologic compensation is used to define the classes of shock, listed in Table 1.

Table 1 Classes of shock

Classes of shock	Total blood volume lost (%)	Clinical presentation
Class I	<15%	No drop in BP No or slight ↓PP No to slight ↑HR Mental status: normal to slightly anxious
Class II	15–30%	Normal to ↓BP ↓PP ↑HR ↑RR Mental status: mildly anxious
Class III	30–40%	↓BP ↓↓PP ↑↑HR ↑↑RR Mental status: anxious, confused
Class IV	>40%	↓↓BP ↓↓PP ↑↑↑HR ↑↑↑RR Mental status: lethargic, confused

The response to transfusion can provide useful clinical information, as a patient whose hemodynamics respond appropriately to the volume of blood given likely have tamponaded the source of bleeding or are bleeding at a slower rate, whereas transient responders or nonresponders have ongoing blood loss, potentially with an element of coagulopathy.

The selection of patients for a minimally invasive approach will depend on the patient's physiologic parameters at the time that intervention is required as well as the pattern of injury and the surgeon's comfort level with such techniques. If a minimally invasive approach is selected, the anesthesia team must be prepared for any number of clinical scenarios in which the patient may decompensate during the operation or at any point during the perioperative period.

Appropriate vascular access must be in place prior to induction. For the injured patient, two peripheral large-bore IVs (at least 18G) are usually placed in the trauma bay; if unable to do so, or if vasopressor or inotrope use is anticipated, then intraosseous or central venous access should be established. The patient's injury pattern can play a role in site selection for central venous catheters (CVCs), and the subclavian vein may be preferrable for its accessibility without ultrasound guidance or in the presence of a pelvic injury or cervical collar.

In patients with significant traumatic injuries or sepsis, an arterial line is essential not only for hemodynamic monitoring; it also allows for frequent blood sampling, including serial ABGs.

Injured patients who are bleeding often invoke a response among care providers to try and give as much fluids as possible in order to achieve a more normal blood pressure; however, this can result in an opposite and untoward effect of causing increasing hemorrhage. Damage control resuscitation is a strategy whereby a patient is given limited to no crystalloids, but rather blood component therapy, to provide oxygen-carrying capacity and coagulation factors. Nested within this strategy is a lower mean arterial pressure (MAP) goal. This restrictive strategy for resuscitation, initially employed in the World War I era [5], is aimed toward preserving local vasoconstriction that decreases hydrostatic pressure on tenuous clots that, if disrupted, would lead to increased hemorrhage. This subsequent hemorrhage would lead to increased fluid resuscitation and worsening coagulopathy, and the cycle would continue. There have been multiple retrospective analyses [6] using hypotensive resuscitation strategies, each showing either improved survival or decreased complications. There have been five prospective randomized controlled trials. One showed improved survival for all, another showed improved survival in a post hoc analysis of blunt trauma patients, and another showed decreased incidence of AKI and a shorter length of stay. Potentially more importantly, none showed harm for hypotensive resuscitation. As a result, the 2013 European Guidelines recommend a target systolic blood pressure (SBP) of 80–90 mmHg until major bleeding has been controlled in the initial phase following trauma without brain injury [7].

Whether or not this strategy could be used in minimally invasive operations for injured patients has not currently been studied. Potential caveats and concerns would revolve around the effect of insufflation on a purposefully low preload, and this may require a higher SBP prior to initiation of pneumoperitoneum. It is important to note that the practice of limiting crystalloid and using whole blood or blood component therapy should be followed, regardless of the surgical approach used.

Communication between the anesthesia and surgery teams is a key component of the success of any surgery, but it becomes even more important when managing an unstable patient. Any bleeding or gross contamination should be conveyed by the surgeon to the anesthesia provider; the anesthesia team must keep the surgeon informed of any persistent hemodynamic instability, acidosis, or hypothermia despite adequate resuscitation that may lead to the decision to convert to an open procedure or even a damage control approach.

3 Positioning

Patient positioning influences the anesthesia plan for the operation and can greatly impact the patient's physiology. In elective thoracic or retroperitoneal operations, the patient will be in lateral decubitus position. The airway and lines must be carefully attended to with any repositioning. Bony prominences must be padded to prevent pressure injuries, and care must be taken to avoid any excessive abduction or extension to protect from possible nerve injury.

In emergency surgery, the need for rapid conversion to an open operation must be taken into consideration. The same principles apply for protection against pressure injuries and excessive body positioning, but a plan for conversion must be in place. The surgeon may utilize rolls or a beanbag to stabilize the patient in a modified lateral decubitus position and airplane the OR table to provide improved body positioning that can be reverted to near decubitus position, should the operation require conversion. Straps must be placed at multiple points along the length of the patient to secure him/her to the operating table; this can both assist in initial positioning and improve safety during the case, as the surgeon will ask the anesthesia team for several table adjustments. An axillary roll should be positioned beneath the dependent axilla in order to decrease the pressure load on the inferior shoulder. The superior arm is extended in order to displace the scapula from the operative field, while the inferior arm is either flexed to no more than 90 degrees or extended out onto a padded arm board.

In the event of a conversion from video-assisted thoracic surgery (VATS) to a thoracotomy, the patient's position should remain the same; however, the patient may need to be repositioned supine, depending on clinical circumstances and surgeon preference. If an emergent repositioning is required, the airway and endotracheal tube must be protected; if there is any concern for tube malposition after movement, a quick bronchoscopy can be performed to evaluate. For an intra-abdominal approach, the patient should be supine with legs either flat on the table or in stirrups if a colorectal anastomosis or sigmoidoscopy/colonoscopy is planned. Adjustable stirrups, such as yellowfins, must be used to allow the surgeon access to both the abdominal and perineal fields. Conversion from laparoscopy to an open procedure should not require must adjustment, if any, to the patient's position.

4   Anatomic and Physiologic Considerations with Insufflation

Several airway considerations for VATS must be reviewed prior to induction. Ventilation to the lung on the operative side will need to be blocked; the choice of endotracheal tube to accomplish single-lung ventilation (SLV) will depend on the provider's preference. There are three ways to accomplish SLV: (1) inserting a standard single-lumen endotracheal tube into a mainstem bronchus on the nonoperative side, (2) use of a single-lumen endotracheal tube with a bronchial blocker, or (3) use of a double-lumen tube.

One advantage of placing a bronchial blocker through a single-lumen tube is that the tube will not have to be exchanged in the event that the patient is to remain intubated postoperatively. While there are many types of blockers, they function in a similar way. They are placed through the single-lumen endotracheal tube under bronchoscopic guidance and passed into the main bronchus of the operative side that requires lung collapse; the balloon is then inflated and lungs auscultated to confirm placement. The blocker catheter itself has a small-diameter channel used to suction out the lung that is to be collapsed. Because the channel is so small, the main disadvantage of utilizing the blocker for SLV is that the blocked lung collapses quite slowly [8] and may not completely collapse. There have been case reports of other complications, including airway obstruction from clots caused by traumatic tube insertion, accidental fracture of the blocker, and inclusion of the blocker in a staple firing across the bronchus [9].

With the double-lumen tube, the longer bronchial lumen enters the right/left mainstem bronchus that is to be occluded, and the shorter tracheal lumen sits in the lower trachea. Tube position can be easily checked with a bronchoscope. For a left-sided tube, the scope is advanced down the tracheal lumen; the carina should be visible, the bronchial lumen should be seen entering the left main bronchus, and the top of the bronchial cuff should be visible but should not reach above the carina. If the bronchial cuff is not visible for a left-sided tube, the tube may have been advanced beyond the left upper or lower lobe orifice and should be withdrawn until the top of the cuff is visible distal to the carina. For a right-sided tube, the bronchoscope is advanced down the bronchial side to confirm that the endobronchial side portal of the tube is aligned with the orifice of the right upper lobe bronchus. When the patient is positioned for surgery, the tube may move relative to the carina; tube position must always be reconfirmed.

Confirming tube position requires several steps: First, the tracheal lumen is clamped, and the patient is checked for unilateral breath sounds. If breath sounds remain present bilaterally, the tube needs to be advanced; if unilateral breath sounds are heard but not on the expected side, then the bronchial lumen has incorrectly entered the opposite bronchus and needs to be repositioned. Once proper placement of the bronchial lumen is confirmed, the tracheal lumen is unclamped and the bronchial lumen clamped. If the bronchial lumen is meant to be in the left main bronchus, for example, when clamped, the provider should only hear breath sounds on the right side. If breath sounds are diminished or absent bilaterally, the tube may be too proximal, with the bronchial cuff occluding the distal trachea.

Complications of double-lumen tube placement include hypoxemia due to tube malpositioning or occlusion as well as traumatic placement or bronchial cuff overinflation resulting in traumatic laryngitis or tracheobronchial rupture. The tube may also be inadvertently sutured to a bronchus during surgery with subsequent inability to withdraw the tube during extubation.

A systematic review and meta-analysis of randomized controlled trials comparing bronchial blockers and double-lumen tubes found that double-lumen tubes were quicker to place and less likely to be incorrectly positioned; bronchial blockers were associated with fewer patients having a sore throat, less hoarseness, and fewer airway injuries than double-lumen tubes [10]. Overall, the choice of tube is most commonly guided by anesthesiologist preference and comfort level with placement as well as patient anatomy.

4.1 Ventilation

Patient positioning alone has a profound effect on physiology, which must be accounted for when an anesthetic plan is created. With lateral decubitus positioning, there is a gravity-dependent increase in pulmonary blood flow (perfusion, Q) to the dependent lung; at the same time, the nondependent lung is preferentially ventilated (V), creating a VQ mismatch and increasing the A-a gradient. There is compression of the dependent lung both by the mediastinum and by abdominal contents pushing up against the diaphragm; the net result for the dependent lung is a decrease in functional residual capacity (FRC), exacerbating the VQ mismatch further.

When both lungs can be ventilated, positive-pressure ventilation can overcome some of these changes. However, when operating in the thorax, the nondependent lung on the operative side is typically collapsed to create working space, and the patient must tolerate single-lung ventilation (SLV). As the collapsed lung continues to be perfused, a large right-to-left intrapulmonary shunt develops. To compensate, blood flow to the collapsed lung is reduced primarily by the intrinsic process of hypoxic pulmonary vasoconstriction (HPV) as well as possibly by physical compression during the procedure. HPV is vital to overcoming the consequences of lateral decubitus positioning and SLV; therefore, it is important to avoid factors known to inhibit HPV, which would again increase the venous admixture and contribute to refractory hypoxemia. Medications that inhibit HPV include vasodilators (i.e., nitric oxide, nitroglycerin, or nitroprusside), phosphodiesterase inhibitors (i.e., milrinone), calcium channel blockers, beta agonists, and inhalation anesthetics with doses greater than one minimum alveolar concentration (MAC) [11]. Physiologic factors that may limit HPV include hypocapnia, alkalosis, hypothermia, and pulmonary hypertension. HPV is therefore augmented by the opposite—hypercapnia, acidosis, and hyperthermia. HPV can also be counteracted by things that decrease the blood flow to the ventilated lung, consequently shunting flow to the collapsed lung, including low FiO_2, which spurs hypoxic pulmonary vasoconstriction in the ventilated lung. Other factors that decrease flow to the ventilated lung include high or intrinsic PEEP, elevated peak inspiratory pressures, or hyperventilation, all of which contribute to high mean airway pressures and decreased perfusion.

If refractory hypoxemia should occur during SLV, several steps should be taken to address the cause. First, the FiO2 should be increased to 1.0 to optimize oxygen delivery. The tube position must be confirmed with a bronchoscope to ensure that surgical manipulation or traction has not changed it. While looking with the bronchoscope, the airway can be checked for secretions or obstruction that may be contributing. Recruitment maneuvers should be performed on the dependent, ventilated lung, and it should be ensured that sufficient—but not excessive—PEEP is being utilized to correct atelectasis without causing barotrauma. Of note, in patients with a history of COPD or bullous emphysematous disease, there should always be concern in cases of refractory hypoxemia for pneumothorax on the dependent side; if the level of concern is high, a chest tube should be placed. If these maneuvers are insufficient to correct hypoxemia, ventilation of the collapsed lung may be necessary. This of course causes limited visualization of the operative field, especially when a VATS approach has been taken, but patient safety must be prioritized. If all other maneuvers have failed to resolve hypoxemia, the aforementioned medications that inhibit HPV can be discontinued.

4.2 Management of Fluids

For patients placed in lateral decubitus position, there are physiologic changes that must be accounted for in order to optimize respiratory function and avoid acute lung injury, which carries an associated mortality or major morbidity risk of about 40% [12]. For instance, excessive fluid administration can cause a gravity-dependent transudation of fluid into the dependent lung or "lower lung syndrome", which then increases shunting and exacerbates hypoxemia. A fluid restrictive strategy is therefore encouraged, although notably there are no definitive studies on an ideal fluid management strategy.

The lung on the operative side, having been collapsed and retracted during the procedure, may be prone to acute lung injury. With re-expansion, the ventilation to that lung is restored; however, flow would have been preferentially shunted to the opposite lung that was being ventilated throughout the case. Therefore, the collapsed lung may experience ischemia-reperfusion injury upon adjustment of the shunt and return of flow. There is some evidence to suggest that this acute lung injury is mediated by free-oxygen radicals derived by xanthine oxidase and tumor necrosis factor (TNF) released from the ischemic or hypoxic lung after reperfusion; these then cause pulmonary capillary injury, characterized by decreased flexibility of the pulmonary vasculature and pulmonary sequestration of neutrophils [13]. Further, there have been reports of ischemia-reperfusion injury extending to the contralateral non-hypoxic lung, as the acute lung injury in the hypoxic lung can cause leukocyte-mediated endothelial injury in the other lung as well as possibly in other organs [14]. Finally, this acute lung injury may be further exacerbated by re-expansion pulmonary edema, a rare but life-threatening complication [15]; this, too, can be seen in the contralateral lung after re-expansion of the collapsed lung by a similar mechanism as that described above [13, 16]. Other causes of bilateral pulmonary edema must also be ruled out, including aspiration, sepsis, heart failure, PE, and transfusion reaction.

4.3 Risk of Arrythmias with Thoracic Manipulation

As in elective thoracic surgery patients, those undergoing urgent or emergent surgical intervention in the thorax are at increased risk of arrhythmias; because of either surgical manipulation of the right atrium or distention secondary to volume reduction of the pulmonary vascular bed, perioperative arrhythmias—particularly supraventricular tachycardias—are quite common, and the risk increases with age [12]. The management of the particular arrythmia should follow ACLS guidelines. Avoidance of volume overload is also key in preventing atrial stretch and consequent atrial arrhythmias.

4.4 Laparoscopy

The physiologic changes that occur during laparoscopy are primarily due to the use of pneumoperitoneum to create working space. With insufflation comes an increase in intra-abdominal pressure (IAP), which has several downstream effects:

1. Venous return is decreased due to compression of the inferior vena cava (IVC) and its tributaries; this also causes peripheral venous pooling and an increased risk of deep vein thrombosis (DVT).
2. Compression of the major arterial vessels in the abdomen creates increased systemic vascular resistance (SVR) as well as decreased delivery of oxygenated blood.

The combination of decreased venous return and increased SVR causes a decrease in cardiac output. Arterial compression by the increased IAP also decreases splanchnic blood flow. Further, renal blood flow is impacted, with downstream consequences including activation of the renin-angiotensin-aldosterone (RAA) system and increased antidiuretic hormone (ADH) in order to increase kidney perfusion.

From a pulmonary standpoint, an increase in IAP reduces lung volumes and causes atelectasis, leading to ventilation-perfusion mismatch. This limitation in gas exchange leads to an increase in the partial pressure of CO_2 and a decreased partial pressure of O_2.

Patient positioning also contributes to these changes. For example, Trendelenburg position is commonly utilized during laparoscopic approaches to lower abdominal or pelvic pathology; the degree of tilt correlates with reduction in lung volumes and risk of atelectasis given the added pressure on the diaphragm. From a cardiovascular standpoint, venous return and cardiac output are preserved in this position.

It has been shown in small studies that laparoscopic surgery is a risk factor for raised intracranial pressure (ICP), with higher CO2 pneumoperitoneum pressure linearly related to the rise in ICP [17, 18]. One retrospective series of nine patients undergoing laparoscopic-assisted ventriculoperitoneal shunt placement found that ICP measured through a ventricular catheter increased in correlation with increasing insufflation pressure [17]. A study of 101 patients undergoing laparoscopic cholecystectomy, randomized to low-pressure (8 mmHg) or high-pressure (14 mmHg) groups, used ultrasound measurements of optic nerve sheath diameter (ONSD) as a surrogate for ICP; at higher insufflation pressures, there was a significant rise in ICP compared to low-pressure pneumoperitoneum [18]. This concern for ICP elevation may become relevant if a polytrauma patient with TBI requires abdominal exploration; there are no current guidelines regarding the use of laparoscopy in this setting, but the surgery and anesthesia teams should take this into account when planning their approach.

4.5   Complications of Laparoscopy

Despite the proposed benefits of minimally invasive surgery, the anesthesia provider must be prepared for untoward complications as they would be for open emergency operations. Just as it can occur in an open operation, the patient's hemodynamic status may suddenly begin to decompensate. The importance of early and continuous communication between the surgical team and the anesthesia teams cannot be understated. It can help identify if the patient is having an untoward response to insufflation and increased compartment pressures or if there is intravascular volume loss. Furthermore, in emergency general surgery cases, it is possible to cause a hemodynamic shift by releasing an abscess or restoring blood supply to an ischemic limb or bowel. This alone is not a reason to convert from laparoscopic to open, but recognition of this process and separating it from the hemodynamic consequences of laparoscopy itself are important.

Although CO2 is far more soluble in blood than oxygen or nitrogen, CO2 embolism can occur. It is an uncommon, yet perilous complication seen with CO2 insufflation during laparoscopy and is important to recognize quickly to avoid severe physiological consequences. The true incidence is not known, as many are clinically insignificant, but estimates range from 17 up to 68% in some case series [19, 20]. For those that do become symptomatic, the mortality rate is believed to be almost 30% [21]; the severity will depend on both the amount of CO2 injected into the systemic circulation and on the ability to eliminate this CO2 by way of the lungs [22]. The most common cause is misplacement of the Veress needle, either directly into a vein or organ, although smaller amounts of CO2 may enter via any injured vessel throughout the case. Patient presentation varies intraoperatively but can include cerebral hypoperfusion, acute hypotension, acute heart failure, myocardial infarction, pulmonary edema, and death. The emboli can be detected on transthoracic or transesophageal echocardiogram, the latter being most sensitive [22]. An abrupt decrease in end-tidal CO2 (ETCO2) may be the first sign, as lung perfusion is compromised and gas exchange is diminished; decreased oxygen saturation is a late sign. If a pulmonary artery catheter is present, the embolism may present as an increase in pulmonary artery pressure. If clinical suspicion of CO2 embolism should arise, immediate action must be taken. The surgeon must quickly release the pneumoperitoneum to prevent further CO2 embolization. The patient must then be positioned in left lateral decubitus position with the head down, known as Durant's maneuver; this position will prevent the venous embolism from lodging in the lungs and instead stay in the right heart until slowly absorbed, as it places the right ventricle superior to the right ventricular outflow tract [23]. Aspiration of the air may be attempted if there is central venous access in place; however, the priority must be to desufflate the abdomen and reposition the patient. The remainder of care is supportive; ACLS protocols should be followed if the embolism were to cause hemodynamic collapse.

5   Postop Pain Control

Pain control can be challenging in the postoperative patient, but it is an essential component of recovery. Uncontrolled pain can lead to decreased splinting and poor respiratory effort, as well as decreased ability to cough for secretion clearance, thereby worsening atelectasis, shunting, and hypoxemia. Further, adequate pain control enables patient ambulation, important for enhanced recovery. Given the worsening opioid epidemic in the United States, limiting the amount of opioids used in the perioperative period has become a top priority across surgical specialties, and the use of multimodal pain regimens (MMPR) has grown considerably with that goal in mind. This approach is based on the premise that the use of multiple nonopioid agents concurrently can have an additive, possibly even synergistic, effect on analgesia while decreasing total opioid intake as well as opioid-related side effects [24]. Ideally, these regimens include a combination of a regional anesthetic (neuraxial or peripheral) with scheduled administration of non-opioid agents including acetaminophen, an NSAID, and a muscle relaxant such as methocarbamol, with or without a gabapentinoid (gabapentin and pregabalin). Usually, tramadol is used initially for breakthrough pain, followed by opioids [24]. Much work on limiting opioid use has also been done in the trauma patient population. A recent randomized clinical trial in patients admitted after trauma demonstrated the utility of a multimodal regimen including oral acetaminophen, naproxen, gabapentin, lidocaine patches, and as-needed opioids in decreasing overall opioid exposure while achieving adequate pain control [25].

Of note, gabapentinoids—previously a component of many Enhanced Recovery After Surgery (ERAS) protocols—have recently lost favor as agents employed in multimodal pain regimens due to concern for increased risk of opioid overdose and respiratory depression. A large cohort study found that those patients given gabapentinoids (gabapentin or pregabalin) coadministered with opioids had higher risk of opioid overdose as well as respiratory complications [26]. Another recent retrospective study in elective colorectal surgery patients found that the use of gabapentinoids was associated with higher odds of noninvasive ventilation and naloxone use after surgery [27]. Because of such findings and reports of adverse events, the FDA issued a warning on serious breathing difficulties associated with gabapentinoids in patients with other respiratory risk factors, including opioid use [28].

Regional blocks can provide excellent analgesia as additions to a multimodal pain regimen (MMPR). Epidurals have been used extensively in elective abdominal and thoracic surgery with great success in providing postoperative analgesia [29]; however, placement may be contraindicated in patients on anticoagulation or anti-platelet agents. The use of erector spinae plane blocks (ESPBs) has grown in popularity in recent years, especially in the trauma population for pain control after rib fractures. One benefit of these blocks is that DVT chemoprophylaxis does not need to be held prior to placement of a catheter [30]; if there is any concern about leaving a catheter in place, a single injection of liposomal bupivacaine can provide pain control for up to 72 h. Of note, the use of liposomal bupivacaine carries higher risk than other local anesthetics; for instance, it cannot be combined with other local anesthetics, and, if injected intravascularly, can reach toxic blood concentrations leading to dysrhythmias and possibly death. As long as attention is paid to proper administration, it is an excellent option for longer-term pain relief in both thoracic and abdominal field blocks.

ERAS protocols have been in place for multiple subsets of elective general surgery for years in order to reduce morbidity, length of stay, and cost. Colorectal surgery was one of the early adopters, followed closely by surgical oncology, hepatobiliary, bariatrics, and thoracic; other surgical fields have followed suit, including urology and gynecology. Various efforts at enhanced recovery protocols have been described for use in emergency general surgery for over a decade [31] in an effort to tackle the much higher morbidity and mortality of emergency cases than that seen in elective general surgery, but no formal guidelines had been established. In early 2021, however, the ERAS society published consensus guidelines for enhanced recovery after emergency laparotomy [32]; although widespread adoption and determination of impact will take time, as it follows the same principles as other ERAS protocols, it holds promise to improve emergency surgical patient outcomes.

---

6   Conclusions

The use of minimally invasive approaches in emergency general surgery and trauma is likely to increase in the years to come. Improved rates of complications and shorter durations of hospital stays have been demonstrated in elective surgery, and early data suggests the same for emergent operations. There are increased layers to consider in these patients including hemorrhagic and septic shock. Furthermore, the systemic inflammatory response in patients with emergency surgery disease processes can increase the hemodynamic lability. However, with solid understanding of these disease processes and constant communication between the anesthesia and surgical teams, these patients can safely undergo minimally invasive operations.

References

1. Madni TD, Nakonezny PA, Barrios E, etal. Prospective validation of the parkland grading scale for cholecystitis. Am J Surg 2019;217(1):90–97.
2. Arnold M, Elhage S, Schiffern L, etal. Use of minimally invasive surgery in emergency general surgery procedures. Surg Endosc 2020;34(5):2258–2265.
3. Evans L, Rhodes A, Alhazzani W, et al. Surviving sepsis campaign: international guidelines for Management of Sepsis and Septic Shock 2021. Crit Care Med. 2021;49(11):e1063–143.
4. Seymour CW, Gesten F, Prescott HC, et al. Time to treatment and mortality during mandated emergency Care for Sepsis. N Engl J Med. 2017;376:2235–44.
5. Cannon WB, Cowell E. The preventive treatment of wound shock. JAMA. 1918;70:618–21.
6. Tran A, Yates J, Lau A, et al. Permissive hypotension versus conventional resuscitation strategies in adult trauma patients with hemorrhagic shock: a systematic review and meta-analysis of randomized controlled trials. J Trauma Acute Care Surg. 2018;84(5):802–8.
7. Rossaint R, Bouillon B, Cerny V, et al. The European guideline on management of major bleeding and coagulopathy following trauma: 4th edition. Crit Care. 2016;20:100.
8. Lu Y, Dai W, Zong Z, et al. Bronchial blocker versus left double-lumen endotracheal tube for one-lung ventilation in right video-assisted Thoracoscopic surgery. J Cardiothorac Vasc Anesth. 2018;32(1):297–301.
9. Niwal N, Ranganathan P, Divatia J. Bronchial blocker for one-lung ventilation: an unanticipated complication. Indian J Anaesth. 2011;55(6):636–7.
10. Clayton-Smith A, Bennett K, Alston RP, et al. A comparison of the efficacy and adverse effects of double-lumen endobronchial tubes and bronchial blockers in thoracic surgery: a systematic review and meta-analysis of randomized controlled trials. J Cardiothorac Vasc Anesth. 2015;29(4):955–66.
11. Farrell S, Curley GF. Respiration: ventilation. Anaesth Intensive Care Med. 2021;22(3):179–84.
12. Butterworth JF, Mackey DC, Wasnick JD. Anesthesia for thoracic surgery. In: Malley J, Naglieri C, editors. Morgan & Mikhail's clinical anesthesiology. 6th ed. New York: McGraw-Hill Education; 2018. p. 553–82.
13. Her C, Mandy S. Acute respiratory distress syndrome of the contralateral lung after Reexpansion pulmonary edema of a collapsed lung. J Clin Anesth. 2004;16:244–50.
14. St. John RC, Mizer LA, Kindt GC, et al. Acid aspiration-induced lung injury causes leukocyte-dependent systemic organ injury. J Appl Physiol. 1993;74:1994–2003.
15. Feller-Kopman D, Berkowitz D, Boiselle P, Ernst A. Large-volume thoracentesis and the risk of Reexpansion pulmonary edema. Ann Thorac Surg. 2007;84:1656–62.
16. Walter JM, Matthay MA, Gillespie CT, Corbridge T. Acute hypoxemic respiratory failure after large-volume thoracentesis: mechanisms of pleural fluid formation and reexpansion pulmonary edema. Ann Am Thorac Soc. 2016;13:438–43.
17. Kamine TH, Papavassiliou E, Schneider BE. Effect of abdominal insufflation for laparoscopy on intracranial pressure. JAMA Surg. 2014;149(4):380–2.
18. Yashwashi T, Kaman L, Kajal K, et al. Effects of low- and high-pressure carbon dioxide pneumoperitoneum on intracranial pressure during laparoscopic cholecystectomy. Surg Endosc. 2020;34:4369–73.
19. Gutt CN, Oniu T, Mehrabi A, et al. Circulatory and respiratory complications of carbon dioxide insufflation. Dig Surg. 2004;21:95–105.
20. Hong JY, Kim WO, Kii HK. Detection of subclinical CO2 embolism by transesophageal echocardiography during laparoscopic radical prostatectomy. Urology. 2010;75(3):581–4.
21. Huntington CR, Prince J, Hazelbaker K, et al. Safety first: significant risk of air embolism in laparoscopic gasketless insufflation systems. Surg Endosc. 2019;33:3964–9.
22. de Jong KIF, Leeuw PW. Venous carbon dioxide embolism during laparoscopic cholecystectomy: a literature review. Eur J Int Med. 2019;60:9–12.
23. Muth CM, Shank ES. Gas embolism. N Engl J Med. 2000;342:476–82.

24. Wick EC, Grant MC, Wu CL. Postoperative multimodal analgesia pain management with nonopioid analgesics and techniques: a review. JAMA Surg. 2017;152(7):691–7.
25. Harvin JA, Albarado R, Truong VT, et al. Multi-modal analgesic strategy for trauma: a pragmatic randomized clinical trial. J Am Coll Surg. 2021;232(3):241–51.
26. Bykov K, Bateman BT, Franklin JM, et al. Association of Gabapentinoids with the risk of opioid-Rlated adverse events in surgical patients in the United States. JAMA Netw Open. 2020;3(12):e2031647.
27. Ohnuma T, Krishnamoorthy V, Ellis AR, et al. Association between gabapentinoids on the day of colorectal surgery and adverse postoperative respiratory outcomes. Ann Surg. 2019;270:e65–7.
28. US Food and Drug Administration. FDA warns about serious breathing problems with seizure and nerve pain medicines gabapentin (Neurontin, Gralise, Horizant) or pregabalin (Lyrica, Lyrica CR) who have respiratory risk factors. 2019. https://www.fda.gov/media/133681/download.
29. Block BM, Liu SS, Rowlingson AJ, et al. Efficacy of postoperative epidural analgesia: a meta-analysis. JAMA. 2003;290(18):2455–63.
30. Dultz LA, Ma R, Dumas RP, et al. Safety of erector spinae plane blocks in patients with Chest Wall trauma on venous thromboembolism prophylaxis. J Surg Res. 2021;263:124–9.
31. Moller MH, Adamsen S, et al. Multicentre trial of a perioperative protocol to reduce mortality in patients with peptic ulcer perforation. Br J Surg. 2011;98:802–10.
32. Peden CJ, Aggarwal G, Aitken RJ, et al. Guidelines for perioperative care for Emergency Laparotomy Enhanced Recovery after Surgery (ERAS) society recommendations: part 1—preoperative: diagnosis, rapid assessment and optimization. World J Surg. 2021;45:1272–90.

Utility of Video-Assisted Thoracoscopic Surgery (VATS) in Acute Care Surgery

Ariel W. Knight and Andre R. Campbell

1   Introduction

Thoracic injuries are directly responsible for approximately 20–25% of trauma mortalities and contribute indirectly to another 25% of trauma-related deaths [1, 2]. Acute mortality is most commonly due to severe airway injury, cardiac injury, or intrathoracic hemorrhage. However, pulmonary complications that manifest later in a patient's post-injury course contribute significantly to both morbidity and mortality due to complications such as pneumonia, ARDS, retained hemothorax, empyema, and missed injury. Ultimately, though, only 10–15% of patients with traumatic chest injuries will require surgical therapy [1, 2]. Emergency thoracotomy can be lifesaving in the trauma setting, but is rarely necessary. Accordingly, the majority of thoracic operations will take place on a less urgent basis with the opportunity for patient stabilization and more thoughtful preoperative planning, including consideration of a minimally invasive approach.

Video-assisted thoracoscopic surgery (VATS) has been increasingly utilized in the treatment of pulmonary and pleural pathology among general and thoracic surgeons. Thoracoscopy was originally utilized to manage pleural effusions, empyema, and thoracic malignancy as early as 1922 in Stockholm, Sweden [3]. It was initially applied to trauma care in 1946 for management of hemothorax secondary to penetrating chest injury [4]. Multiple studies have demonstrated numerous benefits of a VATS-based approach to oncologic pulmonary resection over standard posterolateral thoracotomy, including decreased length of hospital stay, earlier recovery of

A. W. Knight
Department of Surgery, Stanford University, Stanford, CA, USA
e-mail: awknight@stanford.edu

A. R. Campbell (✉)
Department of Surgery, University of California, San Francisco, CA, USA
e-mail: andre.campbell@ucsf.edu

© The Author(s), under exclusive license to Springer Nature Switzerland AG 2023   375
F. Coccolini et al. (eds.), *Mini-invasive Approach in Acute Care Surgery*,
Hot Topics in Acute Care Surgery and Trauma,
https://doi.org/10.1007/978-3-031-39001-2_28

pulmonary function, decreased postoperative pain and subsequent narcotic requirements, decreased incidence of postoperative complications, and lower overall cost [5–8]. Smaller studies have shown similar benefits in trauma patients [1, 9]. Accordingly, thoracoscopy has become increasingly and successfully utilized in both trauma and emergency general surgery settings. This chapter will focus on our general approach to thoracoscopic surgery. Specific management of commonly encountered pathology is discussed elsewhere in this text.

2 VATS Principles

VATS can be both diagnostic and therapeutic when appropriately employed in acute care surgical practice. Careful patient selection is essential for safe and successful thoracoscopic surgery. Common indications for thoracoscopy in the acute care setting are discussed in an earlier chapter. Patients must be sufficiently fit, hemodynamically stable, and adequately resuscitated to be able to tolerate single-lung ventilation. Suspicion for injury in another body cavity must be sufficiently low or previously ruled out, as the lateral decubitus positioning necessary for a standard VATS exploration substantially limits immediate access to the abdomen, retroperitoneum, and extremities. Common contraindications to VATS are discussed later. If a patient who meets one or more of these criteria still requires urgent thoracic surgical intervention, strong consideration should be given to the pursuit of a standard open approach in favor of thoracoscopy.

2.1 Single-Lung Ventilation

Single-lung ventilation (SLV) is almost always required for thoracoscopic surgery. SLV deflates the ipsilateral lung and thus creates increased operating space and improved visibility. Diagnostic thoracoscopy, periodically performed to evaluate for parenchymal or diaphragmatic injury, may be performed with standard double-lung ventilation, often with periodic breath holds. Additionally, in certain clinical scenarios, SLV may protect the contralateral lung from exposure to infectious, bloody, or malignant secretions.

SLV may be achieved by placement of either a double-lumen endotracheal tube or an ipsilateral endobronchial blocker. A double-lumen tube is larger than a standard, single-lumen endotracheal tube and requires bronchoscopic guidance for correct anatomic placement in the proximal right and left mainstem bronchi. Endobronchial blocker positioning requires placement of a size 8.5 or 9.0 endotracheal tube, which may be limited by smaller patient body habitus. The blocker itself has two differently colored balloons and is placed at the carina under bronchoscopic guidance. Selective inflation of the appropriate balloon facilitates blockage of the ipsilateral mainstem bronchus and thus prevents ventilation of the ipsilateral lung. Notably, successful endobronchial blockade of the right lung may be more difficult due to the immediate, acute takeoff of the right upper lobe bronchus, which may preclude adequate isolation. Endobronchial blockade is limited by passive deflation of the ipsilateral lung. While both are safe and effective SLV options, we prefer placement of a double-lumen endotracheal tube as it facilitates more rapid deflation of the ipsilateral lung, allows for pre- and intraoperative flexible bronchoscopy of both lungs, and is less likely to become dislodged during patient positioning. However, neither technique is proven to be superior, and thus, this decision should be made by the responsible anesthesia and surgical teams.

SLV creates a significant ventilation-perfusion mismatch and may lead to hypoxemia. While physiologic hypoxic pulmonary vasoconstriction in the ipsilateral lung offsets some of this phenomenon, hypoxemia may require intraoperative treatment. Common maneuvers include the use of a higher fraction of inspired oxygen or positive end expiratory pressure to facilitate vasodilation and improved ventilation in the contralateral lung, respectively. Recruitment maneuvers may also be utilized. In some circumstances, temporary reversion to double-lung ventilation may be required and is often the safest treatment of persistent or refractory hypoxemia. This circumstance highlights the close, frequent communication needed between the anesthesia and surgical teams to maximize patient safety. Of note, carbon dioxide clearance is seldom affected by SLV so long as minute ventilation remains adequate. Additionally, the singly ventilated lung must be protected from barotrauma and ventilator-associated injury. Maintenance of safe peak inspiratory and plateau pressures is imperative, particularly when larger tidal volumes are utilized to maintain adequate oxygenation. If a patient is ultimately deemed unable to safely tolerate SLV, consideration should be given to proceeding with traditional open thoracotomy.

2.2 Contraindications to Thoracoscopy

Many common contraindications to VATS are listed in Table 1. Importantly, hemodynamic instability is an obvious contraindication and often necessitates conversion to thoracotomy. It may be additionally exacerbated by low flow insufflation that is commonly utilized during thoracoscopy to optimize visualization. The addition of positive intrathoracic pressure can worsen hemodynamic instability by compressing the superior and inferior vena cava and thus decreasing venous return to the heart, as is also observed in laparoscopy. While thoracoscopy may safely be performed

Table 1 Contraindications to video-assisted thoracoscopic surgery in acute care surgery

Hemodynamic instability requiring ongoing medical management
Inability to tolerate single-lung ventilation (due to injury burden or underlying comorbid cardiopulmonary disease)
Multi-compartmental injury requiring concomitant operative management
Clinical indication for exploratory thoracotomy (i.e., massive hemothorax)
Suspected cardiac injury
Contraindication to lateral decubitus positioning
Significant adhesions in the pleural space from prior surgery, infection, inflammation, radiation, etc.

without supplemental insufflation, as SLV often provides sufficient operating space, if adequate visualization cannot be achieved or if treatment of hemodynamic instability is ongoing, the surgeon should have a low threshold to convert to an open approach.

Historic contraindications to VATS include prior thoracic surgery or chest wall instrumentation (including tube thoracostomy) as well as irradiation. As thoracoscopy has become more widely utilized by both thoracic and general surgeons, these factors less commonly preclude a safe VATS approach. Thoracoscopic adhesiolysis may be necessary in these scenarios, but can be safely and effectively performed to free the lung from the parietal pleura. Conversion to thoracotomy may still be required in individual circumstances depending upon intraoperative findings and surgeon discretion.

Lastly, pulmonary function tests are an excellent predictor of tolerance of SLV and magnitude of pulmonary resection. While they commonly inform the decision to proceed with a thoracoscopic versus open approach in elective thoracic surgery, these studies are seldom available in an acute care or traumatic setting. Accordingly, the choice of surgical approach in this circumstance must be dictated by the nature of the planned operation as well as the patient's hemodynamic status, degree of physiologic insult, and comorbidities, if known. If thoracoscopy is pursued, the operative team must be ready to immediately convert to thoracotomy if necessary.

3 Standard Operative Approach

3.1 Operating Room Setup and Equipment

A VATS-capable operating room should include the typical equipment listed in Table 2, with additional instruments being available per individual surgeon preference [10]. Standard thoracotomy equipment should also be immediately available. Typically, the operating surgeon and assistant are positioned on the ventral aspect of

Table 2 Standard VATS equipment

Two standard video monitors
Fiberoptic 5 and 10 mm thoracoscopes
High-resolution video camera
Light source and cable
Image processor
Blunt lung graspers
Curved dissecting forceps
Biopsy forceps
Vascular clamps
Thoracoscopic scissors
Electrocautery
Suction
Trocar selection per surgeon preference

the patient with the scrub nurse or technician opposite the assistant surgeon. The anesthesia team is positioned at the head of the bed.

3.2   Patient Preparation, Positioning, and Bronchoscopy

The patient is initially placed supine on the operating table and general anesthesia is induced. Either a single- or double-lumen endotracheal tube may be placed, depending upon the operating surgeon's preference for preoperative bronchoscopy. However, if a single-lumen tube is placed, it must be exchanged for a double-lumen tube prior to final patient positioning. Large-bore peripheral intravenous access is obtained, and a radial arterial line is typically placed for continuous intraoperative hemodynamic monitoring. A urinary catheter is also commonly placed. An appropriate analgesic plan should be formulated with the anesthesia team, which may include thoracic epidural placement or regional nerve block techniques in addition to the use of local anesthetics.

We begin with a standard video bronchoscopy to the level of the subsegmental bronchi to visualize the tracheobronchial tree and rule out any intraluminal anomalies or occult tracheobronchial injury. Single-lung ventilation is initiated at the conclusion of bronchoscopy. The importance of working with an anesthesia team that is proficient in the management of patients requiring single-lung ventilation in order to maximize the change of successful thoracoscopic surgery with minimal risk of intraoperative complications cannot be overstated. From here, the patient is placed in a standard lateral decubitus position with the ipsilateral shoulder and upper arm suspended on an arm board. All pressure points are adequately padded to prevent nerve injury. We use a bean bag to assist with patient positioning, although gel rolls may be used per surgeon preference.

3.3   Standard Port Placement

We begin by placing a 10 mm camera port in the 7th–8th intercostal space at the posterior axillary line and then proceed with a diagnostic thoracoscopy. Under direct vision, two additional 5 mm working ports are placed, one each in the 4th–5th and 7th intercostal spaces at the anterior axillary line. Further operative management is then dictated by the individual patient's surgical indication. While the specific indications for surgery are discussed in an earlier chapter, this approach allows for successful thoracoscopic treatment of the majority of these acute pathologies [11–13].

4 Conclusion

Acute care surgeons continue to encounter and manage a wide variety of thoracic pathology, a minority of which will require surgical intervention. Multiple studies in both general thoracic and trauma populations confirm the safety, feasibility, and improved clinical outcomes associated with a VATS approach compared to a traditional thoracotomy in appropriately selected patients. As such, non-thoracic, acute care surgeons must remain familiar with diagnostic and therapeutic thoracoscopy as an effective approach to definitively treat multiple injury patterns and benign disease processes.

References

1. Billeter AJ, Druen D, Franklin GA, et al. Video-assisted thoracoscopy as an important tool for trauma surgeons: a systematic review. Langenbeck's Arch Surg. 2013;398(4):515–23.
2. Manlulu AV, Lee TW, Thung KH, Wong R. Curent indications and results of VATS in the evaluation and management of hemodynamically stable thoracic injuries. Eur J Cardiothorac Surg. 2004;25(6):1048–53.
3. Jacobaeus HC. Practical importance of thoracoscopy in surgery of the chest. Surg Gynecol Obstet. 1922;34:289–96.
4. Martins Castello Branco J. Thoracoscopy as a method of exploration in penetrating injuries of the thorax. Dis Chest. 1946;12:330–5.
5. Farjah F, Wood DE, Mulligan MS, et al. Safety and efficacy of video-assisted versus conventional lung resection for lung cancer. J Thorac Cardiovasc Surg. 2009;137(6):1415–21.
6. Onaitis MW, Petersen RP, Balderson SS, et al. Thoracoscopic lobectomy is a safe and versatile procedure: experience with 500 consecutive patients. Ann Surg. 2006;244(3):420–5.
7. Swanson SJ, Meyers BF, Gunnarsson CL, et al. Video-assisted thoracoscopic lobectomy is less costly and morbid than open lobectomy: a retrospective multiinstitutional database analysis. Ann Thorac Surg. 2012;93(4):1027–32.
8. Villamizar NR, Darrabie MD, Burfeind WR, et al. Thoracoscopic lobectomy is associated with lower morbidity compared with thoracotomy. J Thorac Cardiovasc Surg. 2009;138(2):419–25.
9. Ben-Nun A, Orlovsky M, Best LA. Video-assisted thoracoscopic surgery in the treatment of chest trauma: long-term benefit. Ann Thorac Surg. 2007;83(2):383–7.
10. Mehrotra M, D'Cruz JR, Arthur ME. Video-assisted thoracoscopy. In: StatPearls. Treasure Island, FL: StatPearls Publishing; 2021. https://www.ncbi.nlm.nih.gov/books/NBK532952/.
11. Goodman M, Lewis J, Guitron J, et al. Video-assisted thoracoscopic surgery for acute thoracic trauma. J Emerg Trauma Shock. 2013;6(2):106–9.
12. Villavicencio RT, Aucar JA, Wall MJ. Analysis of thoracoscopy in trauma. Surg Endosc. 1999;13(1):3–9.
13. Kong VY, Oosthuizen GV, Clark DL. Selective conservatism in the management of thoracic trauma remains appropriate in the 21st century. Ann R Coll Surg Engl. 2015;97(3):224–8.

MIX
Papier aus verantwortungsvollen Quellen
Paper from responsible sources
FSC® C105338

If you have any concerns about our products,
you can contact us on
ProductSafety@springernature.com

In case Publisher is established outside the EU,
the EU authorized representative is:
Springer Nature Customer Service Center GmbH
Europaplatz 3, 69115 Heidelberg, Germany

Printed by Libri Plureos GmbH
in Hamburg, Germany